AF334097

Acute renal failure:
Diagnosis and management

Rufino C. Pabico, M. D.
University of Rochester
Medical Center
Rochester, N. Y. 14620

Acute renal failure:
Diagnosis and management

ROBERT C. MUEHRCKE, M.D., F.A.C.P.

Director of Medical Education, West Suburban Hospital,
Oak Park, Illinois; Clinical Associate Professor of
Medicine, University of Illinois College of Medicine,
Chicago, Illinois; Consulting Staff, Presbyterian St.
Luke's Hospital, Attending Physician, University of
Illinois Hospital, Consultant Nephrologist, West Side
Veterans Administration Hospital, Chicago, Illinois

With 126 illustrations

Saint Louis

The C. V. Mosby Company

1969

Copyright © 1969 by
The C. V. Mosby Company

All rights reserved. No part of this book may be
reproduced in any manner without written permission
of the publisher.

Printed in the United States of America

Standard Book Number 8016-3577-2

Library of Congress Catalog Card Number 73-80697

Distributed in Great Britain by Henry Kimpton, London

To our past "apostles" of clinical
nephrology: Thomas Addis, A. R.
Cushny, William Bowman, Richard
Bright, Paul Iversen, George Johnson,
John P. Peters, Pierre F. Rayer,
Leonard G. Roundtree, Homer N.
Smith, John R. Squire, and
D. D. Van Slyke

The clinical syndrome [of acute renal failure] may be recapitulated briefly. In most cases the patient has been buried beneath fallen masonry or heavy debris and, on release, may appear well except for swelling of the affected limb. Should shock develop, the blood volume has usually been restored to a normal figure by transfusion and as a rule been well maintained. Some of these patients pass dark-coloured, smoky or red urine which contains albumin and gives a positive benzidine reaction, and on spectroscopic examination shows the absorption bands of myohemoglobin (Bywaters et al). The sediment is full of granular debris and brown pigmented casts, but only rarely shows red blood corpuscles. Subsequently oliguria or anuria may develop, and there is an increase in the concentration of urea, and of phosphate and potassium in the blood. Death may take place about the end of the first week, or recovery may follow upon a diuresis which occurs about this same time. With either course there is a falling off in the excretion of pigment and of casts, which become more cellular in character.

Although in the majority of cases there has been marked crushing injury of muscle, it is to be noted that a similar condition has been found in cases of muscular ischemia of different origin.

E. G. L. Bywaters, and J. Henry Dible
The renal lesion in traumatic anuria,
J. Path. and Bact. **54**:*111, 1942.*

Foreword

Acute renal failure is a central theme of modern nephrology. Richard Bright did not recognize it and Volhard and Fahr did not understand it. Our view of it in 1969, which Dr. Robert Muehrcke presents so well in this book, starts with Eric Bywater's work, in 1940, on the brave fire-fighting citizens of London crushed by the falling walls and debris of buildings blown apart by the Nazi air force during the Battle of Britain. At that time, across the English Channel in Nazi-occupied Holland, a patient and ingenious Dutchman, Willem Kolff, was planning and developing machines that would do the work of the kidneys for the body, while the patients' organs, hopefully, were regenerating cells and lost functions destroyed by one or another of myriad aggravated bodily insults. Soon after 1945, when the war had ended, surgeons, obstetricians, industrial physicians, and toxicologists began to recognize that their patients, ill with acute renal failure, required modern treatment in special centers equipped to deal with their unique problems. These sprang up in Amsterdam, around Borst; in London, around Bull; in Copenhagen, around Iversen and Brun; in Boston, around Merrill; and in Cleveland, around Kolff. Borst and Bull developed conservative dietary regimens to save lives. Merrill and Kolff built practical kidney machines to do the job. The classical histologic studies of Lucké and the nephron dissections of Jean Oliver give no inkling of the early stages of renal pathology in the syndrome. Iverson and Brun developed renal biopsy to look for the common thread of pathophysiology in early or developing cases, and later Danish workers developed the radioactive xenon technique to look into renal blood flow failure as an etiologic factor in the disorder. Meanwhile, Merrill's work on potassium intoxication made nephrologists acutely aware of water and electrolyte disturbances as part of their specialty. By 1959 Doolan had developed a system of peritoneal lavage, which was perfected by nephrologists and anonymous colleagues in the pharmaceutical industry. Peritoneal dialysis brought the treatment of acute renal failure, except for the complicated cases, back to the community hospital.

From these beginnings Merrill and Hume began renal transplantation in twins and revitalized the science of immunology. From these beginnings Scribner developed treatment for patients moribund with end-stage kidney disease by repeated dialysis, and made us ask "What is death?" and "Who shall live?" Dr. Robert Muehrcke in his scholarly book brings to bear his wide research and clinical experience and his deep knowledge of renal pathology to the story of acute renal failure outlined above. He has written a practical book of particular value to doctors in community hospitals, who will help patients by what they will learn from it.

This marvelous story of thirty years of research work and the practical results therefrom—which will continue to save innumerable lives in the future as it has in the past—would not have been written if Dr. Muehrcke's special education in clinical nephrologic research and his research on renal disease had not been supported, since 1950, by funds from the National Institutes of Health. The work could never have been written *now* without past U. S. Governmental research support to Doctors Kolff, Merrill, and Scribner, and particularly to the hundreds of other investigators whose names are listed in the bibliography. We may well ask in this age of restricted funds for renal and other clinical research, "What of the future?"

Robert M. Kark, M.D.

Preface

Since 1960, clinical nephrology has gradually become recognized as a well-established medical specialty. It has been defined as a comprehensive study of renal structure and function in health and disease, including the prevention and treatment of diseases involving the kidney and urinary tract. The development of an important diagnostic tool, the renal biopsy, began a steady, rapid, and burgeoning accumulation of basic knowledge on the kidney. The use of renal biopsy sharpened the physician's diagnostic acumen and established clinical nephrology on a firm footing. The strongest stimulus to the growth of nephrology has been the advent of dialysis and transplantation.

In this book, renal biopsy is applied to a dynamic and vivid correlative cinematographic study of structure and function in patients ill with acute oliguric renal failure. Emphasis is placed on the diagnosis of this well-established clinical syndrome, its meticulous treatment, and its dread consequences. This book is directed to all in medicine interested in patients with renal failure. It is directed particularly to the student, the practicing physician, the internist, the nephrologist, the urologist, and the pathologist.

This book illustrates the vast spectrum of acute oliguric renal failure: the complex etiology, the numerous pathogenic conditions, the tedious management, and varied prognoses in relation to the ever-changing renal morphology. I do not mean for this book to be an encyclopedia on acute oliguric renal failure. It is meant to serve as an illustration of the broad variation in the clinical course of patients with acute oliguric renal failure and to relate these clinical functional abnormalities to the numerous observations on renal structure as made by serial renal biopsy. The book emphasizes the natural history of the numerous ramifications of acute oliguric renal failure and the adverse effects of chemicals and drugs in producing functional and structural changes. Current medical progress in dialysis and transplantation is described in view of beneficial as well as adverse effects on patients with acute renal failure.

I am most grateful to Dr. Robert M. Kark, Dr. Geoffrey Kent, Dr. J. Charles

McMillan, Dr. Conrad L. Pirani, and Dr. Harry Lerner, and to research fellows, residents, interns, nurses, and dietitians on the medical wards of research and educational hospitals of the University of Illinois College of Medicine, Presbyterian–St. Luke's Hospital, Chicago, and West Suburban Hospital, Oak Park, Illinois. Acknowledgment is given these individuals for the care of patients discussed in this book and for their clinical and morphologic data.

Drs. Kark and McMillan made major contributions in reviewing the final manuscript. Dr. Pirani, of the Michael Reese Institute of Pathology, made available special morphologic studies. Mrs. Sofia Michevicius and Johanna Puniska provided technical assistance with electron microscopic studies and special stains. Mrs. JoAnn Cooney typed and edited the manuscript.

Robert C. Muehrcke, M.D.

Contents

Acute renal failure:

Diagnosis and management

Chapter 1

Introduction

Acute oliguric renal failure was first recognized by physicians at least 100 years ago.[252] Like many other clinical disorders, it remained dormant in medical literature except for sporadic reports in the English literature by such pathologists as Councilman[242] and Kimmelsteil[627] or in the German literature by Frankenthal[392] and Minami.[781] However, it was not until World War II that Eric Bywaters (Fig. 1-1) permanently established it as a clinical syndrome.[188-191]

Today acute oliguric renal failure is a well-substantiated clinical syndrome that occurs in a patient with previously healthy kidneys and that is characterized by a sudden decrease below 400 ml (less than 17 ml/hr) in the adult and 50 ml in the child in daily urinary output delivered to the urinary bladder. Acute oliguric renal failure is associated with acute clinical and biochemical manifestations of abnormal renal failure.[375] In some patients acute renal failure may not be associated with oliguria but rather with a "high urinary output" (nonoliguria).[996,1052a] In time both conditions can be reversible, either spontaneously by diuresis or by proper and effective management. On the other hand, acute renal failure can be irreversible, can produce a progressive deterioration in the clinical and biochemical status of the patient, and can lead to death.

The reversibility of acute renal failure depends on several important conditions. The most important is early diagnosis with differentiation from chronic "end-stage" renal disease, renal circulatory failure (prerenal), and obstructive uropathy (postrenal); it can also occur superimposed on chronic renal disease. Once an exact diagnosis is made, prompt and adequate intensive management must follow. An all-important factor in the outcome of the patient with acute renal failure is the pathophysiologic process, especially the specific site and severity of renal damage. There are few clinical disorders that demand of the physician scientific knowledge, practical skill, and clinical common sense as does acute renal failure. The gravity of the disorder and its complete and dramatic reversibility greatly tax physicians' ability; yet, he may experience tremendous gratification once the patient recovers.

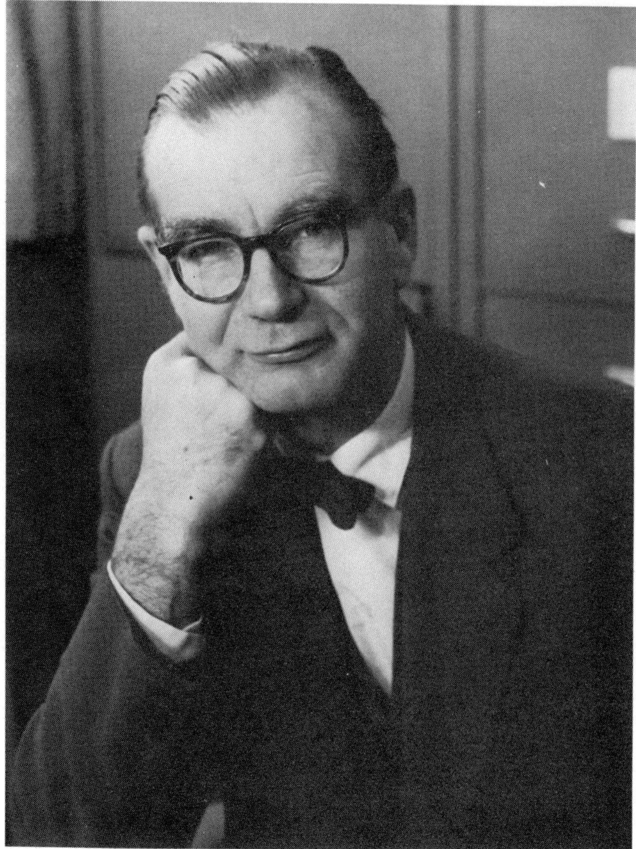

Fig. 1-1. Professor Eric G. L. Bywaters of the Royal Post-Graduate Medical School. In 1942 he described the clinical syndrome of acute oliguric renal failure that roused considerable interest of physicians throughout the world.

Acute oliguric renal failure as known today is a by-product of military and civilian casualty medicine from World Wars I and II. It has long been known to result from shock.[486] Although shock was effectively treated, progressive and fatal renal insufficiency contributed significantly to the final outcome of the battle casualty. During World War I, studies made on combat and civilian casualties with shock revealed the frequent occurrence of renal involvement with progressive azotemia and death.[781] In 1939, Jeghers and Bakst reviewed acute renal failure under the term "extra-renal azotemia."[858] These reports attracted little attention or interest from the medical profession.

During the years 1939-1945, Bywaters and colleagues[188-191,325] aroused considerable attention and stimulated the military physicians' interest in acute oliguric renal failure. During the 1940 bombardment of London, they studied air raid casualties injured by fallen masonry or heavy material. Their patients

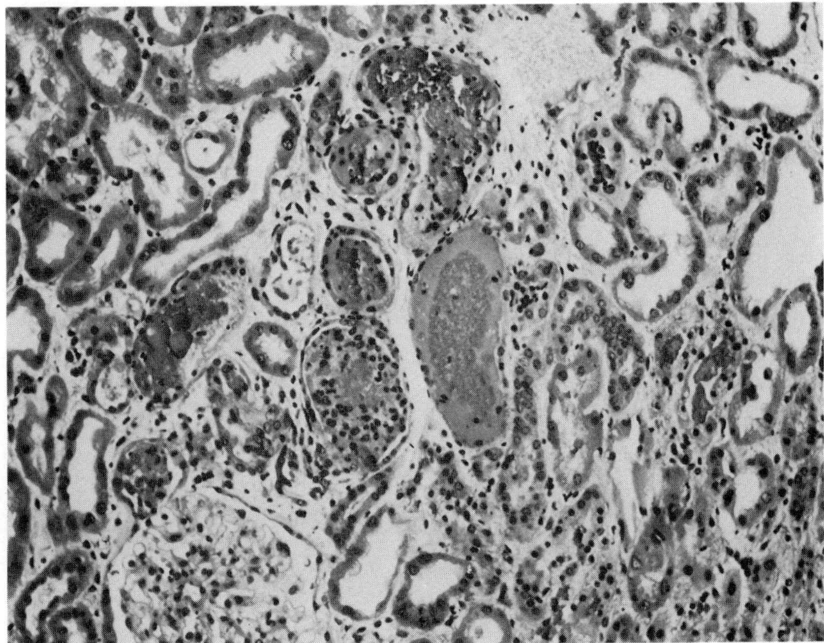

Fig. 1-2. "Crush kidney" described by Bywaters. Patient with acute anuria was found to have acute tubular necrosis. Numerous hemoglobin casts were noted within the renal tubular lumen. Note the necrotic tubules filled with cellular debris and pigmented casts. There were tubules with regenerative changes. There was considerable interstitial edema with mild inflammation. The glomerulus was unremarkable. (H & E × 240.)

recovered from shock but sustained crushing and compressing muscle injuries. Renal insufficiency followed and, in many, was fatal. They designated this disorder the "crush syndrome." At autopsy they found acute necrosis of renal tubules and blanched necrotic muscle. Bywaters' original and accurate drawings of abnormal renal morphologic findings are most impressive and should be reviewed by those interested in this disorder (Fig. 1-2).

Originally Bywaters and associates thought that the crush syndrome was a "hitherto undescribed condition." However, later he called attention to previous reports in the German literature and acknowledged them in a chapter of *History of World War II*, published in 1953.[194] The "compression muscle necrosis with renal failure syndrome" was first described by Frankenthal[392] in 1916 and again 2 years later when he reported a review of thirty patients with muscle necrosis and enlarged kidneys.[393] That same year, Kuttner[657] reviewed the entire subject and added seven patients with compression muscle necrosis. In addition, he referred to Colmers'[229] reports of patients suffering compression muscle necrosis and renal failure in the Messina earthquake of 1909.

The most complete pre–World War II report of acute renal failure was made by Minami in 1923.[781] He suggested that myohemoglobinuria was involved in producing renal abnormalities. Finally, the experience of the German medical corps in World War I was summarized by Kayser.[614] He reported 126 patients with acute renal failure in the official German *Handbuch der arztlichen Erfahrungen im Weltkriege.*

Late in World War II American military physicians became aware of the importance of shock and its association to fatal acute renal failure.[781] For example, they observed acute renal failure in over 40% of a large group of combat casualties and a mortality rate of 90% in those with severe oliguria. Additional observations were made by Mallory, who found acute oliguric renal failure following shock in army battle casualties.[737] He attributed the acute oliguric renal failure to the considerable time that elapsed before the casualty received treatment for shock.

Today, acute oliguric renal failure is still a major problem associated with war and other mass catastrophes.[180] For example, during the 1960 earthquake in Agadir, Morocco, acute oliguric renal failure caused by crushing muscle injuries was a frequent and fatal complication. However, the incidence of acute renal failure in the Vietnam War was greatly reduced. This was attributed to the rapid air evacuation of front line battle casualties to station hospitals for prompt and appropriate treatment. These observations and those made in the Korean War indicate that the incidence of death from battle wounds is directly related to the incidence of acute renal failure. The greater the percentage of acute renal failure the greater the number of deaths from war wounds.

In civilian life acute renal failure is by no means related exclusively to catastrophes. In general, traumatic shock produces an extremely small proportion of acute oliguric renal failure. Because the causes of acute oliguric renal failure are innumerable and diversified, the syndrome becomes very important to physicians in every branch and speciality of medicine.

DIFFERENTIAL DIAGNOSIS OF ACUTE OLIGURIC RENAL FAILURE

The physician must make a prompt differentiation between sudden oliguria or anuria caused by acute renal failure and chronic "end-stage" renal failure.[942] Patients with acute renal failure may not display the typical course, in which there is an onset stage or in which oliguria may not be striking.[339,1037] For further differentiation it seems important to subdivide acute oliguric renal failure into three distinct clinical groups: acute parenchymal disease, acute renal circulatory failure (prerenal),[85] and ureteral obstructive uropathy (postrenal).

Prompt and accurate differential diagnosis is very important for two reasons. First, if acute circulatory failure is not corrected it may progress to parenchymal lesions. Second, hasty and poorly considered management using fluid and electrolytes may be extremely hazardous if parenchymal abnormalities are present. The prerenal disorders include renal circulatory insufficiency due to a variety of causes: acute myocardial infarction, dehydration, and electrolyte and acid-base

Table 1-1. Differential diagnosis of acute renal failure from water and electrolyte depletion

Clinical features	Acute renal failure	Water and electrolyte depletion
History of excessive salt or water loss	Usually absent	Present
Precipitating factor	Present	Absent
Thirst	At first usually absent	Present
Dryness of mouth	Absent	Present
Hyponatremia without evidence of NaCl depletion	If present—diagnostic	Absent
Hypernatremia	Usually absent	If present very helpful
Urinary specific gravity	Usually 1.010 higher in glomerular disease	1.010 usually excludes
Blood urea nitrogen (BUN) BUN/creatinine ratio	High value favor this diagnosis	Usually only slightly elevated
Urinary chloride (mEq/L)	10 to 50	Over 50
Urinary–plasma urea ratio	Less than 5 : 1	Greater than 10

deficiencies such as hyponatremia, hypopotassemia, and acidosis. Clinical features helpful in differentiating dehydration or water depletion from acute oliguric renal failure are listed in Table 1-1.

In the differentiation of prerenal failure from acute oliguric renal failure, 1 liter of 5% glucose in water may be infused over 30 to 45 minutes into a patient not overhydrated or edematous. If the patient has prerenal dehydration, the urinary specific gravity decreases and the urinary volume increases. In patients with prerenal circulatory failure and daily urine volumes less than 400 ml because of dehydration, the urinary specific gravity is approximately 1.030 or greater with an osmolarity of 1,200 milliosmols per liter (mOsm/L). The ratio of urinary urea to plasma urea is usually greater than 10. In "acute tubular necrosis" or severe parenchymal disease the urinary specific gravity approaches 1.010 and the ratio of urinary urea to plasma urea decreases to less than 5 to 1.[454]

First, the physician must exclude all precipitating episodes such as medical and surgical conditions known to be associated with acute renal failure. Then he may concentrate on the possible preexistence of chronic renal disease, which can be done by making careful inquiries into a history of previous renal disease. The best clues are previous hematuria, proteinuria, hypertension, edema, muscle cramping, twitching, toxemia of pregnancy, urine-like taste in the mouth, recurrent renal infections, and the chronic ingestion of nephrotoxic drugs such as analgesic agents.

Physical findings suggestive of chronic renal failure include hypertension, skin discoloration caused by retained urinary chromogen, pallor, ammonia on the breath, red eyes,[99] funduscopic abnormalities, cardiomegaly, pericardial friction rubs, flank pain or tenderness, gross edema, flapping tremor, uremic

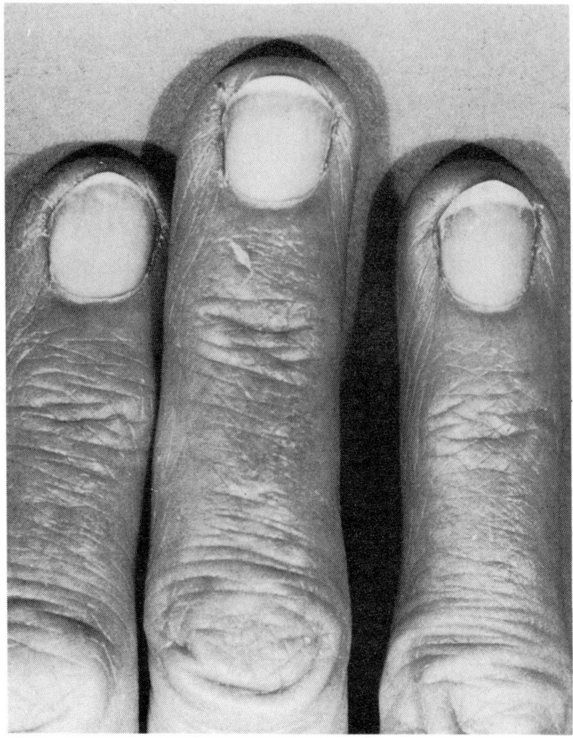

Fig. 1-3. White fingernails, described by Dr. Richard Terry, indicate chronic disease, usually of the liver or the kidney. This clinical finding can be used to distinguish acute from chronic renal failure.

frost, half-and-half nails,[699] white fingernails (Fig. 1-3) or fingernails with a single transverse white band (Fig. 1-4), periorbital edema, and circumflex oral pallor. In prerenal failure caused by dehydration, numerous physical findings are noted. They are decreased turgor of the skin—especially the forehead skin in the elderly—and a dry parched tongue. (Care should be taken to ensure that the dry tongue is not the result of mouth breathing.)

Laboratory findings suggestive of chronic renal diseases are anemia, elevated serum creatinine,[144] elevated serum phosphorus, decreased serum calcium, normal leukocyte counts, and low serum proteins, especially albumin. In prerenal failure caused by dehydration, hematocrit and total protein may be elevated. In addition, the serum uric acid level has been found to be increased out of proportion to the urea nitrogen levels; there has been fixed urinary specific gravity and a serum and urinary urea ratio of more than 10 to 1; and small kidneys have been disclosed by either x-ray studies or by a renal scan study using orthoiodohippurate (Hippuran I[131]).[199] Finally, a percutaneous renal biopsy study may provide the exact renal pathology.[805a]

It must be pointed out that acute oliguric renal failure can be superimposed

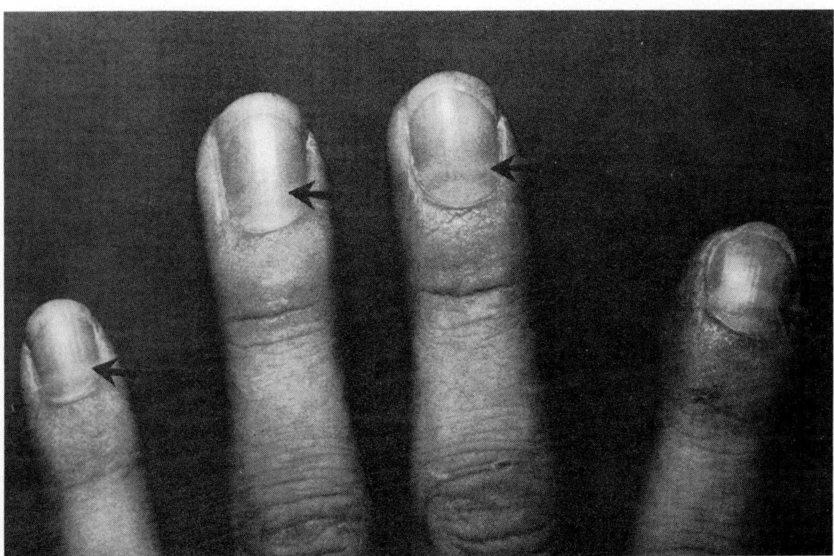

Fig. 1-4. Single transverse white strip in fingernails of 23-year-old student 51 days after onset of oliguria. He sustained a crush injury with intra-abdominal hemorrhage due to fractured liver. Oliguria lasted for 14 days before diuresis occurred.

on chronic renal diseases. For example, patients with advanced renal insufficiency caused by diabetic glomerulosclerosis or by amyloidosis may develop superimposed renal vein thrombosis. This occurs by the abrupt and massive thrombosis of the small intrarenal veins. As a result, the patient develops sudden and absolute anuria.

The clinician should carefully evaluate the patient's chart to appraise intake-output records, blood loss, fall in blood pressure, and the prolonged administration of large quantities of fluids containing glucose. In addition, the physician should check on drugs administered to the patient, surgical reports, hypovolemia, and peripheral vasoconstriction.

The differential diagnosis of acute oliguric renal failure from end-stage renal disease can be most difficult. This is illustrated by the following two cases. In the first patient, chronic end-stage renal diseases could be diagnosed only by percutaneous renal biopsy. Based on a diagnosis of chronic renal disease, prolongation of life by peritoneal dialysis was interrupted. In the second patient, acute anuria resulted from renal vein thrombosis associated with renal cortical necrosis; the nephrotic syndrome was caused by primary amyloidosis.

CASE PRESENTATION

R. S., age 50 years, was transferred to Presbyterian–St. Luke's Hospital on August 1, 1962, with acute oliguric renal failure. He was found to have had "congenital" renal disease in his childhood. On June 15, 1962, he developed fatigue and epigastric pain. His family physician admitted him to a community hospital. He was evaluated and was found to have azotemia.

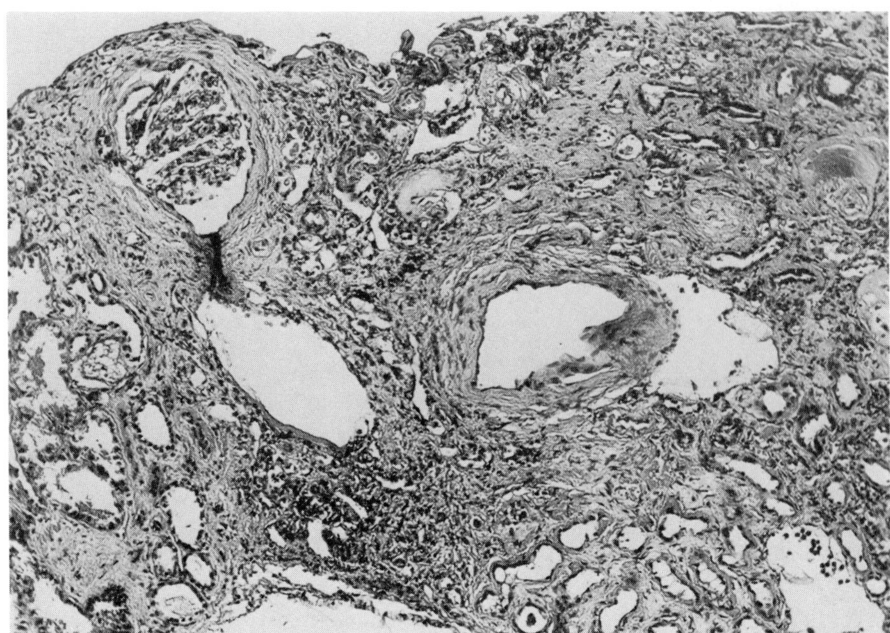

Fig. 1-5. Advanced chronic renal disease. A 50-year-old executive had sudden oliguria. Congenital renal disease was diagnosed in childhood. On the eleventh day of oliguria a renal biopsy study was done to determine the acuteness of renal failure. Chronic renal disease was found. Small cystic lesions were noted with chronic findings of tubular atrophy and interstitial fibrosis. (H&E ×225.)

On physical examination he had marked edema of the neck and face, with periorbital edema and hypertension. His blood pressure was 190/118 to 190/120 mm Hg. His hematocrit was 32%. The leukocyte count was 8,250 per mm^3. Urinalysis revealed gross hematuria, mild proteinuria, and leukocyte casts. The blood CO_2 was 24.5 mM/L. The serum potassium was 5.0 mEq/L. The serum sodium was 135 mEq/L. The blood urea nitrogen (BUN) was 150 mg per 100 ml and rose to 347 mg per 100 ml. The serum creatinine was 9.9 mg per 100 ml and rose to 12 mg per 100 ml.

On admission he received a rapid injection of 25 gm of a 20% mannitol solution without increased urinary output. Peritoneal dialysis was started. The BUN dropped from 150 mg per 100 ml to 96 mg per 100 ml. On August 11, 1962, a percutaneous renal biopsy was done. Chronic pyelonephritis with polycystic renal disease was found (Fig. 1-5). Because of the finding of chronic renal disease, peritoneal dialysis was discontinued. He developed pulmonary edema and was rapidly digitalized. On August 23, 1962, the BUN was 143 mg per 100 ml and the serum creatinine was 16.5 mg per 100 ml. He died on September 5, 1962.

At autopsy the renal biopsy findings were confirmed; bilateral polycystic renal disease was found. On microscopic study there was chronic pyelonephritis.

The following case illustration concerns a patient who presented with all features of the nephrotic syndrome, which was believed to be the result of amyloidosis. He was in shock because of a severe upper intestinal tract hemorrhage. Oliguria followed; a differential diagnosis was between acute tubular necrosis and renal vein thrombosis as the cause of sudden oliguria.

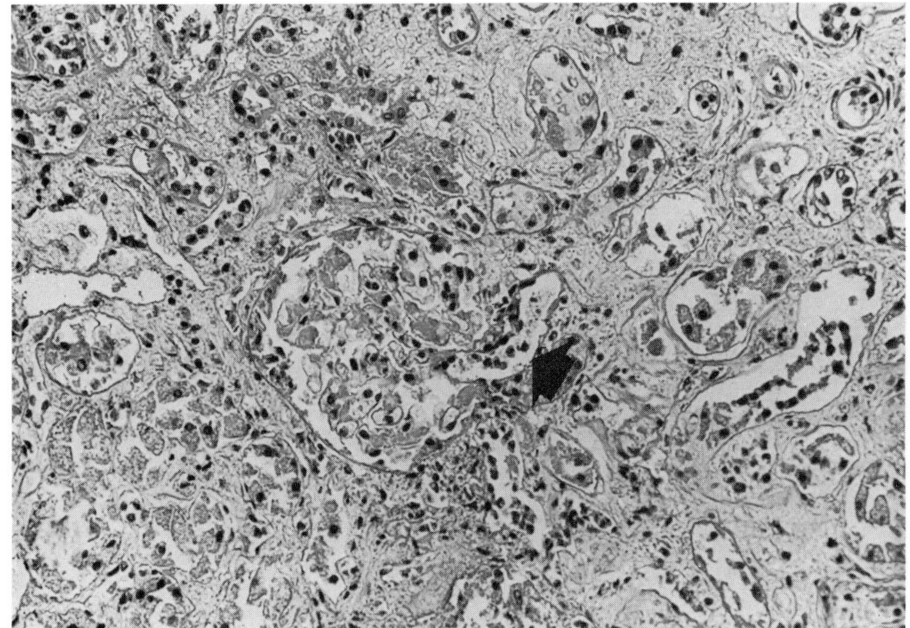

Fig. 1-6. Renal cortical necrosis. A 65-year-old retired executive with the nephrotic syndrome developed shock and subsequent acute oliguric renal failure. Autopsy study of kidney revealed an occlusion of the interlobular arteries and veins. The necrotic glomeruli were involved with amyloidosis. There was marked necrosis of tubules (arrow).

CASE PRESENTATION

On May 12, 1964, C. T., a 65-year-old retired executive with the nephrotic syndrome, was transferred to Presbyterian–St. Luke's Hospital. Gross proteinuria and easy bruising of the skin had been present since August, 1963. His family history revealed a daughter who died at age 34 years of systemic lupus erythematosus.

On physical examination he had marked edema of both legs. His blood pressure was 134/76 to 134/78 mm Hg. Urinalysis revealed proteinuria (4+), a specific gravity of 1.020, and numerous hyaline and granular casts. There was a total of 16 gm of protein in a 24-hour urine specimen. The BUN was 102 mg per 100 ml. The serum cholesterol was 625 mg per 100 ml. The serum albumin was 1.5 gm per 100 ml, and the globulin was 2.2 gm per 100 ml. Because of the nephrotic syndrome, he was treated with adrenal corticosteroids. On May 27, 1964, a massive upper gastrointestinal tract hemorrhage occurred. In spite of blood transfusions and medical management, he continued to hemorrhage. A gastric resection was done. He developed shock for a brief period, and acute oliguric renal failure followed. He died on June 8, 1964.

At autopsy, study of the gross morphology of the kidneys revealed a sharp demarcation of the corticomedullary junction. The cortex was pale, and numerous hemorrhagic infarcts were noted throughout the kidney. There were occlusions of both intralobular arteries and veins. There were mild glomerular lesions of amyloidosis but prominent findings of renal cortical necrosis (Fig. 1-6).

Comment. This patient developed acute oliguric renal failure following a gastrointestinal hemorrhage. Although the nephrotic syndrome was attributed to amyloidosis, the acute oliguric renal failure was the result of vascular thrombosis and cortical necrosis. The histologic finding of renal cortical necrosis was incompatible with recovery and probably resulted from severe hypoxia following the massive gastrointestinal hemorrhage. The reason that renal vein thrombosis occurred in the amyloid kidney is not known.

Ruptured urinary bladder

Absolute anuria can be erroneously diagnosed if the urinary bladder is ruptured and the urine is diverted into the peritoneal cavity. A penetrating injury or blunt trauma in the lower abdomen can result in perforation of the bladder. Extravasation of urine into the peritoneal cavity may produce findings of acute renal failure and, later, peritonitis. This occurs in approximately 60% of the patients with bladder rupture.

Urine trapped inside the peritoneal cavity approaches the osmolarity and chemical composition of the blood. For example, the initial urinary potassium concentration is greater than in the vascular space and would cross the peritoneal membrane into the blood. The overall effects of this "autodialysis" would be a relative loss of sodium and chloride but a gain in BUN and serum potassium.[662,961]

The diagnosis can be based on the characteristic clinical findings of sudden anuria, fever, convulsions and, later, coma. The laboratory findings are leukocytosis, uremia, hyponatremia, and hyperkalemia. Once the diagnosis is made, treatment should be directed to repair of the lacerated urinary bladder. A retention indwelling catheter should be left in the bladder. Urine from the peritoneal cavity should be drained, and the blood biochemical abnormalities should be corrected. By all means, the laceration must be repaired.

Urine and urinary sediment

Today urinalysis remains as much an art as it was centuries ago when first introduced by the Persians. Physicians ritually use urinalysis as an aid in the diagnosis and the management of patients with renal disease. Clinicopathologic correlations made between urinalysis and the vivid and dynamic morphology of renal biopsy are transforming the "art" of urinalysis into a "science."[609] However, there is no specific abnormality to differentiate acute oliguric renal failure from other renal diseases. The findings in the urinary sediment do not reflect the extent of renal damage or the nature of the renal lesion. Moreover, urinalysis is of no value to the physician in making a prognosis during oliguria.

The gross appearance of the urine gives the physician a clue to hematuria, hemoglobinuria, myoglobinuria, and increased bilirubinuria. Gross hematuria occurs with renal infarction such as a renal artery occlusion and renal cortical necrosis. Transitory gross hematuria can occur in renal vein thrombosis and renal cortical necrosis. Hematuria must be distinguished from hemoglobinuria. In patients with intravascular hemolysis, free hemoglobin within the glomerular capillaries is excreted when the serum level of hemoglobin exceeds 135 mg per 100 ml. This excretory rate depends on the plasma haptoglobin level.

The urine may have a coffee color if severe hemolysis occurs, as it does in patients with arsine-induced anuria. Long after hemoglobinuria has subsided, hemosiderinuria persists. The Prussian blue stain is useful in detecting hemosiderinuria. Urine containing myoglobin in both the oxy- and meta- forms is seen in acute oliguric renal failure caused by a crush injury. In some patients with the crush syndrome, myoglobin may exceed 3 gm in 24 hours.

The urine is usually strongly acid in acute glomerular disease, rather than alkaline or slightly acid as in acute tubular necrosis, but this is not always the rule. The urinary pH may vary from 5.5 to 7.5 during oliguria.

The measurement of the urinary, specific gravity in patients with acute oliguria is most helpful in differentiating oliguria caused by parenchymal renal disease from that caused by acute prerenal failure. The urinary specific gravity is fixed in chronic renal disease. The specific gravity is elevated in oliguria caused by dehydration and in acute glomerular lesions that result in acute renal failure. The refractometer, or "TS meter," is a valuable diagnostic tool to measure the urinary specific gravity, especially when only a very small amount of urine is available.

As tubular cells undergo regeneration, the specific gravity first falls below 1.010; later, in the recovery period, it ranges from 1.020 to 1.025. In the recovery period large molecular substances in the urine, such as glucose and protein, may further elevate the urinary specific gravity. A slight proteinuria occurs, probably as a result of the low urinary volume. During the diuretic phase the proteinuria increases and may reach a level as high as 10 gm in 24 hours. In spite of recovery, proteinuria may continue for months or years. This is more likely to occur if acute renal failure is severe or prolonged and if renal interstitial fibrosis develops.

The "histologic biopsy" of the patient's kidney, as referred to by Addis,[8] is the microscopic examination of the fresh urinary sediment. If only a very small amount of urine is available, it can be examined directly by microscopy. To the physician the urinary sediment will be the most valuable of all information obtained from urinalysis.[120] He can base his diagnosis and management on this information.

Hematuria can occur from lesions anywhere along the genitourinary tract. The finding of erythrocyte casts is pathognomonic of renal parenchymal disease (see outline). They are found in patients with renal infarctions following renal artery occlusion, renal vein thrombosis, renal cortical necrosis, lupus glomerulonephritis, sensitivity glomerulonephritis, acute poststreptococcal glomerulonephritis, interstitial nephritis, and ureteral neoplasm. Less serious clinical conditions are renal calculi and pyelonephritis. Leukocytes are noted in the urine of patients with pyelonephritis, lupus nephritis, and papillary necrosis.

Causes of hematuria in the presence of acute oliguric renal failure

    I. Vascular disease
       A. Renal artery occlusion
       B. Renal infarction
       C. Acute renal cortical necrosis

    D. Polyarteritis nodosa
    E. Hypersensitivity angiitis
    F. Necrotizing vasculitis
    G. Scleroderma
    H. Malignant nephrosclerosis
    I. Renal vein thrombosis
 II. Tubular disease
    A. Acute tubular necrosis
III. Glomerular disease
    A. Acute poststreptococcal glomerulonephritis
    B. Hypersensitivity glomerulonephritis
    C. Lupus glomerulonephritis
    D. Thrombotic thrombocytopenic purpura
    E. Hemolytic uremic syndrome
 IV. Interstitial disease
    A. Hypersensitivity interstitial nephritis
    B. Granulomatous interstitial nephritis
    C. Lymphomatous interstitial nephritis
    D. Acute bacterial pyelonephritis
    E. Leptospirosis interstitial nephritis
  V. Pelvic ureteral disease
    A. Ureteral calculi
    B. Ureteral tumor
    C. Crystallization (uric acid or sulfonamides)

Myoglobin and pigmented casts do not stain for free iron. They are found in the urine in traumatic crush syndrome. Large red hemoglobin casts are found in the urine associated with hemoglobinuria. Broad "renal failure" casts, as described by Addis, are frequently seen in acute renal failure.[8] They are renal tubular epithelial cell casts and are identified by the use of Sternheimer-Malbin stain.[10,44] Broad casts in acute renal failure do not portend disaster as they do in chronic renal failure. They are more prone to develop in acute renal failure because of a decreased urinary flow and subsequent cast formation in the largely dilated collecting tubules. This may not be the only explanation, as collecting tubules are not always dilated in renal biopsy material. In the early diuretic phase there are increased numbers of large renal failure casts. They are usually completely gone by the time recovery occurs. Their disappearance indicates that recovery is occurring.

A "telescoped" urinary sediment is characterized by pigmented granular casts, waxy casts, broad casts, and large double refractile oval fat bodies. These findings occur in the presence of glomerular disease such as acute poststreptococcal glomerulonephritis, lupus glomerulonephritis, and sensitivity glomerulonephritis. A telescopic urinary sediment is found in patients with severe lupus glomerulonephritis and in patients with the nephrotic syndrome who develop acute oliguric renal failure.

Obstructive uropathy caused by sulfonamide crystallization within the renal pelvis can be detected by the finding of sulfonamide crystals in the urine. When the obstructive uropathy is caused by uric acid crystallization, uric acid crystals are found in the urine.

Radioisotope renogram

Ureteric catheterization and retrograde pyelography are absolute methods of diagnosing obstructive causes of acute anuria.[587,842a] These methods are not without danger as they can induce fatal retrograde renal infection. Radioisotope renography using sodium orthoiodohippurate (Hippuran) labelled with I^{131} is

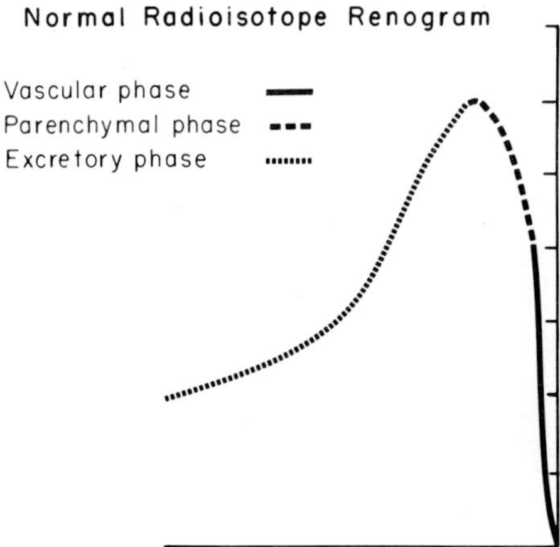

Fig. 1-7. Normal radioisotope renogram. This photograph illustrates the three phases of a normal radioisotope renogram.

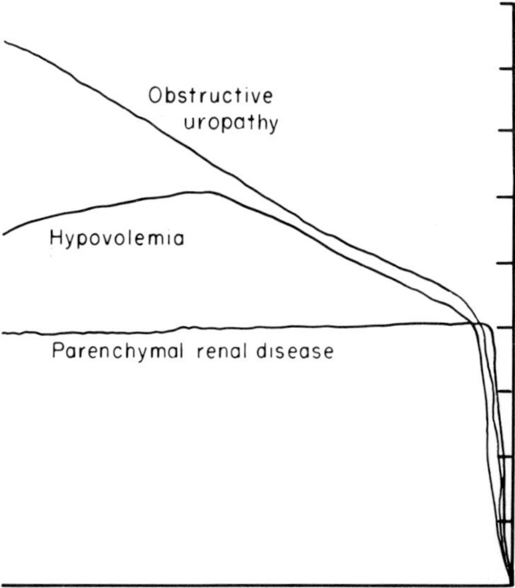

Fig. 1-8. Abnormal radioisotope renogram in acute oliguric renal failure. This photograph illustrates the three specific renograms that may be seen in acute oliguric renal failure. The obstructed uropathy has a continuing rising excretory phase. The hypovolemia curve has an abnormal parenchymal and excretory phase. Acute tubular necrosis can produce abnormalities in the parenchymal phase. Lack of a vascular phase would be suggestive of renal artery occlusion.

a relatively safe and simple test.[119,842a] It can be completed within 10 to 12 minutes and will evaluate the relative function and size of each kidney.[1086]

A renogram using Hippuran I[131] contains three individual segments (Fig. 1-7).[838,1065,1066] The first is the vascular peak, which occurs 20 to 30 seconds after the intravenous injection. The second is the secondary rise resulting from the parenchymal buildup of the radioactive Hippuran. The third is the fall-away, which reflects a combination of diminishing intrarenal concentration and drainage of the Hippuran from the kidney.

Early in ureteral obstruction when the parenchyma is functioning normally, the third segment of the renogram reverses the normal descent with a sharp rise (Fig. 1-8).[1063] In partial obstruction the third segment either falls slowly or rises relatively to the degree of obstruction of the ureter; if renal parenchymal damage occurs, the renogram may be similar to that seen in chronic renal failure.

Role of renal biopsy

Percutaneous renal biopsy is a valuable clinical adjunct to the management of patients with acute oliguric renal failure.[160] It is a relatively safe and painless procedure.[578] Renal biopsy should be done after all other clinical and laboratory investigations fail to differentiate or clarify the underlying renal disorder. Renal biopsy will provide morphologic information on which the physician can base his management and prognosis.

Prior to a renal biopsy, a plain flat plate of the abdomen is taken (Fig. 1-9). This plate is used to help locate the kidney biopsy site. The exact technique of renal biopsy is described in detail elsewhere.[805] In general, percutaneous renal biopsy is done with the patient in a prone position. If the patient has dyspnea it may be necessary to make him sit upright. An 8-inch No. 22 exploring needle is used to locate the kidney, and the biopsy is taken with the Franklin modification of the Vim-Silverman needle (Fig. 1-10).

Caution should be taken not to obtain a biopsy from patients who received heparin while undergoing hemodialysis, from patients with thrombocytopenia, from those in a clinical state of uremia, or from patients about to die. To ensure the safety of the patient, clotting and bleeding times, prothrombin time, and platelet counts should be done. I have found it necessary to improve the clinical fitness of the patient by dialysis before doing a renal biopsy. The renal biopsy is done either on the same day dialysis is completed or on the next day.

The patient with acute oliguric renal failure is a poor risk. It must be stressed that there is a much greater risk in doing a renal biopsy in a patient with severely elevated blood pressure than in a normotensive individual. When severely elevated blood pressure is present I either reduce the blood pressure prior to taking the renal biopsy or take an "open biopsy."

In my laboratory, tissue obtained by renal biopsy is fixed in Helly's solution, which is preferred to buffered formalin solution since it produces less shrinkage of delicate structures, including the tubular epithelial cells. Paraffin sections are

Low circulatory resistance factors

Shock can be associated with low circulatory resistance. It results from toxins (such as gram-negative bacterial endotoxins), anaphylactic reactions induced by drugs, adrenal insufficiency, hyponatremia, and acidosis. Low circulatory resistance is associated with vasodilation and hypotension. Gram-negative bacteria produce an endotoxin that results in a number of reactions. The endotoxin produces an interaction with serum substances such as catecholamines, serotonin, histamines, or adrenal corticosteroids. The arterioles dilate and peripheral stasis follows. The endotoxin may produce either a local or diffuse Shwartzman reaction. The resulting hypotension produces renal hypoxia and subsequent oliguria.

Treatment is directed toward restoration of the internal milieu before renal damage occurs. Anaphylactic shock should be treated by use of adrenal corticosteroids and epinephrine. Shock caused by gram-negative bacterial endotoxin requires large doses of adrenal corticosteroids and antibiotics. The blood pressure should be maintained. Fluid, electrolyte replacement, plasma, and pressor agents are most effective in preventing progression of acute circulatory failure.

Treatment of acute renal circulatory failure

Definitive proof is lacking that acute renal failure can be prevented by use of certain agents or by specific measures.[130,498,690] The incidence and attack rates of prerenal failure and acute parenchymal renal failure are unpredictable and unknown. However, acute renal circulatory failure has been abated through five specific mechanisms. These include: (1) the use of mannitol as an osmotic diuretic agent[62]—it is useful in patients who have acute renal circulatory failure following ischemia or mismatched blood transfusions; (2) the use of hypertonic saline solution, especially in patients with water intoxication and marked sodium deficiency;[113] (3) the use of TRIS-buffer to prevent anuria following acute circulatory failure and acidosis; (4) the use of sodium bicarbonate to correct severe acidosis; and (5) the use of vasopressive agents in combination with adrenal corticosteroids, especially in gram-negative bacteremic endotoxic shock.

In hypovolemic shock the use of low molecular weight dextran has been most effective. However, dextran has produced acute renal failure as a result of marked increase in urine viscosity.[92] Tubular lumen obstruction subsequently occurs. This can be prevented by adding small amounts of mannitol to the solution of low molecular weight dextran.[92] The osmotic effect of added mannitol results in increased water within the tubular lumen, and obstruction does not occur.

It should be pointed out that certain substances and methods can produce further renal damage. For example, the intravenous use of sodium sulfate as an osmotic diuretic may result in congestive heart failure. Furthermore, the physician must avoid a forced diuresis by overexpanding the vascular space with large quantities of saline or osmotic diuretic agents, for this will also produce congestive heart failure.[790,954] Without adequate sodium intake, forced oral fluids can produce water intoxication.

Mannitol

Mannitol is the most extensively used agent in the treatment of acute oliguric renal failure[60,65,139] and drug overdosage. It is the reduced form of the six-carbon sugar mannose. Mannitol is relatively nontoxic and filters through the renal glomerulus without being reabsorbed from the nephron. On intravenous infusion the small molecules equilibrate slowly with the extravascular and extracellular fluids.[170] Within the tubular lumen the particles of mannitol prevent obligatory water reabsorption and carry electrolytes with the unreabsorbed water.[604]

Mannitol was used, as well as inulin, in renal function studies. Homer Smith[1022] noted that some of the patients with posttraumatic anuria developed a diuresis when given mannitol. He speculated that mannitol could have prevented the expected incidence of anuria, and he referred to this relationship as the "osmotic accident." In 1947 Corcoran and Page[234] recommended the use of mannitol in treating acute renal failure.

Mannitol prevents or minimizes the fall in both the renal plasma flow and the glomerular filtration.[61,297] Some physicians believe it has prophylactically prevented acute renal failure in patients undergoing abdominal aortic aneurysmectomy.[46] Early in acute oliguric renal failure mannitol[433] should be used to differentiate prerenal failure from parenchymal disease. Moreover, prolonged renal circulatory failure caused by dehydration or ischemia must be treated before acute tubular necrosis develops.[62] This can be done by using mannitol, especially if hypotension may have occurred.[894] Mannitol was found to be of value as a prophylactic measure against the occurrence of postoperative[351] acute renal failure, such as following trauma,[129,139] in resection of abdominal aortic aneurysm,[63,64] in renal artery occlusion,[79] in jaundiced patients undergoing operations,[270] and after abortion.[285]

When exposed to room air, a 25% supersaturated solution of mannitol is likely to form crystals. This leads to problems with crystallization and plugging of needles, which occur while mannitol is infused and can be remedied by either diluting the mannitol to 20% or by heating the solution. Twenty-five grams of mannitol in a 20% solution should be rapidly given intravenously within 5 to 6 minutes. No other fluid should be infused when mannitol is administered. If within 3 hours the urinary flow exceeds 40 ml per hour, mannitol infusion can be continued to maintain an adequate urinary flow of 100 ml per hour.[63,129]

If the initial mannitol infusion fails to produce a diuresis, an additional 12.5 gm in a 20% solution can be infused. However, one must be guarded in administering excessive quantities. Mannitol can be retained within the intravascular space. This leads to withdrawal of intracellular fluid and may result in acute pulmonary edema.[199] In addition, hyponatremia and acidosis occur.

In patients with acute water retention or refractory water retention 100 gm of mannitol can be given over 90 minutes. It is necessary to replace electrolyte loss by osmotic diuresis.

The exact mechanism of action of mannitol is not well understood—in some patients with prerenal circulatory failure it increases renal blood flow.[66] In addition, mannitol within the tubular lumen may increase the intratubular pressure. Direct micropuncture studies indicate that mannitol, through increased intratubular pressure, can result in compression of the peritubular veins and intratubular veins. This venous compression can lead to diversion of medullary blood to the cortex. When within the limbs of Henle, mannitol may decrease the renal venous resistance. Another characteristic of mannitol is its ability to reverse the fall in urinary oxygen tension.[563] Electron microscopy study of tissue from patients who had received mannitol revealed dense osmiophilic bodies in the cytoplasm of proximal and distal epithelial cells (Fig. 1-11). These bodies appear to be cytolysosomes.

Ethacrynic acid

Ethacrynic acid, an unsaturated ketone derivation of phenoxyacetic acid, is clinically effective as an oral diuretic agent and is readily absorbed by the gut.

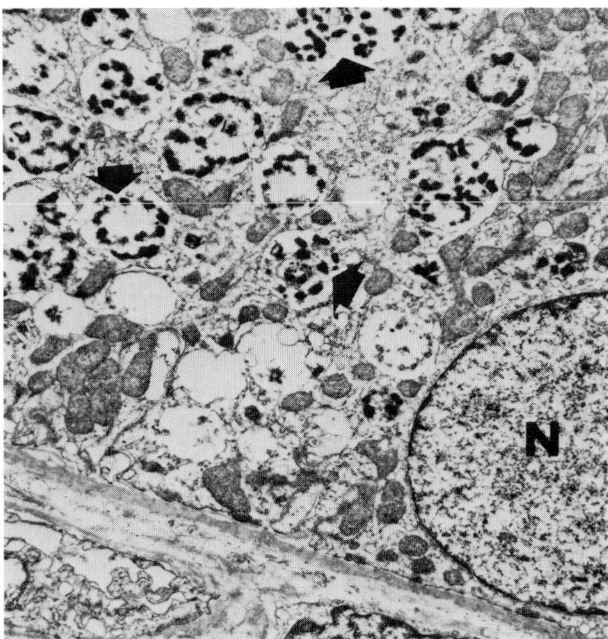

Fig. 1-11. Osmiophilic granular bodies after mannitol infusion. A 15-year-old high school student developed acute renal failure following delivery of a baby girl. Twenty-five grams of a 20% solution of mannitol was given rapidly intravenously. A renal biopsy study was taken 2 hours later. An epithelial cell is illustrated. A nucleus (N) is seen to the right. Numerous bodies containing osmiophilic granules (arrows) fill the cytoplasm. (×6,500.)

It can be injected intravenously and produces a rapid and massive diuresis of water, sodium, and chloride. The peak diuresis occurs in approximately 2 hours and is completed in 6 hours. The major site of ethacrynic acid action is on sodium transport in the ascending limb of Henle's loop.[668]

In plasma, ethacrynic acid is largely bound to serum proteins. A large amount of unbound ethacrynic acid is filtered by the glomerulus. Ethacrynic acid is secreted by tubules, and there is back diffusion of the diuretic agent in the distal nephron.[379]

Mann and Gilmore[740] reversed mannitol-fast oliguria by use of intravenous ethacrynic acid. In eighteen patients with acute oliguric renal failure, mannitol infusion failed to produce a diuresis. However, they had an immediate diuresis up to 285 ml in the first hour following injection of ethacrynic acid (50 mg intravenously). The authors attributed the effect of ethacrynic acid to its ability to reach the tubules without depending on glomerular filtration. Ethacrynic acid can cause deafness that is usually transitory but is sometimes permanent.

Tris buffer

The organic buffer Tham or Tris (hydroxmethyl) aminomethane has two distinguishing mechanisms of action. The foremost is as an osmotic diuretic agent; it is poorly reabsorbed by the normal kidney. Second, it acts as a buffer in correcting metabolic acidosis. Tris can neutralize carbonic acid: $Tris + H_2CO_3 = TrisH+ + HCO_3-$. It is a stronger base than bicarbonate (pH 7.84, compared to 6.10) and yet contains no sodium. Through this mechanism Tris may be especially useful in acute oliguric renal failure following such conditions as hemorrhagic shock, surgical shock, and traumatic shock. Tris is useful in correcting the metabolic acidosis associated with acute renal failure since it is more effective in providing bicarbonate ions than sodium bicarbonate.[636]

Hypertonic saline solution

Hypertonic saline solution is useful in preventing structural renal damage in edema-free patients with marked sodium deficiency and acute renal failure.[113] Marked sodium chloride depletion usually results from persistent and massive vomiting, excessive diarrhea, and fluid loss through the skin caused by burns.[114] The urinary specific gravity ranges between 1.020 and 1.030. Hypertonic saline solution expands the extracellular space. It aids the excretion of urea, sulfates, and phosphates. In addition, it promotes the excretion of hydrogen ions as well as potassium.

Black suggested the use of either undiluted molar sodium lactate or 5% sodium chloride solution.[113] In my experience the intravenous administration of 250 ml of 5% sodium chloride over half an hour to 2 hours has been very successful in inducing diuresis.

Molar sodium lactate has been found to be inferior to sodium bicarbonate or Tris buffer in promoting diuresis. This can be explained on the basis that the

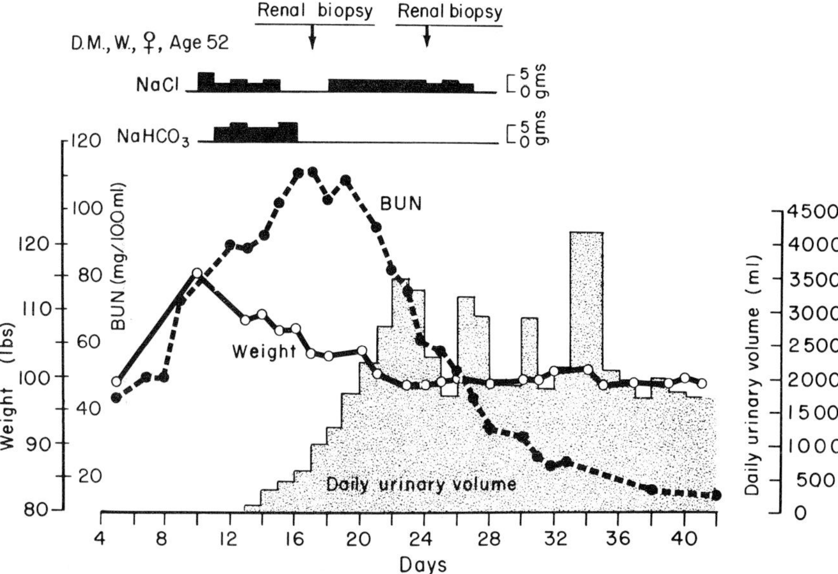

Fig. 1-12. Clinical course of patient with acute renal failure due to acute tubular necrosis. A 52-year-old woman developed acute renal failure without any apparent precipitating factor. Large amounts of sodium chloride and sodium bicarbonate were given. Diuresis occurred on the sixteenth day. Two renal biopsy studies were done, one on the seventeenth day and the other on the twenty-fourth day. Acute tubular necrosis was diagnosed. On the thirty-eighth day the blood urea nitrogen (BUN) was normal.

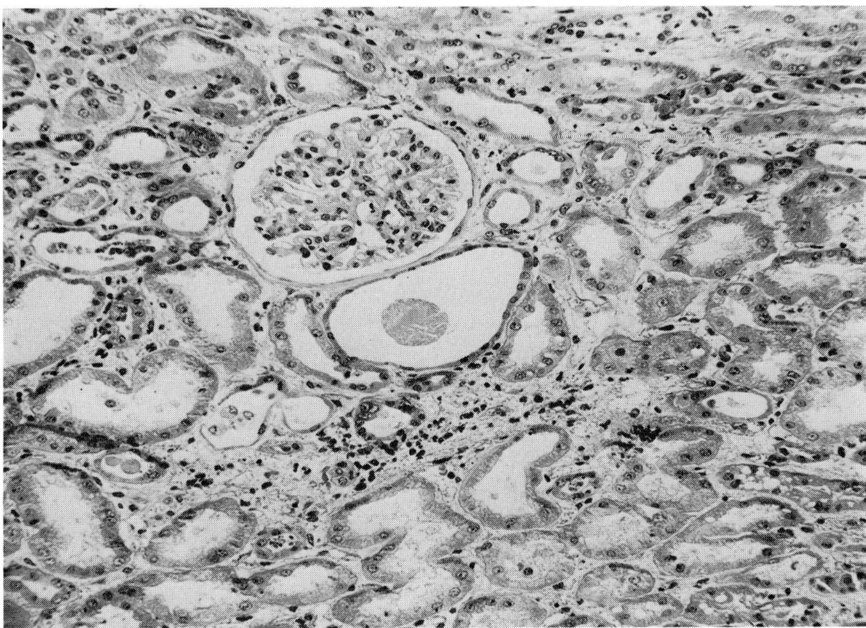

Fig. 1-13. Acute tubular necrosis of unknown etiology. First renal biopsy taken from the patient described in Fig. 1-12. Tissue was obtained at the peak of BUN rise. Tubular regeneration was noted. The striking feature was a diffuse interstitial edema. (H&E ×300.)

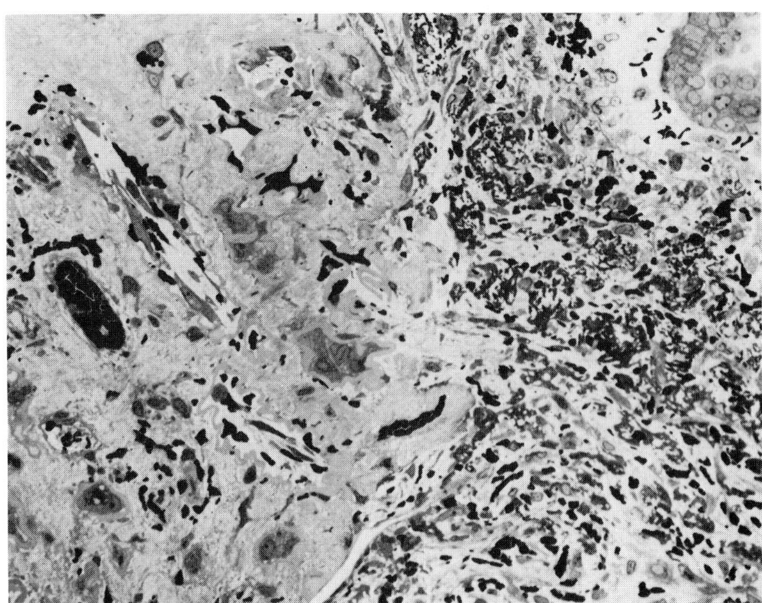

Fig. 1-14. Renopapillary infection. This photograph is a portion of the first renal biopsy of the patient described in Figs. 1-12 and 1-13. The tissue was fixed in osmic acid, cut at 0.5μ, and stained with methylene blue-Azure II. Following the renal biopsy she developed a *Staphylococcus aureus,* coagulase-positive, pyelonephritis. The same organism was cultured in renal tissue obtained by biopsy. Chloramphenicol was given and the infection cleared. The renopapillary interstitium was involved with massive cellular infiltrate of polymorphonucleocytes. The adjacent area appeared fibrosed. (Methylene blue-Azure II ×320.)

lactate ion is metabolized. Lactate solutions can be extremely hazardous if given to patients with lactate acidosis. Care must be taken in establishing the rate of hypertonic saline administration. Patients with hypertension are more prone to develop pulmonary edema.

Hypertonic saline solution is very useful in treating water intoxication resulting from excessive intravenous administration of electrolyte-free fluids. Patients with water intoxication may have marked disorientation, various neurologic complications, oliguria, and marked edema. When the urinary output increases following the administration of 250 ml of hypertonic saline solution, a second 250 ml of hypertonic saline should be given. Frequent observations should be made of the urinary output, the serum sodium, and the BUN. If marked sodium deficiency remains uncorrected, acute tubular necrosis can result. This is discussed in the following case presentation.

CASE PRESENTATION

On June 28, 1964, D. M., a 51-year-old woman, developed sudden nausea followed by epigastric pain and "explosive vomiting." Although the pain lasted several hours, the severe vomiting persisted for 24 hours. Complete anuria followed and she collapsed. On July 2 she was hospitalized at Gottlieb Memorial Hospital. (Her clinical course is plotted in Fig. 1-12.)

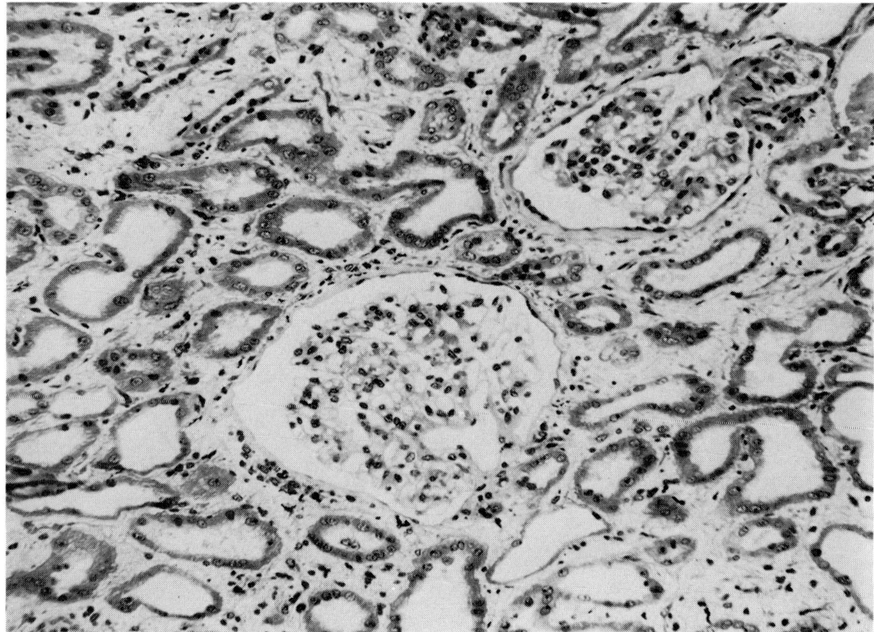

Fig. 1-15. Tubular regeneration with interstitial fibrosis. This photomicrograph illustrates the second renal biopsy taken from the patient described in Figs. 1-12, 1-13, and 1-14. Tissue was obtained at the height of diuresis when the BUN was 48 mg%. The tubular epithelial cells are flat and tubule repair is noted. A permanent diffuse interstitial edema and fibrosis are striking. The glomeruli appear normal. (H&E ×300.)

She was dehydrated and was given intravenous fluids. Oliguria persisted for 10 days and she was transferred to Presbyterian–St. Luke's Hospital for possible hemodialysis. Her blood pressure was 180/88 mm Hg, and pretibial pitting edema was noted. Urinalysis revealed a specific gravity of 1.011, proteinuria (3+), and 30 to 40 WBC per high power field (hpf). The serum sodium was 123 mEq/L, the serum potassium was 4.3 mEq/L, and the CO_2 combining power was 15.8 mM/L. BUN was 110 mg per 100 ml. Urine culture revealed over 100,000 colonies of *Staphylococcus aureus*, coagulase-positive.

Treatment consisted of limited fluid intake containing hypertonic saline solution, oral sodium bicarbonate, and a protein-free, high-calorie diet. On July 13, when the urinary output was 450 ml, a percutaneous renal biopsy study revealed acute tubular necrosis (Fig. 1-13). In addition, there was a marked papillary interstitial infiltrate of polymorphonuclear cells (Fig. 1-14). *Staphylococcus aureus*, coagulase-positive, was grown from the renal tissue. Methicillin sodium was given and the kidney infection abated. The urinary output increased, and on July 19 the output was 3,000 ml. The BUN fell, and on the forty-second day of illness was 25 mg per 100 ml. On the twenty-fourth day of illness a repeat renal biopsy revealed that the tubules were still not normal. There was interstitial fibrosis with basement membrane thickening of collecting tubules and Henle's loops, especially in the medulla of the kidney (Fig. 1-15).

Comment. Acute oliguric renal failure resulted from marked dehydration associated with severe hyponatremia and acidosis. Early in the course of her illness the patient may have had prerenal failure. Rapid replacement of fluids and electrolytes and the correction of acidosis did not prevent the development of tubular necrosis. Once tubular necrosis occurred the clinical features of acute oliguric renal failure followed. The illness was complicated by a *Staphy-*

lococcus aureus, coagulase-positive, kidney infection. Morphologic findings of papillary interstitial nephritis may have represented renal infection and could have been correlated with the culture of *Staphylococcus aureus,* coagulase-positive, from both the kidney and the urine. Diffuse interstitial fibrosis in the postrecovery period from acute oliguric renal failure is a common finding in biopsy material.

POSTRENAL FAILURE

The complexity and distance from the renal pelvis to the urinary bladder predisposes the ureter to a variety of pathologic conditions that lead to obstructive uropathy.[822] The diagnosis of obstructive causes of acute renal failure is very important; its management is completely different from that for parenchymal involvement. In the past acute, oliguric renal failure caused by mechanical obstructive uropathy was referred to as "surgical anuria," and the only treatment was surgical intervention with the purpose of relieving the obstruction.[778] Mechanical obstruction of the ureter and subsequent acute anuria usually present diagnostic difficulties and not conceptual problems.

Clinical features

Although some patients with ureteral obstructive uropathy may experience mild pain, others experience severe pain in the flank, lower quadrant of the abdomen, and suprapubic area. On examination a large tender kidney may be palpated and flank tenderness may be found. Patients with obstructive uropathy will usually have an associated hypertension accompanying the obstructive process. This has been observed in patients with previously normal blood pressure and a subsequent sudden ureteral obstruction. When the obstructive process was removed or the urinary flow was diverted, the blood pressure returned to normal. One explanation for the hypertension is that damage to the renal medullae interfered with or prevented the production of the renal medullary antihypertensive factor of Grollman. A neutral lipid hormone called "Medullin" has been isolated from the renal medulla.[810] This hormone has the ability to reduce an elevated blood pressure.

When urinary flow is established either by removal of the obstruction or by diversion of the urinary stream, a marked diuresis occurs within the first few hours. The diuresis is excessive and apparently results in massive loss of sodium and potasium. It is very important to evaluate fluid and electrolytes at 6-hour intervals, rather than daily, as is usual. Spontaneous improvement occurs within several weeks to months. When improvement is maximum, the kidneys regain their ability to regulate extracellular and intravascular fluid composition.

Diagnosis

The diagnosis of obstructive uropathy[822] must be made as quickly as possible to relieve the obstructive process before irreversible parenchymal damage occurs.[53] Some patients will have no symptoms related to ureteral obstruction, although the foremost diagnostic clue is usually a sudden and complete anuria. Total anuria over 24 hours is rare and should make the physician suspicious of obstructive uropathy. However, total anuria can occur in a patient with acute tubular necrosis, such as in arsine-induced anuria; this condition is rare. In addition, total anuria can occur in severe acute glomerular afflictions and in diffuse necrotizing vasculitis. These glomerular diseases include acute post-streptococcal glomerulonephritis, hypersensitivity glomerulonephritis, lupus glomerulonephritis, acute thrombotic thrombocytopenic purpura (TTP), and bilateral renal cortical necrosis. Erythrocyte casts and subsequent absolute anuria that develop in a patient receiving sulfonamides usually indicate an underlying renal vasculitis.

Obstructive uropathy can be characterized by intermittent anuria alternating with periods of polyuria.[328] The urinary osmolarity during periods of polyuria would increase above that seen in acute tubular necrosis. The indisputable diagnosis of ureteral obstruction can only be made by ascertaining the patency of the urinary tract from renal pelvis to urinary bladder.

Etiology

The commonest etiology of obstructive uropathy in a patient with a single kidney is ureteral obstruction by urinary calculi, a blood clot, or a necrotic papilla. These causes also occur in patients in whom the contralateral kidney is completely functionless. A rare condition known as "reflex calculus anuria" occurs when calculus is in one ureter and bilateral ureteral obstruction re-

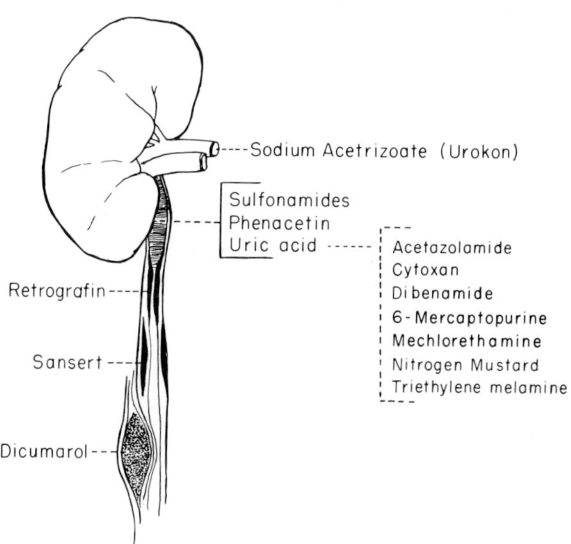

Fig. 1-16. Drug-induced obstructive uropathy. This schematic drawing illustrates the morphologic sites of drugs that produce acute oliguric renal failure from obstructive uropathy.

sults.[788,1085] Previous attacks of ureteral colic caused by renal calculi may have occurred.[691] One must consider hyperparathyroidism, excessive vitamin D ingestion,[5,479] excessive ingestion of alkaline salts, gout, metabolic bone disease, and vitamin A deficiency.

Carcinoma, either metastatic or by direct extension, can involve both ureters. The uterus, stomach, and prostate are the most common primary sites. Rare causes of obstructive uropathy include carcinoma of the urinary bladder trigone, spontaneous perivesicle or retroperitoneal hematoma, hematoma following pelvic surgery, abdominal aortic aneurysm, intra-abdominal pregnancy, and accidental ureter injury or ligation during pelvic surgery. Accidental ligation of a single ureter can result in "absolute anuria" if the contralateral kidney is either absent or functionless.

Drug-induced uropathy (Fig. 1-16) can follow treatment with sulfonamides,[533] alkylating chemotherapeutic agents,[378] urocosuric drugs,[67] anticoagulants,[596] or methysergide maleate (Sansert);[460] it can also follow prolonged phenacetin ingestion[36] and iodinated radiopaque pyelography.[19]

Renal calculi

Patients with ureteral obstruction and anuria caused by urinary calculi are usually seen by the urologist. Although some authors believe this condition to be common, I have observed it infrequently.

Renal colic, flank pain, and hematuria caused by renal calculi usually occur prior to anuria. Because renal pain and colic can occur with other conditions, a differentiation must be made between renal artery occlusion, acute glomerulonephritis, renal vein thrombosis, acute renal infarction, necrotizing papillitis, pyelonephritis, blood clots, and retroperitoneal hematomas.

In general, renal calculi are usually multiple, and a history of previous renal calculi may be obtained. The serum chloride may be elevated.[363] A flat plate of the abdomen that reveals the opaque calculus usually confirms the diagnosis. The calculi should be removed.

Retrograde pyelography

Ureteral obstructive uropathy can result following retrograde pyelography. It results from direct trauma at the ureterovesical orifice,[1017] hypersensitivity reaction of the ureteral mucosa, or papillary necrosis caused by infection introduced by the ureteral catheter. It is more likely to occur in patients with a small kidney or with a completely functionless contralateral kidney.

Ureteral obstruction following ureteral catheterization occurs predominantly in males.[613] The reason males are afflicted more frequently than females is not entirely known. In males the urinary bladder neck is fixed and rigid. It is located more ventral to the ureteral orifices than the urinary bladder neck in women. It may cause a greater bowing of the ureteral catheter and stretching of the ureterovesical orifices, with subsequent local trauma.[520] This is more likely to occur in males, in whom the ureterovesical orifice has a stronger trigonal musculature and greater supporting effect from the vas deferens, seminal vesicles, and supporting fascia.

Radiologic studies indicate that partial distal ureteral obstruction can follow retrograde catheterization. Postoperative pyelogram studies have revealed pyelectasia and ureteral dilatation down to the ureterovesical area. Ureterovesical edema with ureteral obstruction is more likely to follow use of a large catheter resting against the intramural ureter. This usually occurs in males undergoing evaluation for renal hypertension when minimal leakage is essential.

Hypersensitivity edema can follow use of all types of ureteral catheters, including those made of nylon, polyethylene, and woven silk. The ureteral edema involves the entire ureter. In addition, one must consider sensitivity reactions to detergents, iodinated radiographic material, and formalin. Once postureteral catheterization-induced obstructive uropathy is diagnosed, conservative medical management is used. Antibiotics may be given, the biochemical abnormalities should be corrected, and, if necessary, the urinary stream should be diverted. Complications of obstructive uropathy are acute pyelonephritis, pyonephrosis, and septicemia. The use of Teflon ureteral catheters in studying split renal function has reduced the occurrence of obstructive uropathy.

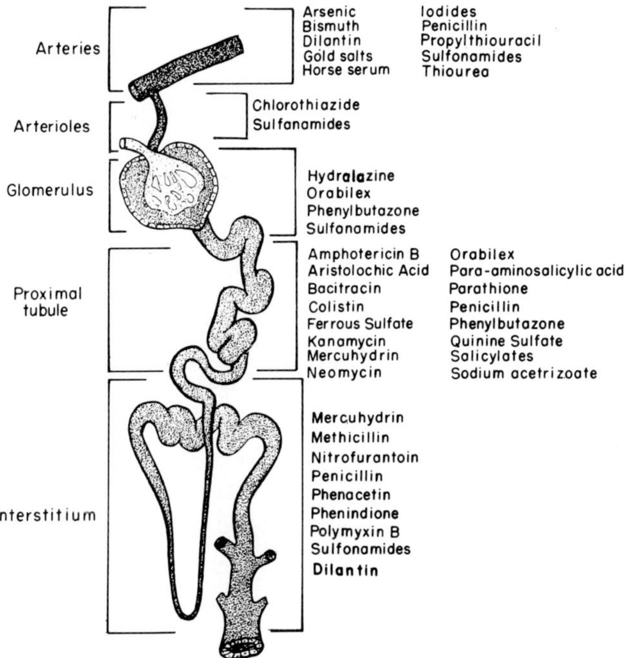

Fig. 1-17. Drug-induced acute oliguric renal failure. Schematic representation of morphologic site of drug-induced acute renal failure. In this photograph the nephron is divided into the arterioles, the glomerulus, the tubules, and the interstitium. Illustrated are the morphologic sites damaged by drugs when the agents induce acute renal failure.

Drug-induced obstructive uropathy

Drug-induced renal disease, like other iatrogenic disorders, annoys the patient and humbles the physician when he finds that he has done harm at the time he thought he was doing good. Over the past several years, physicians have become more and more aware of the adverse effects of drug therapy. The kidney with its rich blood supply and superior excreting function is especially vulnerable to the adverse effects of drugs.

Drug-induced obstructive uropathy occurs either directly or indirectly through one of three renal pathopharmacologic mechanisms. These include hypersensitivity, nephrotoxicity, and mechanical mechanisms. The exact site of pathopharmacologic action is schematically represented in Fig. 1-17. Drugs may induce ureteral obstruction by blocking the urinary flow within the renal pelvis by crystals, both sulfonamide and uric acid,[378] by local inflammation of ureter mucosa (Retrografin), and by periureteral obstruction (methysergide).[460]

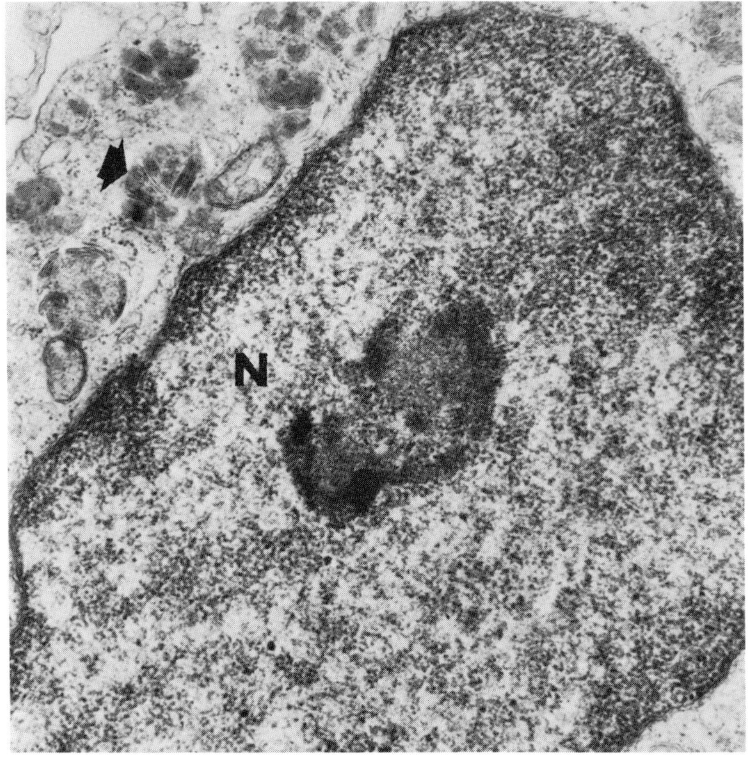

Fig. 1-18. Renomedullary interstitial cell containing crystalline structure. Renomedullary interstitial cells were studied from a renal biopsy of a 44-year-old physician with chronic phenacetin nephritis. The interstitial cells contain dark laminated sac-like structures (arrow) near the Golgi apparatus. These crystalline structures require identification. A large nucleus (N) contains a nucleolus. ($\times$28,710.) This cell resembles a basophil or mass cell.

Nephrotoxicity. Chronic nephrotoxicity may be induced by prolonged phenacetin abuse, and a chronic interstitial (fibrosis) nephritis results.* It is indistinguishable from chronic pyelonephritis. By electron microscope, the medullary and papillary interstitial areas contain many basophils (Fig. 1-18). Renal papillary necrosis is associated with "phenacetin nephritis"; when necrotic papillae "slough off," ureteral obstruction occurs.† Patients have developed obstructive uropathy in a single ureter by necrotic papillae, but bilateral ureteral obstruction may occur.

Mechanical mechanisms. Crystallinization of either uric acid or of sulfonamides is an excellent example of a mechanical mechanism of drug-induced obstructive uropathy.[322] At present, sulfonamide crystallinization in the renal pelvis is uncommon. In the past it was a more common cause of obstruction, but sulfonamides are not used as frequently today as they were previously. Instead, physicians are more inclined to use broad-spectrum antibiotics. At present, sulfonamide crystallinization occurs in dehydrated patients who are receiving large doses of sulfadiazine.

Sulfonamide crystals can be found in the urinary sediment. Once the condition is diagnosed, the forcing of alkaline fluids has promoted a diuresis. In a patient with sulfonamide crystal obstruction, a rare condition, treatment consists of gentle retrograde lavage of the renal pelvis with warm solution of 10% sodium bicarbonate. In addition, sulfonamides can induce acute renal failure by sensitivity polyarteritis nodosa, sensitivity glomerulonephritis, hemoglobinuria, and acute tubular necrosis. These renal lesions will be discussed in drug-induced parenchymal lesions.

If sulfonamides are used, a combination of three sulfonamides decreases considerably the probability of crystallinization and ureteral obstruction. If sulfadiazine is used, fluids should be forced and sodium bicarbonate administered to alkalinize the urine. However, sulfisoxazole (Gantrisin) and sulfamethoxazole (Gantanol) are very soluble in urine and such measures are not necessary when these two are used.

Hyperuricemia with hyperuricosuria can occur on a metabolic basis following treatment of lymphomas.[647] Uric acid is the end-product of purine metabolism, and the major pathway of excretion is through the kidneys. The serum uric acid is filtered through the glomerular capillaries into the renal tubules. It is also actively excreted across the distal tubules. As a result of proliferation and destruction of leukemic and lymphomatous cells there is increased uric acid filtering through into the tubular lumen. This supersaturation may produce uric acid crystallinization in the renal pelvis and subsequent mechanical obstruction to urine flow. The mechanical obstruction usually occurs in patients with lymphoma or leukemia following treatment with radiation, alkylating agents, or uricosuric

---

*See references 360, 365, 1033, and 1062.
†See references 521, 697, 1039, and 1052.

agents. In the past, uric acid crystallinization was induced by acetazolamide (Diamox),[876,1142] methotrexate, triethylenemelamine,[647] mechlorethamine, mercaptopurine, cyclophosphamide (Cytoxan), nitrogen mustard,[926] dibenamide, and by radiation therapy.[679]

Obstructive uric acid uropathy is more likely to occur if the patient is dehydrated, which usually occurs as the result of anorexia or systemic toxicity. This is explained on the basis that the urinary output is insufficient to prevent the formation of a supersaturated solution. Obstructive uropathy from uric acid occurs when alkalinization in the renal pelvis is unusual, such as in patients with chronic renal failure.[201] These patients' kidneys are incapable of secreting a concentrated urine; therefore, uric acid uropathy may develop. Findings of dysuria, flank tenderness, ureteral colic, and uric acid crystals in the urine, and a history of administration of an agent described previously or of chlorothiazide[424] would help establish the etiology of acute oliguric renal failure. The renal pelvis and ureter should be washed down with a warm 10% solution of sodium bicarbonate until the urinary flow is adequate.

Another example of the mechanical action of drug-induced ureteral obstruction is a hematoma induced by use of anticoagulants.[596] Heparin and bishydroxycoumarin (Dicumarol) can produce acute oliguric renal failure by producing a large hematoma that obstructs urine flow. Spontaneous retroperitoneal hematomas may dissect anteriorly toward the urinary bladder, and obstruction to the urine flow follows. The ureteral obstruction is usually characterized by intermittent anuria.

This disturbance can be differentiated from parenchymal causes of acute oliguric renal failure on the basis of palpation of the intra-abdominal mass. In addition, the urinary osmolarity is near normal. This indicates that kidney function is above that level found in renal parenchymal disease—for example, acute tubular necrosis. A flat film of the abdomen may aid in locating the hematoma. A perivesicular hematoma may produce an hourglass appearance of the urinary bladder. The prothrombin time may be normal or prolonged. Treatment should be directed toward prevention of hypotension and ischemia and toward restoration of the prothrombin time to normal, and ureteral catheterization should be done to mechanically reestablish the urine flow.

Hypersensitivity (periureteral fibrosis). An example of drug hypersensitivity is the production of retroperitoneal fibrosis by methysergide. This condition can progress despite cessation of the drug.[460]

Since 1961, methysergide (Sansert) has been effective in the prophylactic treatment of migraine and other vascular headaches. The drug's mode of action is not clearly known. It may produce antagonism to neurokinin or to serotonin. More recently it has been used in treating patients with the carcinoid syndrome.[765] It is better known as a serotonin antagonist, as are the ergot preparations. Methysergide has no direct vasoconstrictor actions such as angiotensin, nicotine, ergotamine, and catecholamines. The side effects are usually mild and transient.[258] The chronic use of methysergide may lead to retroperitoneal fibrosis,[460,1094] mesenteric arterial lesions, pulmonary inflammation with fibrosis, and vascular lesions of the heart.[460] Although the process has regressed with the aid of adrenal corticosteroids or spontaneously after the drug is discontinued, one must emphasize that retroperitoneal fibrosis may have progressed despite stoppage of methysergide.

Graham reported twenty-seven patients[460] with retroperitoneal fibrosis following treatment with methysergide. Hydronephrosis eventually developed; when the obstruction was complete, there was absolute anuria. The fibrotic process has involved other retroperitoneal structures, such as the aorta and its branches;

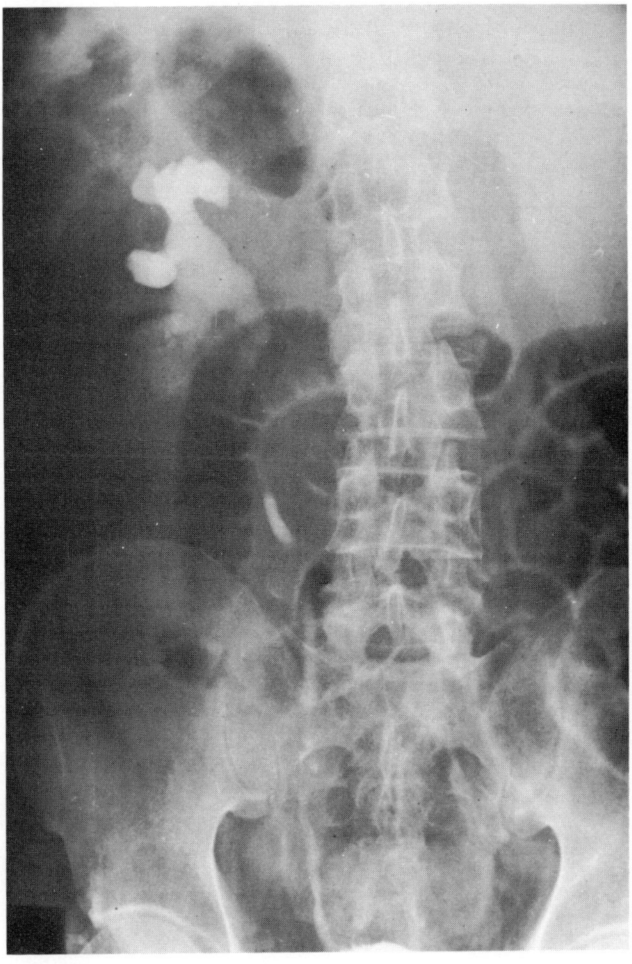

Fig. 1-19. Sansert-induced hydronephrosis. A 47-year-old woman took Sansert for migraine headaches. She developed pain over both kidneys. A retrograde pyelogram study revealed bilateral hydronephrosis. The hydronephrosis disappeared when Sansert was stopped. The etiology of the hydronephrosis was retroperitoneal (periureteral) fibrosis.

it has also produced venous obstruction.[792,902] On retrograde pyelography the ureter was narrowed at the pelvic brim and was deviated medially (Fig. 1-19).

In some incidences ureteral catheterization may not disclose an obstructive lesion. Furthermore, the diagnosis may become apparent only after the radiographic opaque material is injected, following the ureteral catheter removal, or by Braasch bulb retrograde ureterography. The treatment is catheterization of the ureter and then complete release of the ureters from the fibrosed tunnel. Obstruction does not usually recur. In 1958, Ormand[852] first described retroperitoneal fibrosis as a condition in which the ureter and other retroperitoneal structures become surrounded in masses of thick fibrous tissue. The pathologic physiology is unknown.[746a] There is a relationship to other fibrosing and sclerosing processes. These include mediastinal fibrosis, Dupuytren's contraction, sclerosing cholangitis, Peyronie's disease, and Riedel's struma. Should one of these diseases be found, a clinical search should be made for the presence of others.

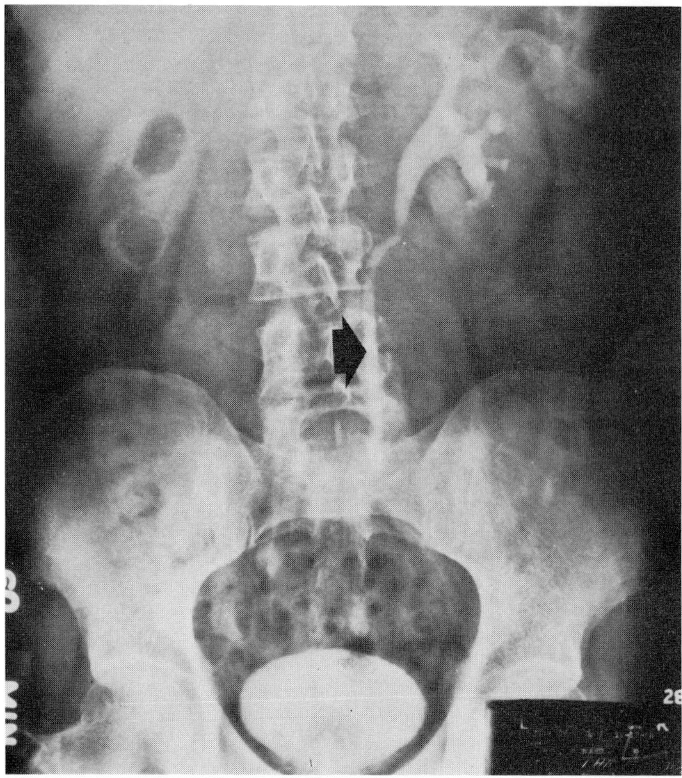

Fig. 1-20. Obstructive uropathy caused by periureteral fibrosis. This photograph illustrates an intravenous pyelogram taken from a patient with acute renal failure due to periureteral fibrosis following administration of Sansert. The left kidney is enlarged and its ureter (arrow) is fixed toward the midline. The right hydronephrotic kidney is small.

Retroperitoneal fibrosis resulted from a variety of causes other than methysergide,[154] including systemic lupus erythematosus, malignant neoplasm (either primary or metastatic), trauma, radiation, and infection. Necrotizing arterial lesions[460] have been found within fibrous tissue. Fetal retroperitoneal fibroses were reported with hydramnios.[323] The sclerosing processes of retroperitoneal fibrosis in some aspects resemble Weber-Christian syndrome in that the process begins as an inflammatory[782] disorder of adipose tissue. It is also possible that retroperitoneal fibrosis develops as a result of a chronic infectious process such as histoplasmosis. Because retroperitoneal fibrosis has no specific features of a single etiology, the physician must exclude all causes before accepting a diagnosis of idiopathic retroperitoneal fibrosis.[906,912] Shelly's in vitro methysergide maleate–induced degranulation of basophils may be of help to the clinician in detecting drug reactions.[1006] The clinical features of retroperitoneal fibrosis in a patient taking methysergide are discussed in the following case illustration.

CASE PRESENTATION

A 59-year-old male had migraine headaches for 30 years and was treated with methysergide (2 to 8 mg daily) for 3 years. For 6 months he developed increasing weakness, fatigue, and

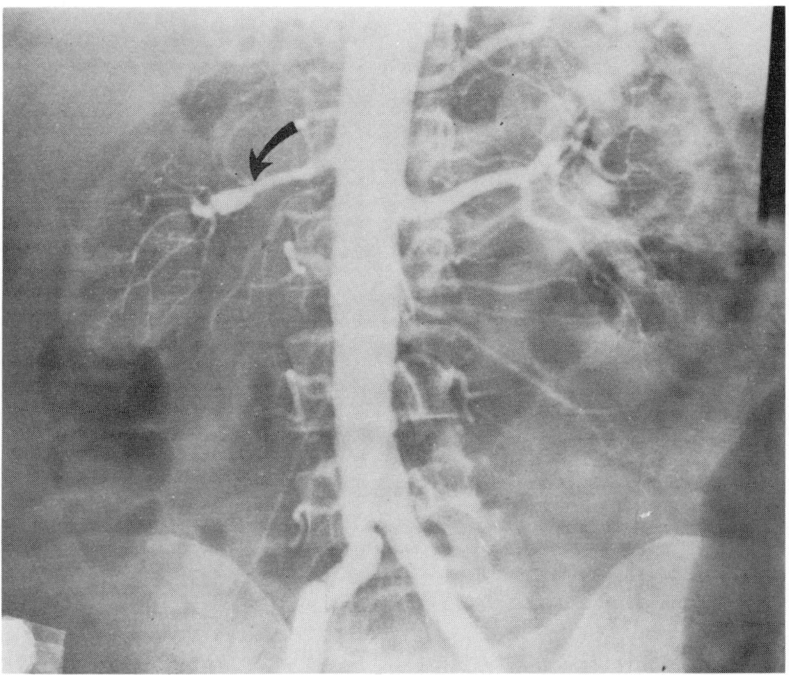

Fig. 1-21. Renal artery stenosis in a patient taking Sansert. This photograph illustrates a renal arteriogram from the patient described in Figs. 1-22 and 1-23. The right kidney was hydronephrotic and had a renal artery stenosis (arrow). On nephrectomy the blood pressure returned to normal.

nocturia. Anuria and hypertension were present for 2 weeks. After a 17-pound weight gain he spontaneously entered the diuretic stage.

Physical examination revealed an alert white male. His blood pressure was 200/110 mm Hg. Findings from funduscopic examination were normal. There was slight cardiomegaly. A small right pleural effusion, some ascites, and peripheral edema were present. The hematocrit was 40%. Urinalysis revealed a specific gravity of 1.010, proteinuria (1+), and numerous erythrocytes.

On admission the BUN was 179 mg per 100 ml and after diuresis it was 15 mg per 100 ml. The serum creatinine dropped from 19.7 mg per 100 ml to 1.5 mg per 100 ml. The CO_2 combining power was 17.1 mM/L. The serum potassium was 6.9 mEq/L. Intravenous pyelography showed a small, poorly functioning, right hydronephrotic kidney. The left kidney was large and appeared normal. There was tortuosity of the ureter (Fig. 1-20). Because of the sustained hypertension, percutaneous femoral aortography was done. A stenosis of the right renal artery was found to be associated with a poststenotic dilation (Fig. 1-21).

In December, 1964, a small hydronephrotic and ischemic right kidney was removed (Fig. 1-22). The right renal artery was narrowed over a distance of 4 cm by an arteriosclerotic plaque. There was no retroperitoneal fibrosis. The patient was symptom-free, and his blood pressure became normal.

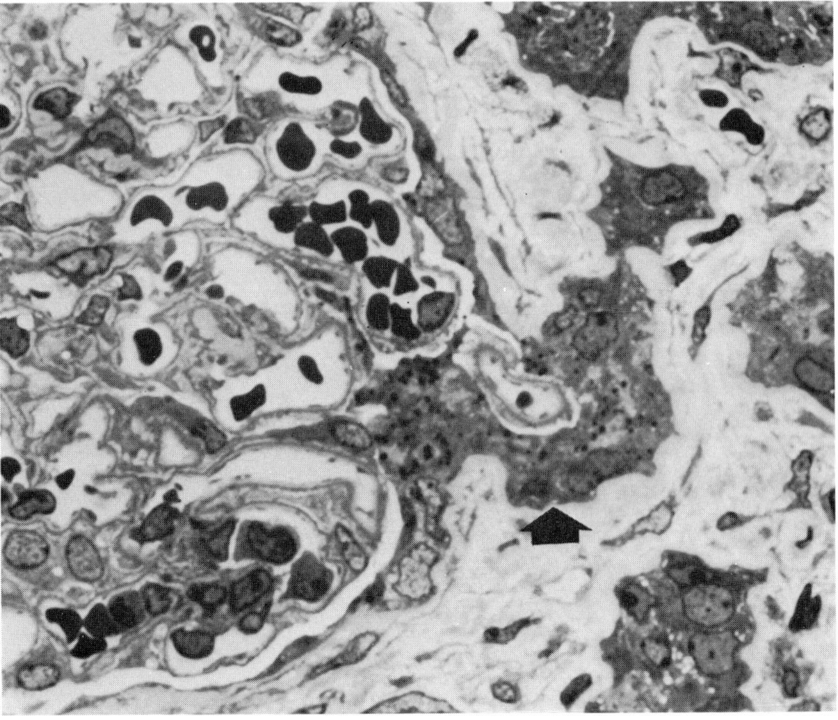

Fig. 1-22. Hydronephrotic kidney caused by obstructive uropathy. This microphotograph illustrates the right kidney of a 59-year-old man who took Sansert for migraine headache. Periureteral fibrosis produced hydronephrosis and renal artery stenosis produced severe hypertension. On removal of the kidney the blood pressure returned to normal. There is a portion of the glomerulus with a prominent juxtaglomerular apparatus (JGA). Increased granularity is seen of the JGA cells at the glomerular base. Adjacent tubules are atrophied. (Methylene blue-Azure II ×1,200.)

In April, 1965, the patient developed headaches and vomiting. His blood pressure was 220/118 mm Hg. Funduscopic examination revealed a Keith-Waganer Grade III retinopathy. There was mild cardiomegaly. Urinalysis revealed a trace of protein and numerous erythrocytes. The hematocrit was 40%. The BUN was 117 mg per 100 ml. A retrograde pyelography study on the left side revealed marked calyectosis and dilatation of a medial deviated ureter with narrowing at the pelvic brim by extrinsic pressure.

A retrograde catheter was retained in the left pelvis. Diuresis followed, and 5 days later the BUN was 54 mg per 100 ml and the blood pressure was normal. Seven days later the left ureter was freed from its tunnel within a dense fibrosis tissue (Fig. 1-23). In a follow-up several months later the patient was normotensive and in good health.

Comment. Methysergide produced progressive ureteral obstruction—first, hydronephrosis and, later, complete anuria. Because of the obstruction, the right kidney became almost functionless. The initial hypertension was probably the result of the renal artery stenosis. The second hypertensive state was probably the result of the obstructive uropathy. This phenomenon has been observed in numerous other individuals with obstruction. Once the obstruction was relieved the patient's blood pressure returned to normal.

The progression of retroperitoneal fibrosis once methysergide was discontinued is difficult to explain. It is possible that the patient had a hereditary predisposition to a sensitive or toxic condition that was triggered by methysergide. This reaction was continuous and may have been arrested by use of adrenal corticosteroids. Methysergide should be used with great caution and should be avoided in patients with cardiovascular disease, those with liver and renal disease, and those with a collagen disease diathesis. Once the drug is discontinued the patient should be followed at periodic intervals to ensure against a latent development of retroperitoneal fibrosis.[987]

The management and clinicopathologic correlation of Retrografin-induced ureteral obstruction is discussed in the following case presentation.

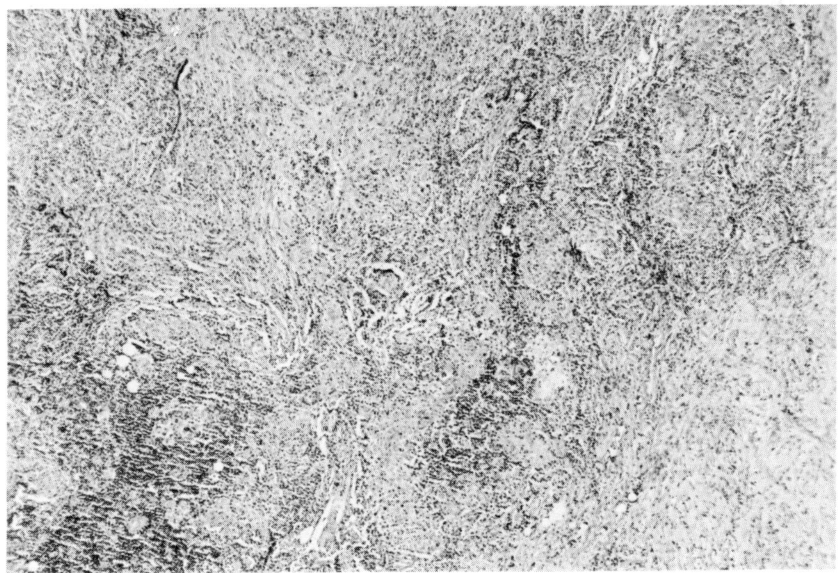

Fig. 1-23. Sansert-induced periureteral fibrosis. This microphotograph illustrates the morphologic lesions of periureteral fibrosis from the patient described in Figs. 1-20 and 1-21. The tissue was obtained when the left ureter was set free from the fibrosis bed. The tissue was fibrotic and contained numerous monocytes, lymphocytes, and eosinophils. (H&E ×64.)

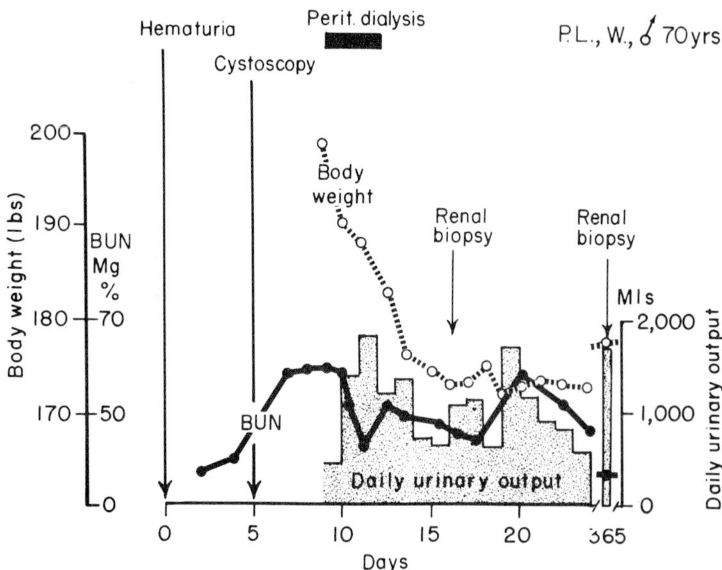

Fig. 1-24. Clinical course of patient with obstructive uropathy. A 70-year-old man had hematuria. Following retrograde pyelography using retrografin he developed obstructive uropathy. Peritoneal dialysis improved the patient. A renal biopsy was done on the eleventh day after oliguria developed. One year later a second renal biopsy was taken.

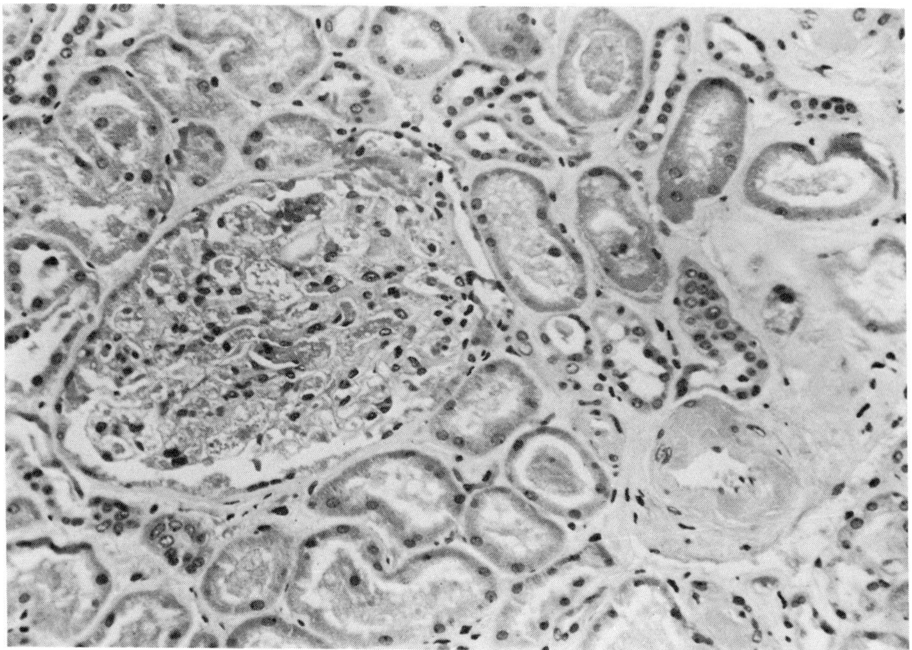

Fig. 1-25. Retrografin-induced renal failure. This microphotograph illustrates the first renal biopsy from patient described in Fig. 1-24. Tissue was obtained on the eleventh day after the onset of anuria when the daily urinary output was 1,150 ml. The tubules were normal by electron microscopic study. There was mild interstitial fibrosis and striking nephrosclerosis. (H&E ×340.)

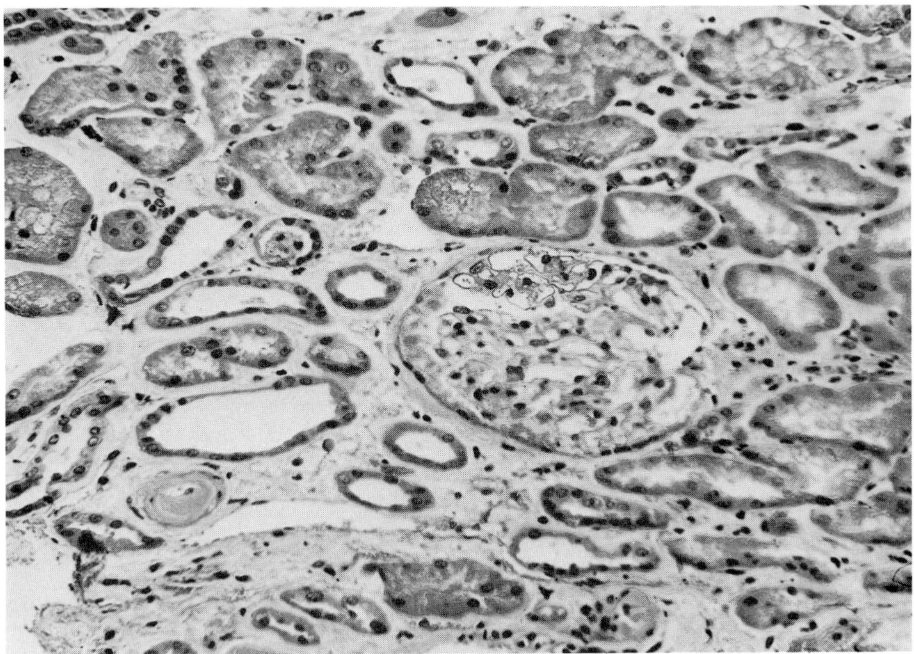

Fig. 1-26. Repeat renal biopsy 1 year after obstructive uropathy. This microphotograph illustrates the second biopsy obtained from the patient described in Figs. 1-24 and 1-25. One year after acute renal failure, the striking feature was a diffuse interstitial fibrosis. (H&E ×340.)

CASE PRESENTATION

A 70-year-old elderly male was admitted to the hospital with gross hematuria of 2 days' duration. Retrograde pyelograms were performed with Retrografin as a contrast media. No abnormalities were noted in the size and configuration of the renal pelvis. However, anuria followed retrograde catheterization. Over the next 4 days, his fluid intake was excessive and he developed water intoxication.

Urinalysis revealed proteinuria (3+) and numerous erythrocytes in the urinary sediment. The hematocrit was 42%. The BUN was 70 mg per 100 ml. The serum sodium was 117 mEq/L, serum chloride was 83 mEq/L, and CO_2 combining power was 15.3 mM/L. (His clinical course while in the hospital is plotted in Fig. 1-24.) A peritoneal dialysis was done, using twenty-seven exchanges.

The patient entered the diuretic stage on the sixth day after anuria. A percutaneous renal biopsy was done during early diuresis and 1 year later. The glomeruli and tubules appeared normal. A diffuse interstitial edema and fibrosis were noted.

Comment. The patient developed absolute anuria following retrograde ureteral catheterization using Retrografin. Following excessive fluids he developed water intoxication and required peritoneal dialysis. Although the glomeruli and tubules were apparently normal, a diffuse interstitial edema occurred (Fig. 1-25). One year later diffuse interstitial fibrosis was noted (Fig. 1-26). This lesion was probably the result of the previous acute renal failure.

Obstructive uropathy associated with a single kidney

Obstructive uropathy is more prone to occur in an individual with a single functioning kidney that suddenly becomes obstructed. Ureteral obstruction can occur as a result of tumor, calculi, papillary necrosis,[221] or a hematoma. In the following case presentation are illustrated the diagnostic difficulties that resulted from ureteral obstruction caused by a metastatic tumor in a patient with a previously undiagnosed single kidney.

CASE PRESENTATION

On August 14, 1965, C. R., a 56-year-old male, developed persistent and severe diarrhea while vacationing in Michigan. Frequent watery diarrhea lasted for 10 days; during this period he developed edema of his legs. A physician was consulted and he made a diagnosis of congestive heart failure. In spite of digitalization the patient continued to deteriorate.

On returning home he consulted his family physician, who hospitalized him. In the hospital the patient was found to have renal failure. On August 29, 1965, when the BUN reached 134 mg per 100 ml, he was transferred to Presbyterian–St. Luke's Hospital. Physical examination revealed an obese, pale, middle-aged male who was lethargic and in a semicoma. His respiration rate was deep and rapid. There was edema of the leg and face. The blood pressure was 210/108 to 210/140 mm Hg. The pulse was 104 and regular, the respiration rate was 28

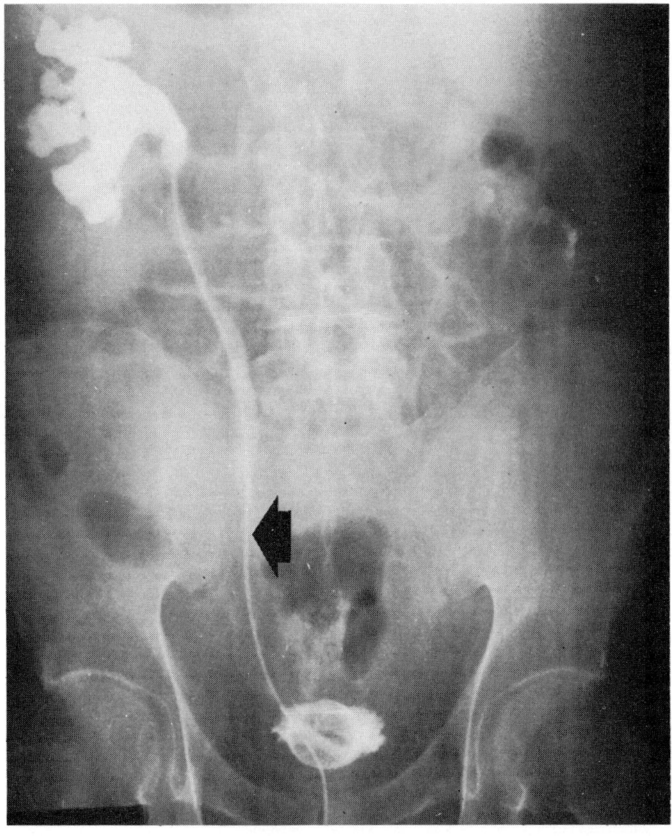

Fig. 1-27. Obstructive uropathy caused by neoplasm in a patient with a single kidney. This retrograde pyelogram study revealed a single right kidney. There was ureteral obstruction at the lower third of the right ureter (arrow)

per minute, and the temperature was 99.6° F. Funduscopic examination revealed a Grade II hypertensive retinopathy. The neck veins were distended. The heart was enlarged to the anterior axillary line. The abdomen was protruded. There was pitting edema (4+) to the knees. The right lobe of the prostate was extremely firm and enlarged.

On admission the BUN was 144 mg per 100 ml, the serum potassium was 8.2 mEq/L, and the CO_2 combining power was 10.4 mM/L. Peritoneal dialysis was started and continued for 36 hours. The BUN fell to 50 mg per 100 ml. After 24 hours of absolute anuria, the daily urinary output increased; after 1 week, it rose to a peak of 4,000 ml. The blood chemistries returned to normal and his clinical state greatly improved. Drip intravenous pyelogram demonstrated an absent left kidney and a rather large right kidney. The collecting system was found to be somewhat dilated. During retrograde cystoscopy hydronephrosis and ureteral obstruction were found approximately 10 cm from the ureterovesical junction (Fig. 1-27 and 1-28).

On September 20, 1965, a transabdominal exploration was done. A tumor mass was found to be partially obstructing the right ureter. This was described as a glandular tumor that was possibly arising from the prostate. A T-tube was inserted to divert the urinary stream and to allow urinary drainage. On October 3, 1965, when he was completely asymptomatic and his BUN was 20 mg per 100 ml, he was discharged.

Comment. Acute oliguric renal failure occurred while the patient was on vacation and was

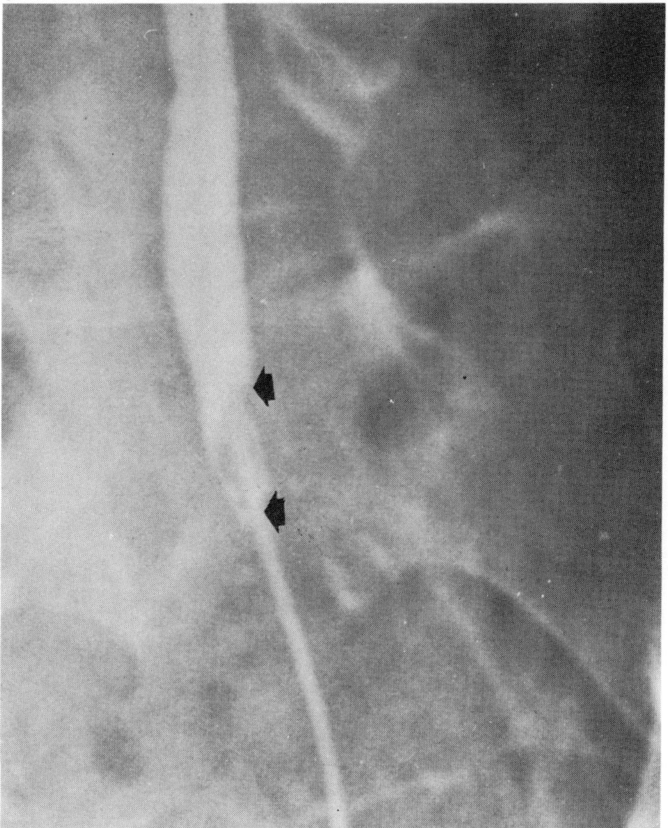

Fig. 1-28. High magnification of tumor producing obstructive uropathy. This high magnification of a retrograde pyelogram illustrates the obstructive lesion (arrows). A metastatic adenocarcinoma of the prostate was found to have obstructed the ureter of a single kidney.

not correctly recognized until he was hospitalized. The development of absolute anuria suggested a ureteral obstructive process. On spontaneous diuresis, acute tubular necrosis was diagnosed incorrectly. A drip intravenous pyelogram aided in establishing the correct diagnosis of obstructive uropathy in a single kidney. The finding of a metastatic lesion producing the obstruction was not unusual. However, the finding that the metastatic lesion originated in the prostate was most rare. Once a diagnosis was established, treatment was to divert the urinary stream and to treat the patient for adenocarcinoma of the prostate.

Renal papillary necrosis

The clinical features of ureteral obstructive renal failure caused by papillary necrosis are similar to other forms of obstructive uropathy.[36,783] The patient experiences abdominal pain—usually colicky because of passage of the papillae down the ureter.[787,903,907] The papillae slough off and may lodge in the ureter and produce an obstructive uropathy.[837] In addition, the patient may have fever, chills, sweats, pyuria, leukocytosis, and azotemia. Diagnosis may be established when the necrotic papillae are recovered in the urine (Fig. 1-29). Therefore, the urine should be strained through gauze to recover the papillae. All tissue-colored material should be fixed in formalin solution and examined.

Retrograde pyelography is very useful in demonstrating the roentgenologic findings of renal necrotizing papillitis. These include the "signet ring" defect, calyceal blunting, and mottled filling defects in the calyces.[1076] The absolute diagnosis is finding the sloughed necrotic papillae in the urine. Treatment should

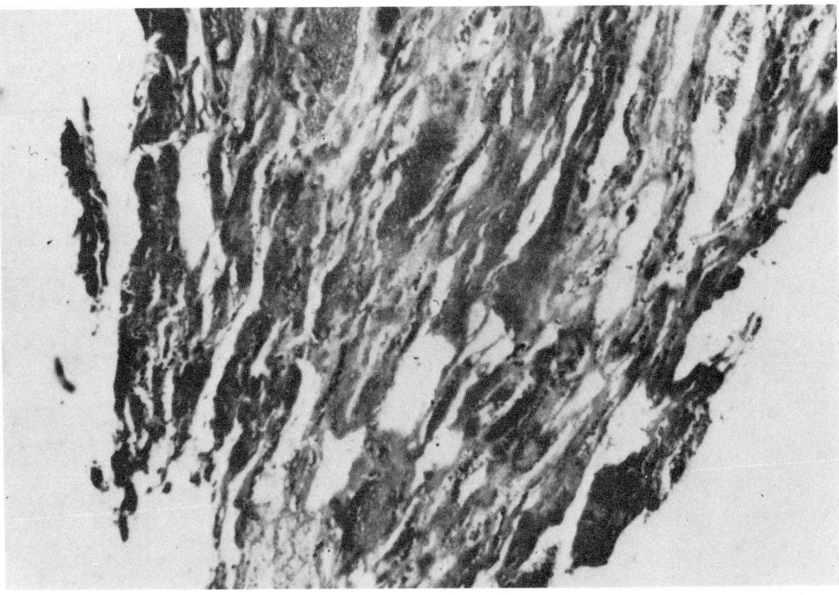

Fig. 1-29. Necrotic papillae found in urine of patient with analgesic nephritis. This microphotograph illustrates a necrotic papillary tip passed in the urine from a 44-year-old physician with analgesic nephropathy. The papillary anatomic structure appears to be lost. The parallel collecting tubules and limbs of Henle are identified. (H&E ×400.)

be directed to the removal of the necrotic papillae and toward eradication of the infection at the base of the necrotic papilla. Chloramphenicol and tetracycline have been effective if used adequately and aggressively early in the course of the illness.

Renal papillary necrosis is more likely to occur in the patient over 40 years of age with diabetes mellitus and urinary tract infection.[42] For example, Mandel[739] observed 153 patients with papillary necrosis and found it to be associated with diabetes mellitus and urinary obstruction in 90% of them. The percentage of patients (5 to 6%) with diabetes mellitus and papillary necrosis at necropsy has changed very little over the past 25 years.[1128] These patients are extremely ill, and bacterial shock usually supervenes. Renal function may deteriorate rapidly, and the patient dies from renal failure. Renal papillary necrosis has been reported to occur in patients with chronic alcoholism. It is usually diagnosed at autopsy. When diagnosed during life, the prognosis is very poor.

Prolonged phenacetin abuse can produce interstitial fibrosis indistinguishable from pyelonephritis (Fig. 1-30) and it is usually associated with papillary necrosis. It has resulted in bilateral ureteral obstruction caused by lodged necrotic papillae within ureters. In recent years increasing reports have appeared on

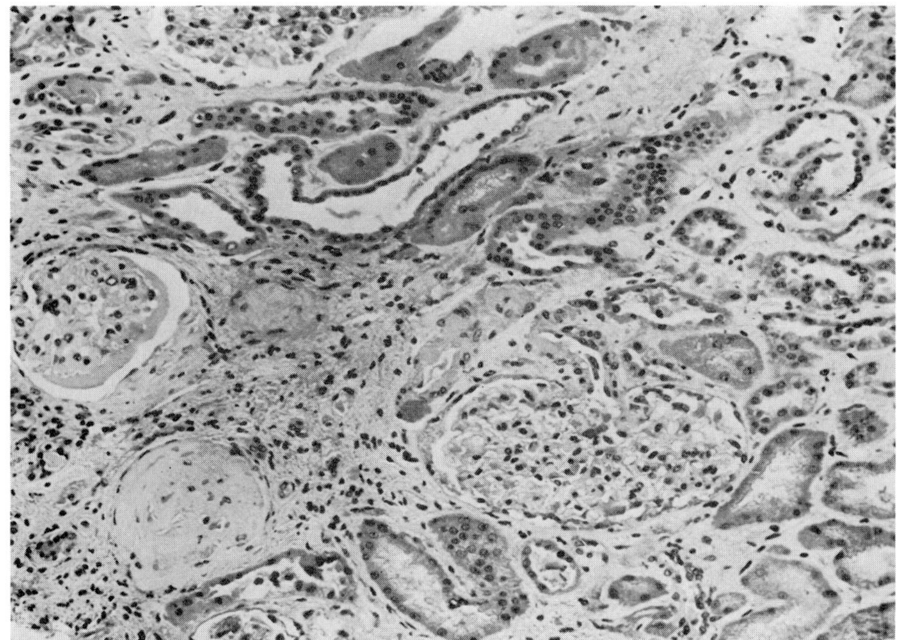

Fig. 1-30. Chronic "phenacetin nephritis." A 44-year-old physician took large quantities of phenacetin-containing analgesic drugs for 5 years. He passed eleven necrotic papillae. He developed acute oliguria from ureteral obstruction. The papillae were spontaneously passed. A diuresis followed and the patient improved when he overcame his analgesic addiction. Dense interstitial fibrosis is noted with tubular atrophy and periglomerular fibrosis.

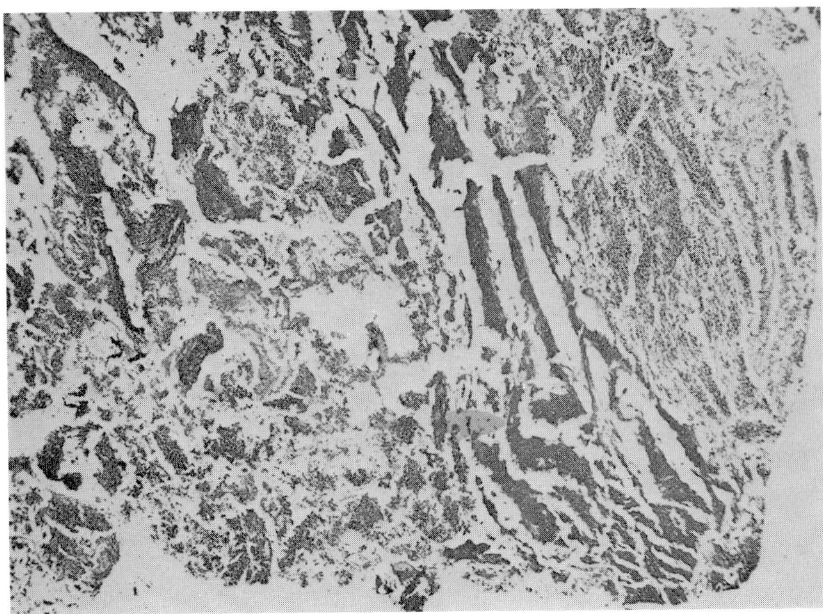

Fig. 1-31. Papillary necrosis and analgesic nephritis. This photograph illustrates a necrotic renal papillae. A 54-year-old housewife with rheumatoid arthritis ingested twelve to fourteen APC tablets daily for over 8 years. She died in uremia. Eight of eleven papillae of her right kidney were damaged. Bacterial culture of a papillary tip was sterile. Note the demarcation line at the papillary base. (H&E ×25.)

obstructive uropathy due to phenacetin-induced papillary necrosis (Fig. 1-31). The patients usually do not have as severe a urinary tract infection as diabetic patients and therefore have neither fever nor pyuria. In general, the prognosis is better in a patient with phenacetin-induced papillary necrosis than in the diabetic patient or the patient with chronic alcoholism.

Treatment

It is imperative that retrograde pyelography be done as early in the course of obstructive uropathy as is clinically possible. The longer the duration of ureteral obstruction the less likely is complete recovery of the renal parenchyma.

Some clinicians suggest that each ureter be catheterized singly and that the catheter be removed from one ureter before examining the other. This should prevent "reflex anuria." This has not been my experience. Individuals with retroperitoneal fibrosis and absolute anuria have had both catheters left in place without adverse sequelae.

Cystoscopy and bilateral ureteric retrograde catherization must be performed on all patients with ureteric obstructions, especially when crystallization occurs in the renal pelvis. When ureteral blockage results from crystalluria following treatment with sulfonamide, uricosuric agents, radiation, or alkylating agents, retrograde flushing of the renal pelvis with warm sodium bicarbonate solution can wash away both uric acid crystals and sulfonamide crystals.

Bilateral simultaneous necrotic papillae sloughing from the kidney caused by chronic phenacetin nephritis has been successfully treated by retrograde flushing. If the obstruction is caused by retroperitoneal fibrosis the ureter will remain near the vertebrae and will appear stiff (Fig. 1-20). It may be necessary to leave the ureteral catheter in place. When the clinical condition of the patient improves, surgical intervention with tunneling frees the ureter from the fibrotic periureteral bed. If surgical correction is not possible the urinary stream must be diverted.

Chapter 2

Intrinsic renal disease

Fifteen years ago much of the morphologic knowledge associated with acute renal failure was based on innumerable case reports describing the classic morbid anatomy. Since 1952 freshly harvested tissue, obtained by serial renal biopsy, has provided a dynamic and vivid cinematographic image of the exact structural lesions of acute renal failure. In addition, serial electron microscopic studies have further clarified this dynamic morphology. The complex clinical, biochemical, and renal functional abnormalities of acute renal failure can be attributed to a wide range of renal structural findings.[294,395]

Numerous morphologic findings must be considered. They vary from apparently normal and mild to severe and progressive irreversible damage. These findings involve all four anatomic segments of the kidney—the interstitium,[543] the tubules, the glomeruli, and the vasculature. In the past emphasis was placed on each of these segments, either singly or in combination, regarding the specific site producing acute renal failure. It is very likely that many of these morphologic changes are accessories that accompany acute renal failure but do not produce it.

ACUTE INTERSTITIAL NEPHRITIS

The earliest description of interstitial involvement was reported by Biermer in 1860.[107] He studied a patient with absolute anuria of 10 days' duration. At autopsy he found acute interstitial nephritis. Councilman[242] in 1898, and 40 years later, Kimmelstiel,[627] related acute hematogenous interstitial nephritis to acute renal failure.

The first outstanding morphologic study of acute interstitial nephritis was that of Councilman[242] (Fig. 2-1). He described the disease as an acute inflammation of the kidney characterized by interstitial cellular infiltrates and interstitial edema. In the majority of his patients, lymphocytes, eosinophils, plasma cells, and histocytes infiltrated the interstitium. Today eosinophils are the predominant infiltrators of the interstitium in acute renal failure induced by such drugs as phenindione,[86] methicillin,[148] or meralluride (Mercuhydrin). The finding of

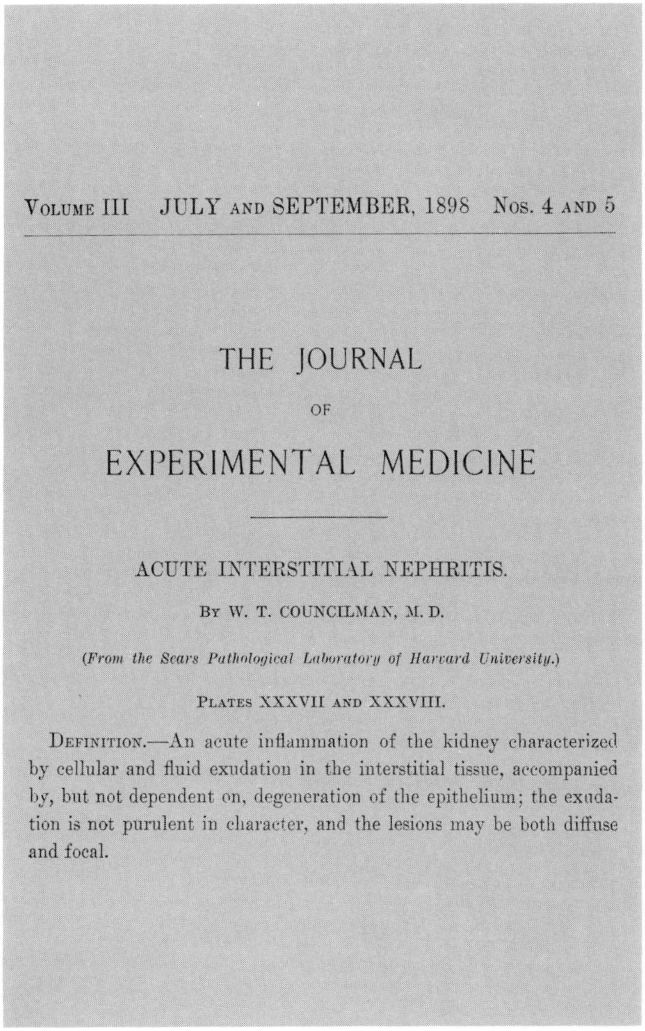

VOLUME III   JULY AND SEPTEMBER, 1898   NOS. 4 AND 5

THE JOURNAL

OF

EXPERIMENTAL MEDICINE

ACUTE INTERSTITIAL NEPHRITIS.

BY W. T. COUNCILMAN, M. D.

(From the Sears Pathological Laboratory of Harvard University.)

PLATES XXXVII AND XXXVIII.

DEFINITION.—An acute inflammation of the kidney characterized by cellular and fluid exudation in the interstitial tissue, accompanied by, but not dependent on, degeneration of the epithelium; the exudation is not purulent in character, and the lesions may be both diffuse and focal.

Fig. 2-1. Councilman's description of acute interstitial nephritis. In 1898, Councilman described the pathologic finding of acute interstitial fibrosis in a schoolgirl with fatal acute oliguric renal failure.

interstitial nephritis is usually associated with but is not preceded by tubular epithelium degeneration.[1077]

Acute hematogenous interstitial nephritis

Kimmelstiel observed acute hematogenous interstitial nephritis in association with hemolytic reactions following blood transfusions and in the hepatorenal syndrome.[627] He described the renal morphology in patients with anuria as a "cellular infiltration, interstitial edema, hematin casts within the tubular lumen, tubular dilation and epithelial cell degeneration." He pointed out that these changes could be present simultaneously or that any one of these processes could be absent. He differentiated acute hematogenous interstitial nephritis from the lymphogenic ascending type of interstitial nephritis; he regarded it as an allergic hyperergic response to either foreign proteins or protein breakdown products. Moreover, he pointed out that the renal interstitium was an area where hypersensitivity reactions can occur. Time has proved his postulate to be true. We know now that drugs such as methicillin, phenindione, and meralluride can produce hypersensitivity reactions of the interstitium. This reaction is reversible when the drug is stopped and adrenocortical steroids are administered. Patients with acute renal failure caused by a drug-induced interstitial nephritis have cellular infiltrates of eosinophils, small lymphocytes, and plasma cells. The cellular infiltrates occur at the corticomedullary junction with a much more extensive involvement of the cortex. After treatment with adrenocortical steroids the interstitial cellular infiltrates disappear and the patient may recover.

Councilman interstitial nephritis

Neither Councilman nor Kimmelsteil attributed acute interstitial nephritis to direct bacterial invasion. They based this on finding a diffuse lesion rather than a focal interstitial lesion. However, Munk believed that the interstitial lesion was not a primary kidney disease but a general cellular exudation caused by bacterial or viral infection of the interstitium such as complicating streptococcal infections or smallpox.[813]

The gross appearance of the kidney on cut sections reveals an obscured architecture of the cortex ill defined from the medulla. In interstitial nephritis the cortex is glistening, in contrast to its dull surface when acute tubular necrosis is present.

Diffuse interstitial cellular infiltrates of plasma cells and eosinophils are the striking histologic findings of a Councilman interstitial nephritis. The glomeruli are usually normal and the intrarenal vessels are not involved with the hypersensitivity reaction. The tubules may have undergone an associated tubular change varying from normal to tubular degeneration. In addition, the interstitium is edematous and contains numerous bundles of collagen (Fig. 2-2) and additional cellular infiltrates of lymphocytes, histiocytes, and fibroblasts.

A drug-induced (methicillin) Councilman type of interstitial nephritis is discussed in the following case presentation.

CASE PRESENTATION

On December 12, 1966, L. M., a 30-year-old Negro postman, developed fever, shaking chills, and pustules on his trunk and extremities. On December 15, 1966, he was admitted to Municipal Contagious Disease Hospital. He was found to be acutely ill and had a fever of 104° F (Fig. 2-3).

Staphylococcus aureus, coagulase-negative, was cultured from his skin and from one of three blood cultures. A diagnosis was made of staphylococcal septicemia secondary to a staphylococcal dermatitis. Findings from the admission throat culture were negative and from the

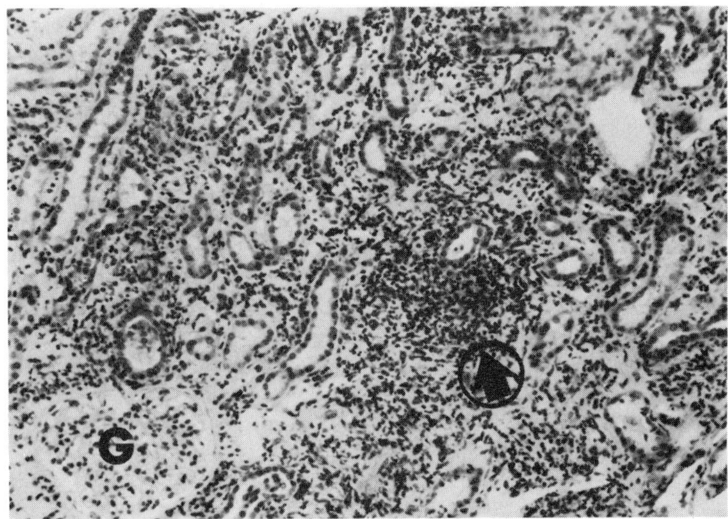

Fig. 2-2. Councilman's acute interstitial nephritis. This microphotograph illustrates the kidney of the 30-year-old man described in Fig. 2-3. The tubules were separated apart by interstitial edema, fibrosis, and cellular infiltrates. The one glomerulus (G) in the field appeared normal. Interstitial infiltrates (arrow) contained plasma cells, eosinophils, and lymphocytes. (H&E ×100.)

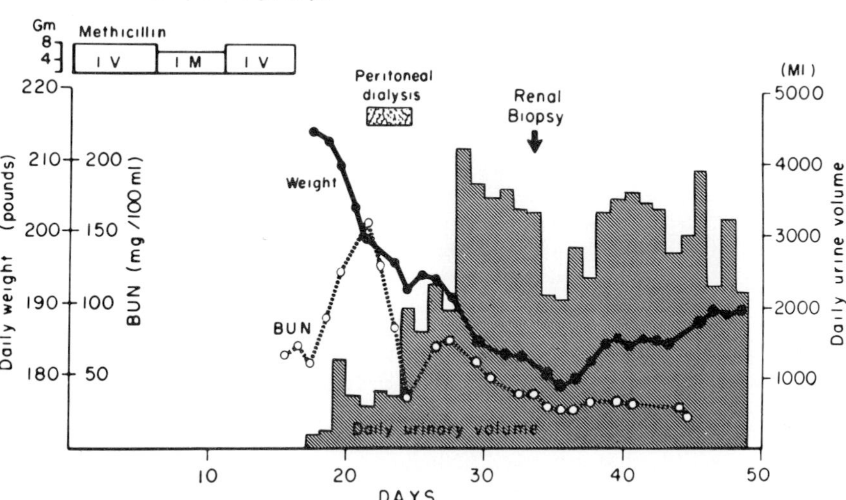

Fig. 2-3. Clinical findings of patient with methicillin-induced acute renal failure caused by acute interstitial nephritis. This patient developed fever, dermatitis, eosinophilia, and acute oliguric renal failure. Methicillin was given for 16 days before oliguria was diagnosed. The BUN (dotted line) rapidly increased from 50 to 159 mg per 100 ml, and it fell to 45 mg per 100 ml. A step-wise profuse diuresis occurred on the twenty-fourth day. Urinary output markedly increased and reached a peak of 4,250 ml on the twenty-seventh day. The body weight rapidly declined from over 200 pounds to 180 pounds and was 187 pounds when he was discharged. A renal biopsy study was done on the thirty-fourth day and revealed an acute interstitial nephritis with mild tubular regeneration. Culture of the renal tissue was sterile.

urinalysis were normal. On December 15 the patient was treated with erythromycin and novobiocin. From December 15 to December 21, 2 gm of methicillin was given intravenously every 4 hours. From December 21 to December 25, 1 gm of methicillin was given intramuscularly every 4 hours. On December 26 and for 3 days following, 2 gm of methicillin was given intravenously every 4 hours.

On December 20 he was afebrile. On December 25 he had fever. The next day he experienced dysuria, urinary frequency, and urgency. On December 30 gross hematuria without erythrocyte casts was noted. He had proteinuria (4+), and many leukocytes were seen in the spun urinary sediment. The BUN was 73 mg per 100 ml and the daily urinary volume was 200 cc. Acute oliguric renal failure was diagnosed.

On January 1, 1967, he was transferred to The Research and Educational Hospital of the University of Illinois. (His clinical course is plotted in Fig. 2-3.) On physical examination the patient was found to be a large, well-developed Negro male who appeared weak and lethargic. His blood pressure was 150/70 mm Hg, his pulse was 80 per minute and regular, and he was afebrile. Findings from funduscopic examination were normal. A few prominent soft anterior cervical lymph nodes were found. There was slight tenderness in the right upper quadrant on deep palpation. Tenderness was noted over the left kidney. No peripheral edema was noted.

Admission laboratory study revealed a hematocrit of 35%, hemoglobin of 12.2 gm %, and a leukocyte count of 16,500 per mm^3. The differential cell count revealed 8% eosinophils. Urinalysis revealed a specific gravity of 1.010, a pH of 6, proteinuria (4+), numerous erythrocytes, and 40 to 50 leukocytes per hpf of the spun urine sediment. No erythrocyte casts were noted.

Methicillin was stopped on January 1, 1967. Oliguria continued until January 2, when diuresis started and the 24-hour urine output was 1,250 ml. On January 5 the 24-hour urinary output was 800 cc. The BUN was 159 mg per 100 ml, and the serum potassium was 7.5 mEq/L. Peritoneal dialysis was started and continued for 72 hours. Diuresis continued and on January 11 the peak daily urinary output was 4,252 ml. The BUN was 72 mg per 100 ml, and 20% eosinophils were found on a peripheral blood smear.

On January 17, when the BUN was 38 mg per 100 ml and the 24-hour urinary output was 3,320 ml, a percutaneous renal biopsy was done. An interstitial nephritis was found. This was characterized by diffuse interstitial edema, fibrosis, and cellular infiltrates of plasma cells, eosinophils, fibroblasts, and lymphocytes. The glomeruli, tubules, and vessels were normal (Fig. 2-4). A diagnosis was made of methicillin-induced acute oliguric renal failure. On January 23, 1967, the BUN was 24 mg per 100 ml. On February 2, 1967, the patient was discharged. He felt well and his urine was free of protein and casts.

Comment. Methicillin induced a hypersensitivity interstitial nephritis of the Councilman type. The disease initially produced gross hematuria without erythrocyte casts. The interstitial disease progressed in severity to produce an oliguria. An eosinophilia is most unusual in acute renal failure caused by tubular necrosis or by a poststreptococcal glomerulonephritis. However, an eosinophilia[1034] developing in a patient during acute oliguric renal failure strongly suggests

---

Fig. 2-4. A, Acute interstitial nephritis assoicated with acute oliguric renal failure. A renal biopsy was obtained during the diuretic stage of acute oliguric renal failure caused by methicillin-induced acute interstitial nephritis. This microphotograph illustrates a portion of renal tubules and an accumulation of cellular infiltrates. The interstitium was edematous and contained polymorphonucleocytes, plasma cells, eosinophils, and small lymphocytes. (H&E ×600.) **B,** This electron microphotograph illustrates Councilman's acute interstitial nephritis. The patient developed fever, hematuria, oliguria, and eosinophilia following treatment with methicillin. Acute interstitial nephritis was diagnosed on renal biopsy. Above is a normal glomerular capillary loop. Proteineous material fills the urinary space (US). Bowman's membrane (BM) is thickened. The interstitium is edematous and contains a plasma cell (P), eosinophil (E), and small lymphocyte (L).

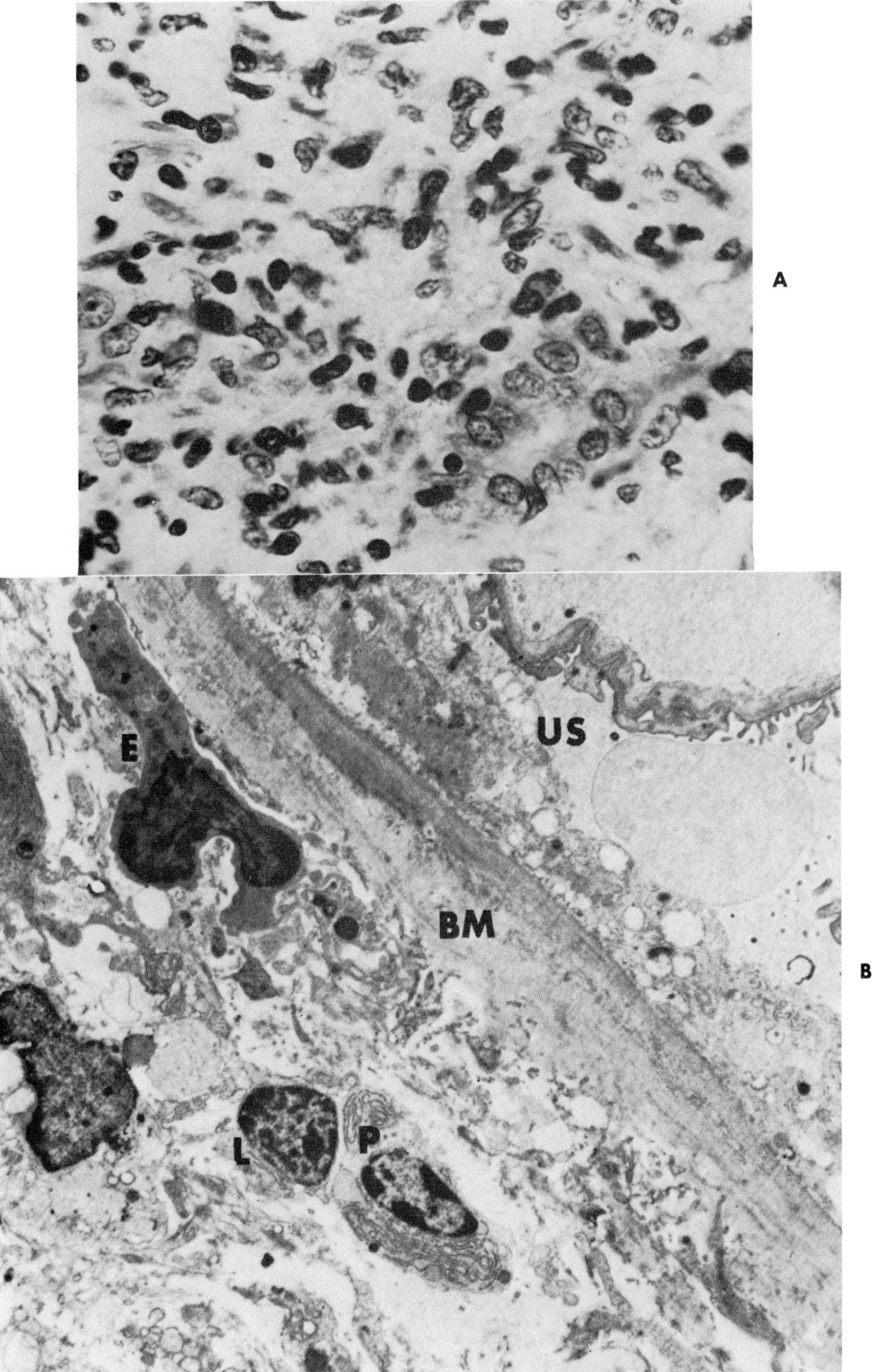

Fig. 2-4. For legend see opposite page.

a hypersensitivity lesion such as a hypersensitivity polyarteritis nodosa or a hypersensitivity interstitial nephritis.

The morphologic presence within the interstitium of large numbers of plasma cells and eosinophils reflected the hyperallergic response of the kidney (Fig. 2-4). Renal biopsy was of great value in verifying the clinical diagnosis of hypersensitivity interstitial nephritis.

Interstitial fibrosis

I reported a clinicopathologic renal biopsy study of seventy-six patients with interstitial nephritis that revealed a variety of etiologic groups.[806] Bacterial cultures of their renal tissue were sterile. From this study it was concluded that the morphologic changes started with interstitial edema and progressed to either diffuse or focal interstitial fibrosis.

Renal biopsy studies by Brun of patients with acute renal failure indicate the association of normal glomeruli with focal or diffuse interstitial edema and

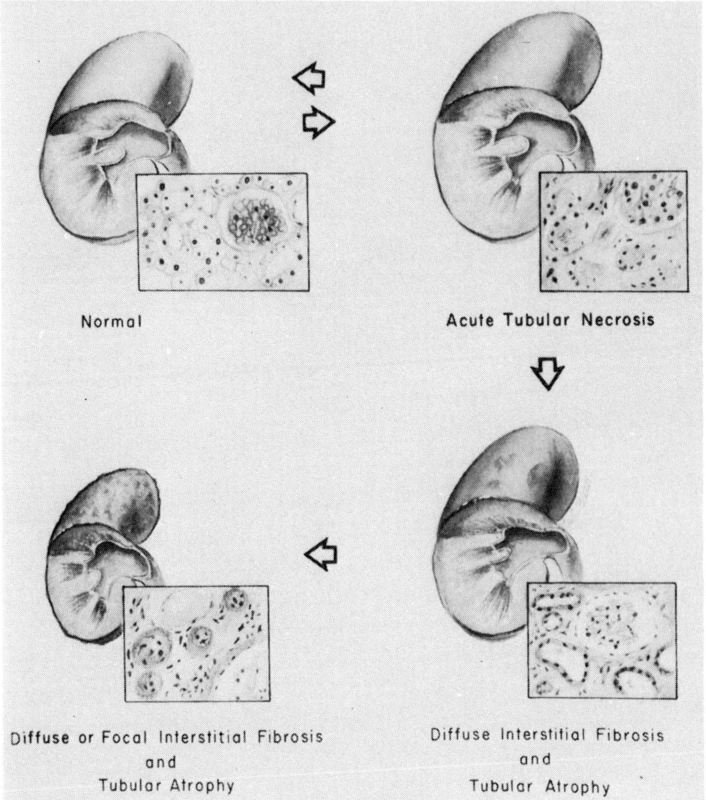

Fig. 2-5. Evolution of kidney changes following acute tubular necrosis. This photograph illustrates the evolution of renal changes in patients with acute renal failure. The normal kidney increases in size when damaged by tubular necrosis. Interstitial edema and, later, fibrosis occur. If oliguria is severe and prolonged a diffuse interstitial edema and fibrosis follow. This diffuse lesion may be irreversible and can progress on to a contracted kidney with diffuse or focal interstitial fibrosis and tubular atrophy.

tubular damage.[160] He therefore coined the term "tubulo-interstitial nephritis" to describe his histologic finding. He observed a flattening of proximal tubular epithelial cells with tubular dilatation. The distal tubules and ascending Henle's loops were dilated. In our laboratory acute interstitial edema has always been observed in kidneys of patients with acute renal failure. It appeared to be associated with tubular damage and was much greater in the cortex than in the medullae. In 7 to 12 days interstitial fibrosis developed. This progressed by a gradual replacement of the edema until interstitial fibrosis was uniform and diffuse throughout the kidney. If the initial insult is mild and if oliguria is short, the kidney returns to normal. If the insult is severe and if oliguria is prolonged, diffuse interstitial fibrosis develops; in some patients acute renal failure may progress to a contracted kidney with chronic renal failure (Fig. 2-5).

The Councilman type of interstitial nephritis leading to acute renal failure is discussed in the following case presentation.

CASE PRESENTATION

In August, 1965, A. D., a 38-year-old Negro male, was admitted to Research and Educational Hospital with fever of undetermined origin.

In February, 1965, the patient had started to work in a meat packing plant, which exposed

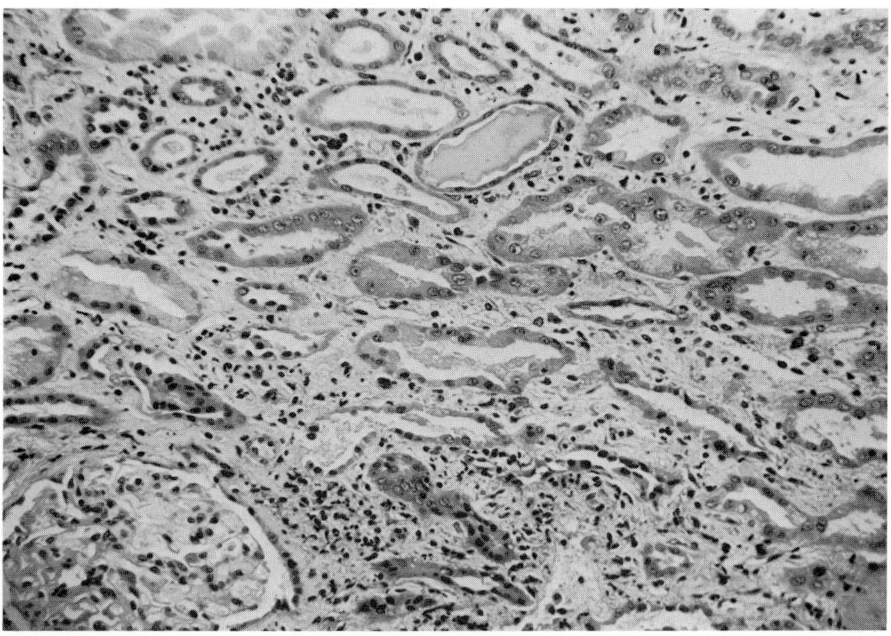

Fig. 2-6. Acute interstitial nephritis caused by brucellosis hypersensitivity. This microphotograph illustrates a renal biopsy obtained from a 38-year-old meat packing plant worker. Renal biopsy was done before he was treated for an infection with *Brucella suis*, when he had gross proteinuria and a BUN of 62 mg per 100 ml. There was diffuse interstitial edema and fibrosis with cellular infiltrates of plasma cells and small lymphocytes. Electron microscopic study revealed normal glomeruli and tubules. (H&E ×300.)

him to hog carcasses. In June, weakness, arthralgia, and a brief erythematous rash developed and he was forced to quit work. In July, chills, fever, and sweating first occurred, and soon thereafter he became bedridden. At the time of admission he had a dry cough, a mild polyuria, dysuria, pain, and weakness in the arms and legs. In addition, he had lost approximately 30 pounds.

Examination revealed an ill-appearing febrile Negro male. Blood pressure was 120/78 mm Hg. The liver was palpable 5 cm below the right costal margin and was smooth and firm. The spleen was not enlarged. There were no other abnormal physical findings. Urinalysis revealed gross proteinuria, 10 to 12 WBC per hpf, 2 to 3 RBC per hpf, and leukocytes and hyaline casts.

Findings from eight blood cultures were positive for *Brucella suis,* and *Brucella* agglutinins were found in a titre of 1:2,560. Hemoglobin was 12.6 gm per 100 ml, white blood cell count was 5,250 per mm^3, and the corrected erythrocyte sedimentation rate was 52 mm per hour. The BUN was 62 mg per 100 ml, and the serum creatinine was 2.9 mg per 100 ml. The total serum protein was 5.4 gm per 100 ml (albumin 1.3 and globulin 4.1). The serum cholesterol was 250 mg per 100 ml, the serum alkaline phosphatase was 5.3 units (normal range 2 to 4), the latex fixation test was 1:5,120, and the indirect Coombs test was positive. The serum bilirubin, serum electrolytes (potassium, sodium, chloride, calcium, and phosphate), serum amylase, and serum glutamic oxalacetic transaminase were normal. Liver biopsy study revealed a mild hepatitis with small areas of focal necrosis, Kupffer cell hyperplasia, and mild round cell infiltration.

Tetracycline (2 gm daily) was begun and continued for a month. In addition, streptomycin

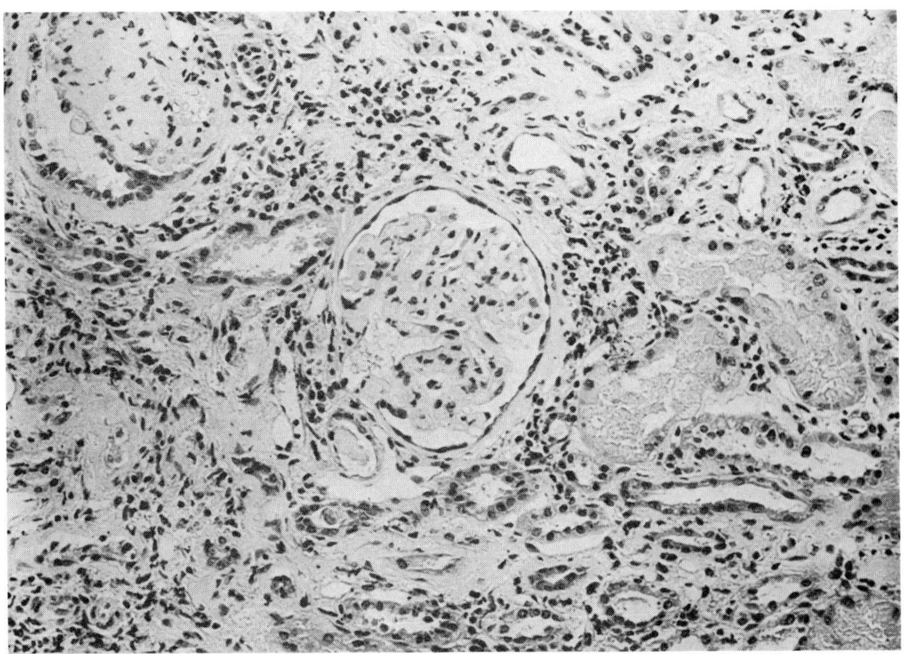

Fig. 2-7. Progression of interstitial nephritis caused by brucellosis hypersensitivity. This microphotograph illustrates the second renal biopsy taken from the patient described in Fig. 2-6. The second biopsy study was done 9 months after treatment was started. Although the BUN returned to normal, the 24-hour proteinuria varied between 7 and 12 gm. The striking change was an increase in the interstitial fibrosis. In addition, cellular infiltrates were prominently fibroblasts and monocytes. (H&E ×320.)

(1 gm daily) was administered for the first week but was subsequently discontinued because of the renal impairment. Gradual improvement occurred, the fever abated, and renal function became normal. Because of persisting proteinuria, a percutaneous renal biopsy was done (Fig. 2-6). The prominent histologic abnormalities were found in the renal interstitium. There was edema, round cell infiltration, and fibrosis. Electron microscopy study revealed fusion of the glomerular epithelial foot processes; the glomeruli were otherwise normal.

The patient was discharged from the hospital in September. His strength and appetite returned and he gained weight. However, proteinuria persisted and nocturia and frequency developed a few weeks later. He was readmitted to the hospital in October, 1965.

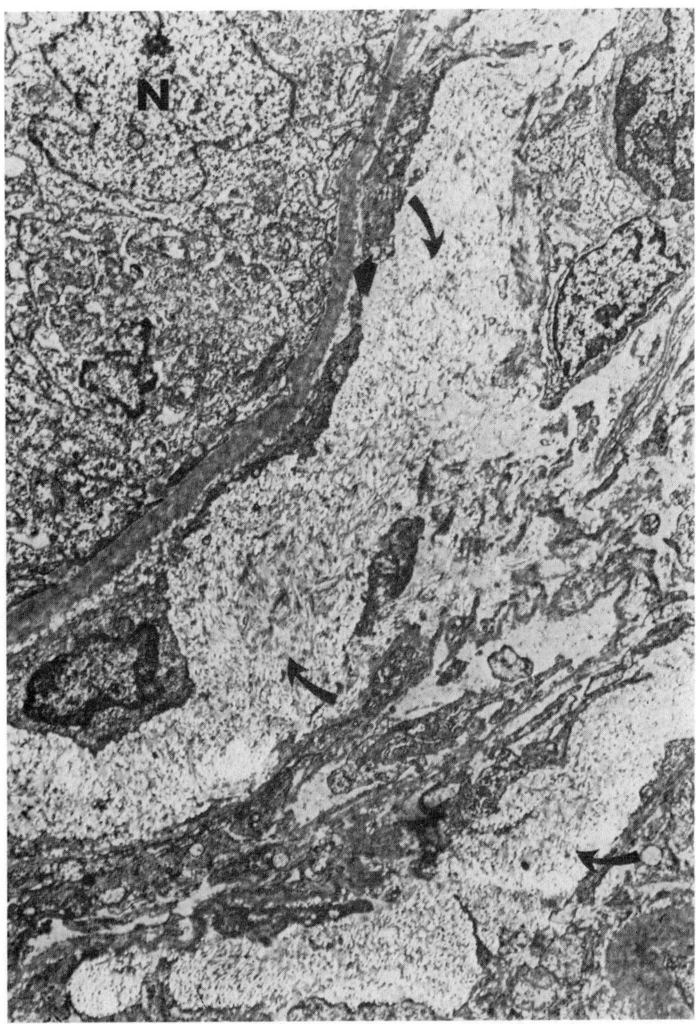

Fig. 2-8. Ultrastructure of progressive acute interstitial nephritis. This electron microphotograph illustrates the progression of acute interstitial nephritis in the second renal biopsy of the patient described in Figs. 2-6 and 2-7. A portion of cortical tubule was seen at upper left. The cell nucleus (N) was irregular. The tubular basement membrane (straight arrow) was thickened. Numerous bundles of collagen fibers (curved arrows) were seen in the interstitium. ($\times$7,256.)

Physical examination revealed a healthy-looking man. Although he was afebrile, he had excessive sweating and mild hypertension ranging from 180/90 to 210/110 mm Hg. A white transverse line in the fingernails was present. There were no other abnormal physical findings. Urinalysis revealed gross proteinuria and pyuria.

Laboratory findings showed hemoglobin was 15 gm per 100 ml, the leukocyte count was 9,700 per mm³, and the corrected erythrocyte sedimentation rate was 34 mm per hour. The BUN was 15 mg per 100 ml, the serum creatinine was 1.3 mg per 100 ml, the total serum protein was 7.7 gm per 100 ml (albumin 2.9 and globulin 4.8), and the serum cholesterol was 265 mg per 100 ml. The latex fixation test was 1:5,120, the indirect Coombs test was positive, and tests of liver function were normal. The serum electrolytes (potassium, sodium, chloride, and calcium) were normal. The *Brucella* agglutinin titre was positive (1:1,280), and several blood cultures were again positive for *Brucella suis*.

The 24-hour creatinine clearance was 114 ml per minute, the 15-minute excretion of PSP was 36%, the 24-hour urinary protein varied from 7 to 13 gm, and the maximum urinary concentration was 733 mOsm/L (specific gravity 1.022). The acidification test (Wrong and Davies) resulted in a drop in urinary pH to 5.0; the maximum titratable acidity was 76 μEq per minute, and the maximal ammonium production was 76 μEq per minute. Findings from the intravenous pyelogram were normal and a second percutaneous renal biopsy was done (Fig. 2-7). There was extensive peritubular fibrosis, and a severe infiltrate of lymphocytes was present. Some glomeruli were completely hyalinized in focal areas. The diagnosis was interstitial nephritis.

Prolonged treatment was begun with 2 gm of tetracycline per day and 1 gm of streptomycin per day. The patient had remained asymptomatic and the daily proteinuria had decreased to 3.7 gm. Renal function had remained normal. Serum albumin was now 3.7 gm per 100 ml. Pyuria and mild hypertension persisted.

Comment. The renal morphologic abnormalities in the patient just discussed resemble the lesions seen in other patients with *Brucella* endocarditis. Severe interstitial infiltrates of lymphocytes and plasma cells were the most striking lesions. No granulomas were seen. Renal tubules had undergone atrophy and had dilated. Although most glomeruli were normal, a few had patchy lesions, again reminiscent of bacterial endocarditis. The repeat renal biopsy examination revealed an apparent progression of the interstitial lesions in spite of improved renal function and in spite of the patient being apparently well. Many glomeruli were normal and a few had prominent focal lesions of hypercellularity. Fusion of the glomerular foot processes was the most striking lesion seen on electron microscopy.

The interstitial findings of edema and cellular infiltrates resemble a Councilman interstitial nephritis (Fig. 2-8). Bacteria were absent on Gram's stain of the renal tissue, and culture of renal tissue was sterile. This would support the impression that the etiology of the interstitial nephritis was not caused directly by bacterial infection but was a result of an immunologic process. This is suggested by a generalized immunologic setting such as the positive Coombs test, a positive latex fixation test, and an elevated serum globulin level. This same immunologic mechanism may be reflected in the response of the renal interstitium in the subsequent evaluation of a Councilman type of interstitial nephritis.

Lymphomatous interstitial nephritis

In patients with malignant lymphoma or with multiple myeloma,[528] acute oliguric renal failure may result either from secondary obstructive uropathy caused by retroperitoneal lymph node involvement or from direct infiltration of the renal parenchyma,[35] mainly the interstitium.[1032]

Uric acid obstructive uropathy is far more common in producing acute renal failure than parenchymal interstitial lymphomatous involvement. The clinical feature produced by lymphomatous involvement of the interstitium is one of progressive renal failure.[844,927,1002] Initially anemia, fatigue, and weight loss may precede oliguria or anuria. Acute renal failure can occur without peripheral

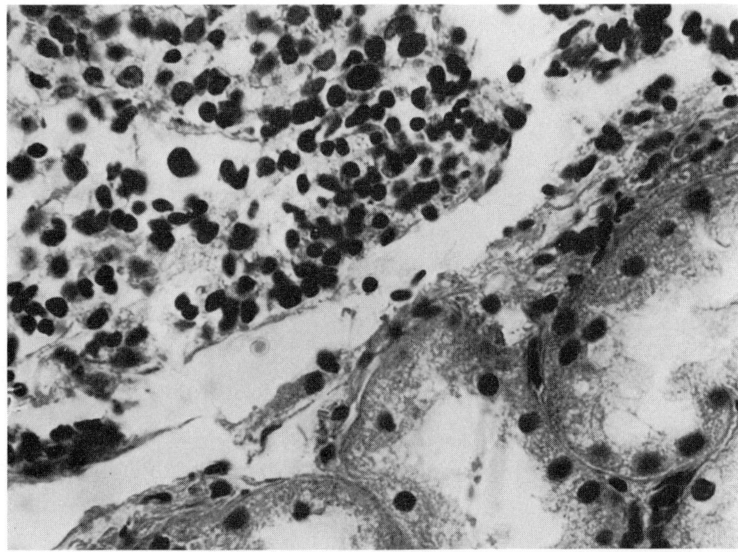

Fig. 2-9. Lymphomatous interstitial nephritis. Renal biopsy study of a 48-year-old woman with acute renal failure due to a malignant lymphoma revealed large interstitial infiltrations of malignant lymphocytes. An area of apparent normal tubules is noted to the lower right. (H&E ×470.) (Courtesy Dr. R. Smith, Utica, New York.)

lymphadenopathy, hepatosplenomegaly, or other clinical features of malignant lymphoma or other malignancies.[1111] The urine usually contains small quantities of protein, microscopic to gross hematuria, numerous leukocytes, and broad casts. The urinary specific gravity is usually fixed at 1.010. Bence Jones protein may be associated with myelomatosis or with lymphosarcoma.[1030]

The kidneys are enlarged and the renal parenchyma becomes replaced by lymphomatous masses. A diagnosis can be made by renal biopsy, as was done by Dr. R. Smith of Utica, New York (Fig. 2-9). His patient was a 48-year-old woman with fatal acute renal failure. The interstitium and subsequently the tubules and glomeruli became infiltrated with lymphomatous cells. The finding of lymphomatous cells aided the pathologist in making the diagnosis of malignant lymphoma. In some areas the kidney was entirely free of lymphoma and cellular infiltrates, and the tubules appeared adjacent to one another (Fig. 2-9).

In the few patients treated for acute oliguric renal failure caused by malignant lymphoma the prognosis was most grave—none has survived. Treatment with x-ray radiation, adrenocortical steroids, and alkylating agents has had no beneficial effect. In fact, the use of alkylating agents has increased the nitrogen load in the kidneys and has been extremely hazardous to the failing kidneys.

Interstitial infection

Interstitial infections caused by bacteria, leptospirosis, and candidiasis[992] have individually produced acute renal failure. Significant bacterial growth from urine cultures or findings of leptospira in the urine have helped in diagnosing such an infection.

Homograft kidney transplant rejection

Rejection of a homograft kidney transplant may produce acute oliguric renal failure because of a well-known primary rejection reaction at one of two anatomic sites—either the renovascular[273] or the interstitial. Acute tubular necrosis can occur in a transplanted kidney. Renal biopsy study can aid in this diagnosis.

Arterial lesions

When a renovascular rejection of a renal transplant occurs, the clinical features are oliguria, increase in the systemic blood pressure, increase in urinary osmolarity, and decrease in urinary sodium concentration. The predominant morphologic abnormalities occur in the renal arteries. This pathologic change is an acute polyarteritis of the major renal arteries. In addition, proliferative glomerulonephritis occurs. These clinicopathologic abnormalities are almost completely reversed by effective treatment of the transplant rejection process. Treatment consists of adrenocortical steroids in large doses such as prednisone and the so-called immunosuppressive agents such as azathioprine. After the rejection phenomenon is suppressed, a chronic obliterative healed arteritis occurs.

Interstitium

The rejection process caused by interstitial nephritis is rapid in onset. The patient develops oliguria with a fixed, low osmolarity and a high urinary sodium excretion. The patient is usually afebrile, and an abnormal urinary sediment is noted.

The kidney becomes enlarged by the hypersensitivity interstitial nephritis. The interstitium is edematous and is infiltrated by polymorphonucleocytes and mature lymphocytes. On effective treatment with high doses of prednisone, immunosuppressive agents, and anti–small lymphocyte serum, the renal size gradually returns to normal.

As the patient recovers the urinary output increases; the hematuria, proteinuria, and abnormal renal sediment return toward normal. A focal to diffuse interstitial fibrosis may result at the final stage of interstitial healing.

ACUTE TUBULAR NECROSIS

Acute tubular necrosis can result from trauma,[188] hemorrhage,[712] hemolysis,[166,202] water and electrolyte depletion,[90] nephrotoxic chemicals,[849] drugs,[176] and numerous other situations and substances.* These will be discussed in detail in the next chapter.

Morphologic findings of tubular necrosis were first described by Hackradt[486]

---

*See references 807, 807a, 1012, and 1017.

and later by Minami.[781] Although tubular necrosis was not commonly recognized, it was in 1942 that the lesion was fully established by Bywaters.[188-190] He described the lesion in patients with traumatic anuria as an involvement of the distal convoluted tubules and the ascending limb of Henle's loop. He emphasized the intense catarrh of the proximal tubular epithelium. He observed that the most severe damage occurred in small areas of Henle's loop and secondarily in convoluted tubules. He also emphasized the findings of metaplasia in the parietal epithelial cells of Bowman's capsule with cuboidal cell formation adjacent to the tubular entrance. In addition, he associated interstitial cellular infiltrates and interstitial fibrosis with tubule repair. These observations received support by renal biopsy studies from our laboratory.

Lower "nephron nephrosis"

In 1946, Lucke studied material at the Army Institute of Pathology.[712] He reemphasized necrosis of the lower reaches of the nephron as the principal renal lesion in traumatic acute renal failure. It was this lower nephron selectivity that led him to coin the phrase "lower nephron nephrosis." Mallory believed the morphologic changes in the lower nephron segment to be reactive.[737]

Lucke found that acute tubular necrosis undergoes complete repair within 10 days.[744] Serial renal biopsy studies of tubular repair in acute necrosis do not support his autopsy observations. Recent electron microscopic studies of patients with acute renal failure revealed patchy necrosis of the nephron and failure of tubular repair to be complete up to 6 months after injury. Oliver used a three-dimensional approach in microdissecting entire nephrons; his investigations revealed that widespread and random tubular necrosis can occur anywhere along the nephron.[846,847] On the basis of Oliver's observations and recent renal biopsy studies, the term "lower nephron nephrosis" is an inappropriate and incorrect term. It has long been dropped by many nephrologists.

Nephrotoxic vs tubulorrhexic lesions

Oliver's classic studies in renal morphology and function in acute renal failure described two distinct histologic abnormalities occurring in the nephrons of patients with acute tubular necrosis.[849] These lesions varied considerably from nephron to nephron and within single nephrons. The first abnormality was termed a "nephrotoxic lesion" and was characterized by a select-desquamation and necrosis of the proximal tubule down to the tubular basement membrane but not including it.

The secondary abnormality was called a "tubulorrhexic lesion" and followed renal ischemia. The lesion was characterized by a destructive, disruptive, and necrotic tubular lesion anywhere along the nephron and fragmentation of the tubular basement membrane.[672] Oliver believed that a complete disintegration of the tubular structure led to leakage of the tubular contents into the interstitium with subsequent formation of interstitial edema.[847]

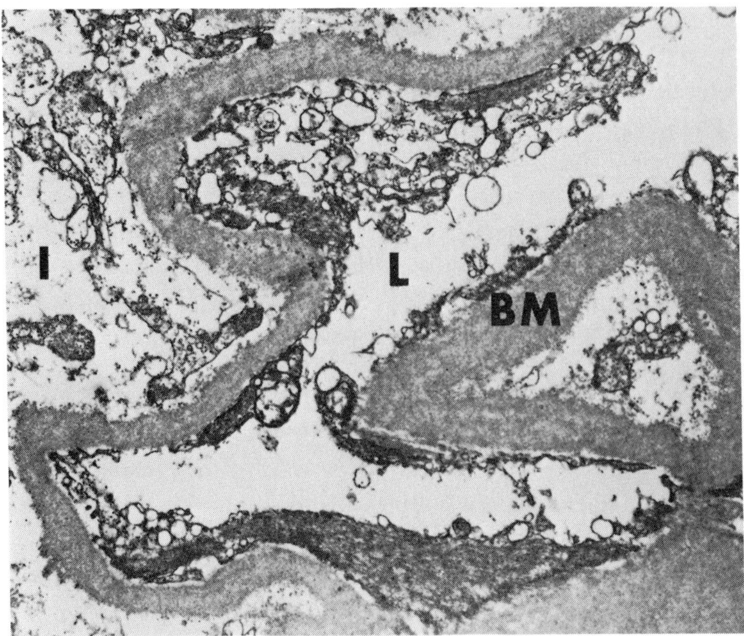

Fig. 2-10. Severe acute tubular necrosis. This electron microphotograph illustrates severe tubular cell necrosis extending down to the tubular basement membrane (BM). The tubular lumen (L) contains cellular debris. The interstitium (I) is edematous. (×13,000.)

Serial renal biopsy studies of a large group of patients with acute tubular necrosis due to a variety of causes revealed exceptions to this hypothesis. Some patients with acute tubular necrosis caused by nephrotoxic agents had marked disruption of the tubular basement membrane (Fig. 2-10). On the other hand, patients with acute renal failure caused by ischemia had no apparent or very mild tubular changes even by electron microscopy (Fig. 2-11).

Nephron population differences

Microdissection studies of entire nephrons have indicated that in certain situations two nephron populations exist—damaged and undamaged nephrons. Histologic normal nephrons were found interspaced among damaged nephrons.[197] This observation may explain discrepancies found between renal morphology and the clinical syndrome of acute oliguric renal failure. As mentioned previously, for example, acute renal failure has occurred without abnormal renal morphology. It was Kimmelstiel who first made mention that no renal abnormal morphologic finding may be detected in kidneys of patients with anuria.[627] Twenty-five years later, electron microscopy studies of renal biopsy specimens have supported his observations. In some patients with acute oliguric renal failure, the tubules, the glomeruli, and renal vessels have been completely normal by electron microscopy.

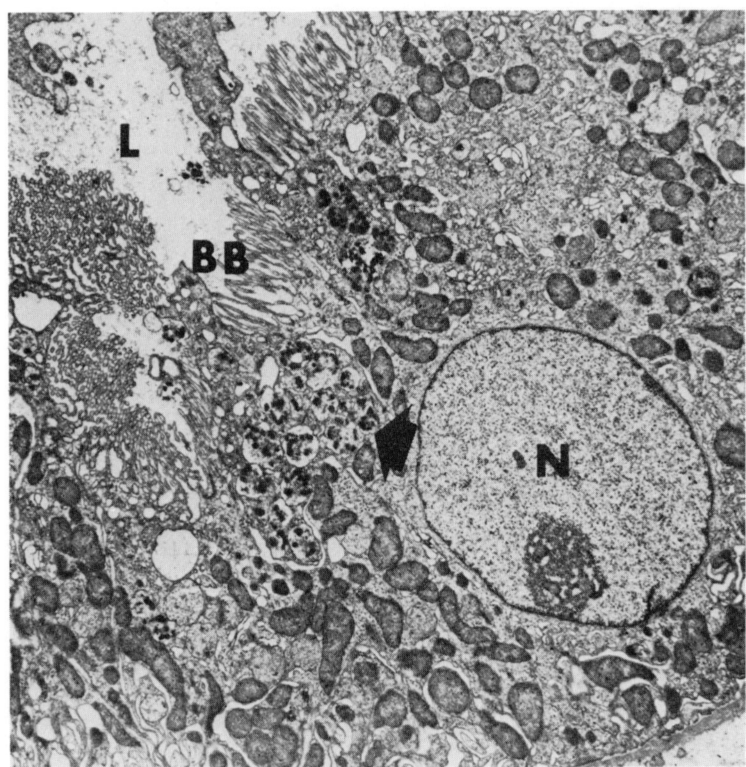

Fig. 2-11. Normal tubules associated with acute oliguric renal failure. A 54-year-old housewife developed acute oliguria. Her BUN rose to 114 mg per 100 ml. She was given intravenous mannitol and ethacrynic acid without a diuresis. A clinical diagnosis was made of acute oliguric renal failure due to "acute tubular necrosis." A renal biopsy study was done on the fourth day of oliguria. The tubules appeared normal by light and electron microscopy. A large oval nucleus (N) was seen. Normal brush border (BB) extended into the tubular lumen (L). Numerous electron dense granular bodies were noted (arrows). These bodies are believed to be the result of mannitol infusion. ($\times$6,090.)

Renal interstitial edema appears to be the most universal parenchymal abnormality of acute renal failure and probably is responsible for the increased size of the kidney. It is usually noted in the kidney of patients with oliguria or anuria when no other parenchymal abnormality is found.

Complicated acute tubular necrosis

On a morphologic basis, acute tubular necrosis can be subdivided into uncomplicated acute tubular necrosis and complicated acute tubular necrosis. The latter is defined as acute tubular necrosis complicated by an additional morphologic lesion such as calcium deposits in the tubules associated with ethylene glycol toxicity or hemoglobin or myoglobin pigment within the tubular lumen, within the tubular epithelial cells, or within the interstitium.

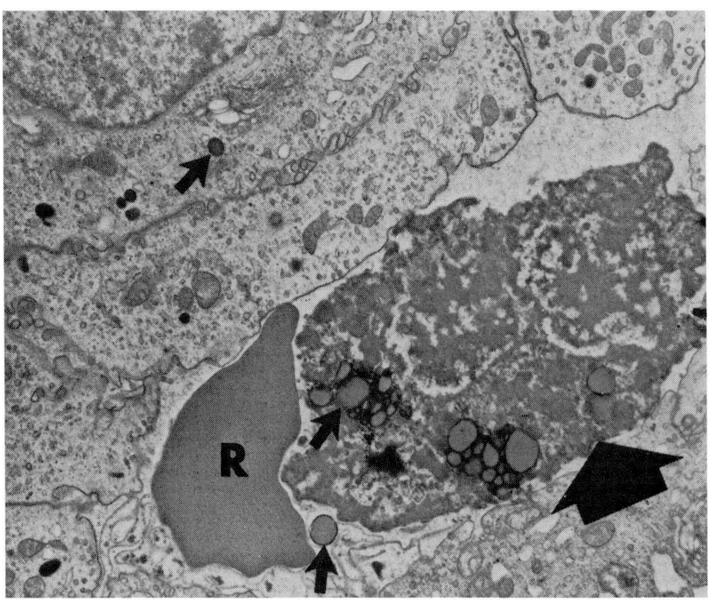

Fig. 2-12. Degeneration of erythrocyte cast within tubular lumen. This electron microphotograph illustrates degeneration of an erythrocyte cast (large arrow) within distal tubular lumen. Renal biopsy was taken during acute anuria following a severe and massive hemorrhage. In addition, the patient had a severe hemolytic anemia with a transitory thrombocytopenia. Several small homogeneous bodies (small arrow) are noted. One body is free in the tubular lumen (left bottom), another body is in the epithelial cell above. Note the intact erythrocyte (R) adjacent to the degenerating erythrocyte cast. ($\times$9,100.)

Acute tubular necrosis complicated by intravascular hemolysis or myoglobinuria was originally described by Bywaters[196] and later by Mallory,[737] who studied army casualties resuscitated from shock. In addition to the effects of pigmented casts on the tubular epithelium, one must consider the additive effects of hypoxia that result from the hemolytic anemia.[202] This additional factor by itself could produce tubular necrosis. Acute tubular necrosis with hemolysis was called "hemoglobinuric nephrosis" by Mallory.

In both subdivisions of acute tubular necrosis, the kidneys are usually enlarged, heavy, and swollen. The capsule is tight but strips with ease. When the kidney is cut the moist parenchyma bulges through. The differentiation between cortex and medullary area is well delineated. The cortex is salmon pink and the medullary area appears congested and dark.

In some instances, when acute tubular necrosis is associated with hemolysis, numerous hemoglobin or erythrocyte casts can be seen in the tubular lumen (Fig. 2-12). Later, degraded erythrocytes and hemoglobin breakdown products can be found within the renal tubular cytoplasm, the tubular lumen, and the interstitial cells (Fig. 2-13). Special stains for iron and hemoglobin can trace the breakdown and reabsorption of these segments. Iron in the form of ferritin

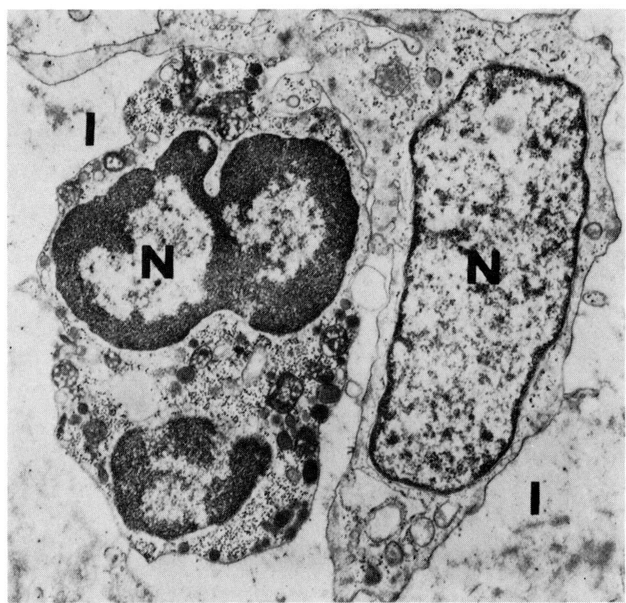

Fig. 2-13. Hemoglobin pigment within an interstitial cell following severe hemolysis and acute anuria. A renal biopsy was obtained from a patient during acute anuria following massive hemolysis. Two interstitial cells were seen surrounded by an edematous interstitium (I). The nuclei (N) occupied much of the cell. The left interstitial cell contains numerous electron dense granules. Thick sections (0.5μ) were stained for hemoglobin and were positive for hemoglobin pigment. ($\times 12,500$.)

can be found in the regenerating renal tubules as late as 6 months after the initial insult.

Acute tubular necrosis complicated by massive hemolysis is discussed in the following case presentation. Massive hemolysis resulted from the direct effect of arsine on the erythrocytes.

CASE PRESENTATION

On November 9, 1962, a 32-year-old husky truck driver delivered a solution containing sodium hydroxide and arsenic trioxide in an aluminum tank trailer truck. He emptied the tank, crawled into it, and for approximately 30 minutes flushed out the residual liquid with water. Arsine was determined to have evolved by the reaction of the aluminum wall of the truck with sodium hydroxide and arsenic trioxide. Two hours later the patient felt "sick." Four hours after arsine exposure he vomited and was jaundiced. Eight hours later he had costovertebral angle pain and a few hours later he passed dark urine. Twenty-four hours after exposure he had complete anuria.

On the second day of his illness he was transferred to Presbyterian–St. Luke's Hospital. He was semicomatose; his skin was an unusual bronze color tinged with blue. His pulse rate, temperature, and blood pressure were normal. His liver was enlarged and tender. Marked tenderness was also noted over both costovertebral angles. His hemoglobin was 7.5 gm per 100 ml, one-third of which had been liberated into the serum as free hemoglobin (2.5 gm per 100 ml of blood). The serum sodium, chloride, potassium, and CO_2 combining power were all normal. The BUN was 135 mg per 100 ml. (The patient's hospital and clinical course over the next 74 days is illustrated in Fig. 2-14.)

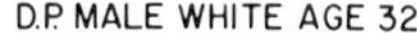
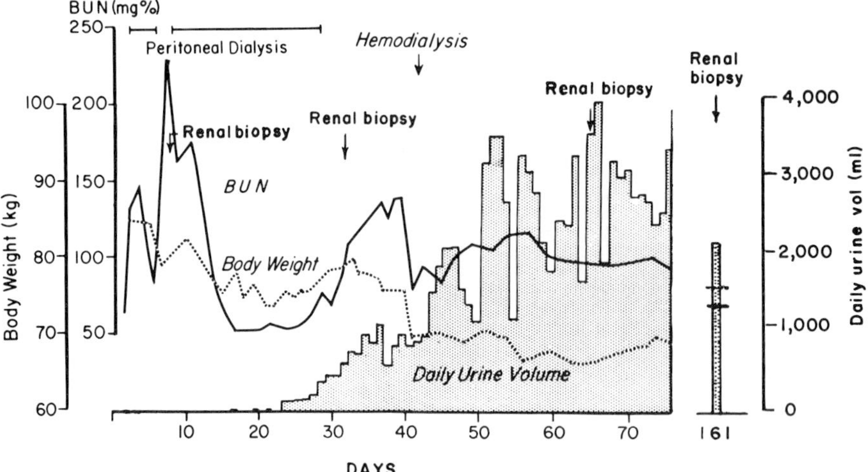

Fig. 2-14. Hospital course of patient with arsine-induced anuria. The 74-day hospital course is plotted of a 32-year-old truck driver with arsine-induced anuria. The patient was treated with exchange transfusions, peritoneal dialysis, and hemodialysis. Renal biopsies were obtained during anuria, early diuresis, late diuresis, and later during the recovery period.

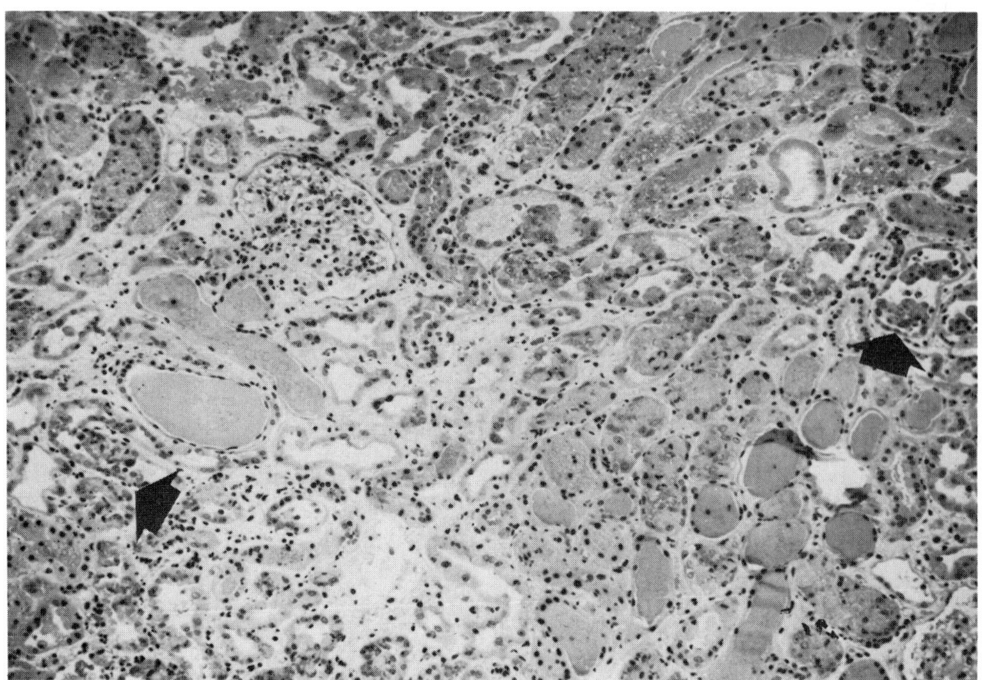

Fig. 2-15. Acute tubular necrosis caused by arsine. The first renal biopsy of the patient described in Fig. 2-14 was taken on the seventh day after exposure to arsine. There were areas of tubular necrosis and regeneration (arrows). Hemoglobin casts filled many of the tubular lumen. The glomeruli appeared normal. (H&E ×110.)

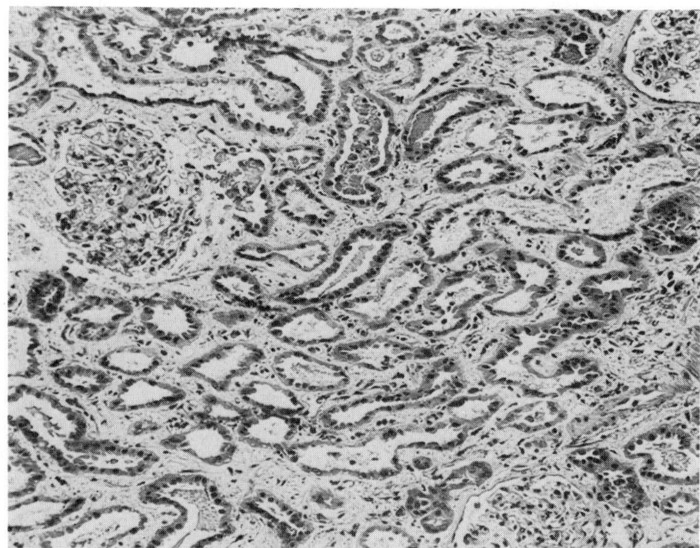

Fig. 2-16. Acute tubular regeneration during early diuresis. The second renal biopsy of the patient described in Figs. 2-14 and 2-15 was taken on the thirty-third day of acute arsine-induced renal failure. There was striking diffuse interstitial edema with mild interstitial fibrosis. (H&E ×110.)

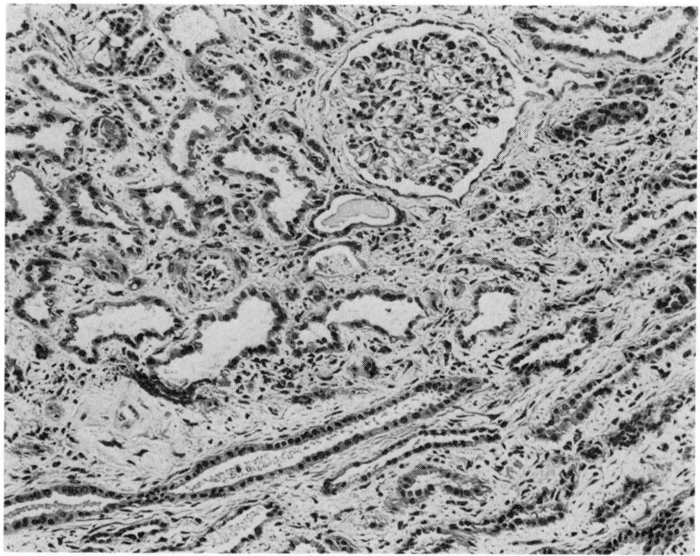

Fig. 2-17. Repair of acute tubular necrosis at the height of diuresis. This microphotograph illustrates the renal biopsy obtained on the sixty-sixth day after onset of anuria when the patient had a "peak diuresis." The tubular epithelial cells were still in a process of regeneration. The interstitium was diffusely fibrosed. The glomeruli appeared normal. Hemoglobin casts were still present. (H&E ×100.)

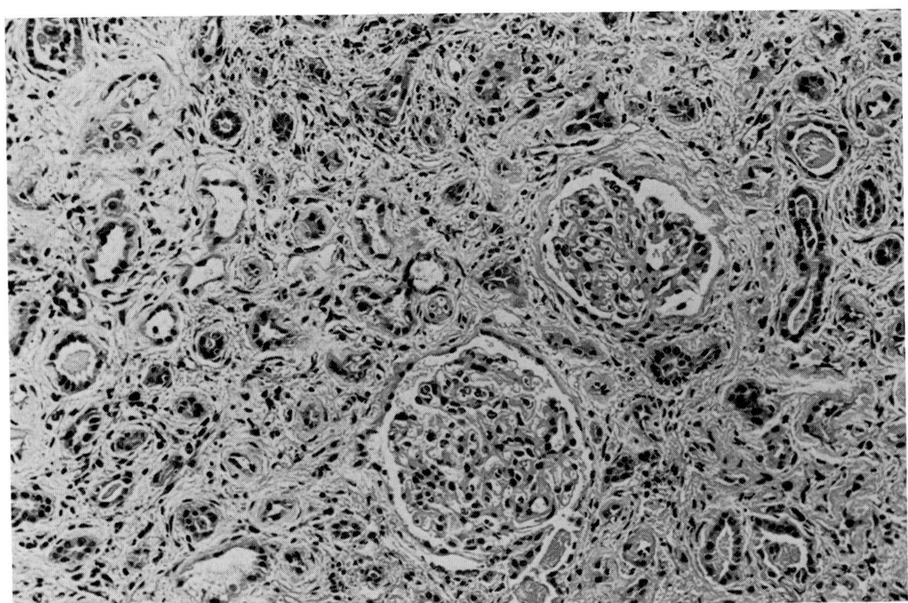

Fig. 2-18. Tubular regeneration following acute necrosis. Renal biopsy taken during recovery from acute tubular necrosis. The striking morphologic finding was a diffuse interstitial fibrosis associated with thickening of the cortical tubular basement membrane. (H&E ×210.)

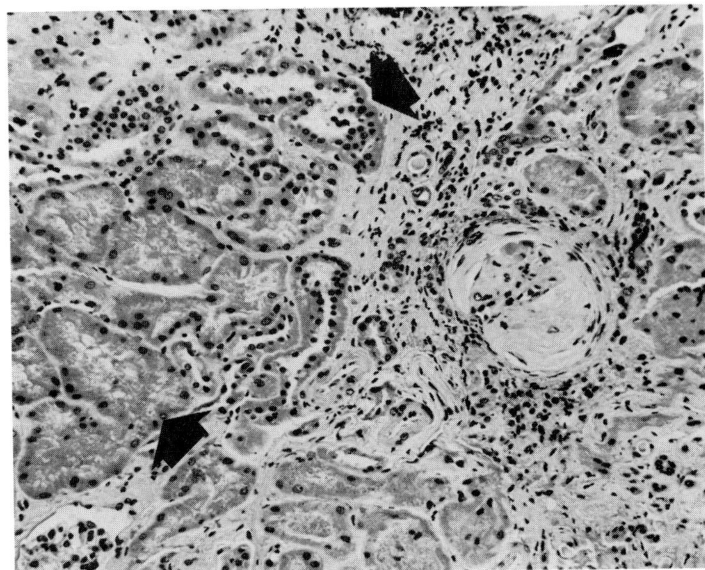

Fig. 2-19. Three years after recovery from acute tubular necrosis. A fifth renal biopsy was obtained from the patient described in Figs. 2-14 to 2-18. The study was made 3 years after arsine-induced acute tubular necrosis was found. The patient had chronic renal failure and anemia. Small microvilli were noted in a few areas. Cellular debris were noted in some areas (arrows); the tubules were normal and free of interstitial fibrosis. In other areas the interstitial fibrosis was focal. (H&E ×110.)

Peritoneal dialysis was started and an exchange of whole blood was given—one unit of blood was removed and one unit was administered. In all, nineteen units were given. This removed large quantities of the "arsenic-hemoglobin complex" and greatly improved the clinical state of the patient. The next morning he appeared alert and active. The hematocrit and tests of hepatic functions (bromosulfalein, thymol turbidity, prothrombin time, and serum proteins) were normal. Abnormally high levels of arsenic were found in the blood obtained during the exchange transfusion. On the fifth hospital day peritoneal dialysis was stopped and a right percutaneous renal biopsy was done (Fig. 2-15).

On the seventh day of hospitalization peritoneal dialysis was restarted and was continued up to the twenty-eighth hospital day. There were no abnormal levels of arsenic in the fluid removed during the first three days of peritoneal dialysis. Throughout the period of peritoneal dialysis the patient received a high-carbohydrate, high-fat, low-protein, low-phosphorus, low-potassium diet. On the thirty-first day diuresis occurred.

The serum albumin fell to 2.2 gm per 100 ml and the prothrombin time was 5% of normal. In addition to intramuscular injections of vitamin K, 200 gm of salt-poor human serum albumin was infused. The serum albumin levels were raised toward normal and the prothrombin time returned to normal.

On the thirty-first hospital day, when early diuresis occurred, a second renal biopsy was done. Renal tissue was studied by light and electron microscopy (Fig. 2-16).

On the thirty-eighth hospital day uremic pneumonitis developed and there was a rapid deterioration of the patient's clinical state. After 6 hours of extracorporeal diuresis a third renal biopsy was done (Fig. 2-17).

On the seventy-fourth hospital day the patient was discharged. His blood pressure was normal. The BUN was 79 mg per 100 ml, the hematocrit was 24%, and the 15-minute excretion of intravenous injected PSP was 0.

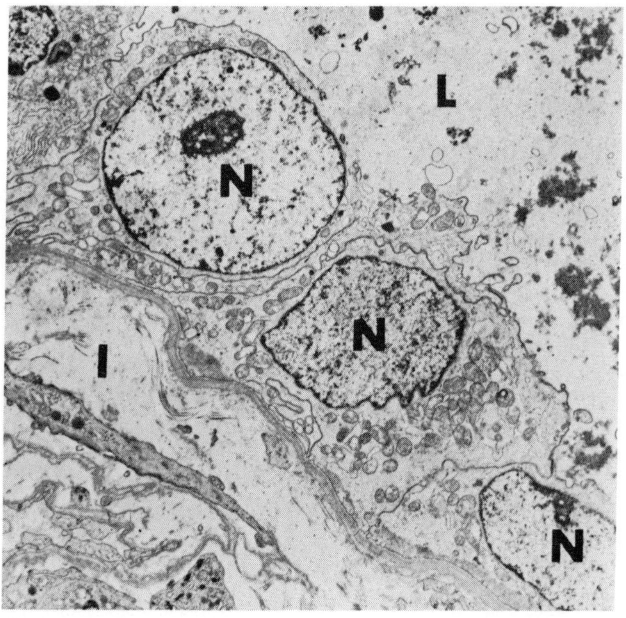

Fig. 2-20. Acute tubular necrosis with regeneration. This electron microphotograph was taken of the second renal biopsy from patient described in Fig. 2-14. Large nuclei (N) filled much of the cell. Small microvilli were noted in a few areas. Cellular debri was noted in the tubular lumen (L). The interstitium (I) was edematous. (×3,600.)

Five months after his first admission he was readmitted to the hospital. He was symptom-free, his blood pressure was 110/88 mm Hg, and no edema was noted. A 24-hour urine specimen contained 2.7 gm of protein. The urinary specific gravity was 1.013, and several hyaline and granular casts were found in a high power field of the spun urine sediment. The BUN was 61 mg per 100 ml, the hematocrit was 30%, and the 24-hour creatinine clearance was 15 ml per minute. A fourth renal biopsy was done (Fig. 2-18).

On October 3, 1964, he was readmitted to the hospital for reevaluation. His weight was 140 pounds, his blood pressure was 110/68 to 110/70 mm Hg, and he had peripheral edema. Urinalysis revealed a specific gravity of 1.010 and a trace of proteinuria. There were 2 to 30 erythrocytes and a rare granular cast per hpf. The 24-hour proteinuria was 88 mg. The hematocrit was 40%. The BUN was 42 mg per 100 ml, and the 15-minute excretion of intravenous injected PSP was 13%. The 24-hour creatinine clearance was 24 ml per minute. Culture of the urine was sterile. A timed nephrogram study revealed symmetrical and bilateral visualization of the collecting system at 3 minutes. There was bilateral thinning of the renal cortices. This was best noted at the upper pole of the right kidney. There was no blunting of the calyces. On October 6, 1964, a percutaneous renal biopsy was done (Fig. 2-19).

The morphologic light and electron microscopic findings are grouped together in the following paragraphs.

The first renal biopsy study revealed adequate renal cortex but no medulla was present (Fig. 2-15). The glomeruli were essentially normal. The cortical convolutions of tubules were lined by necrotic or markedly degenerated cells. Their lumina were often filled by

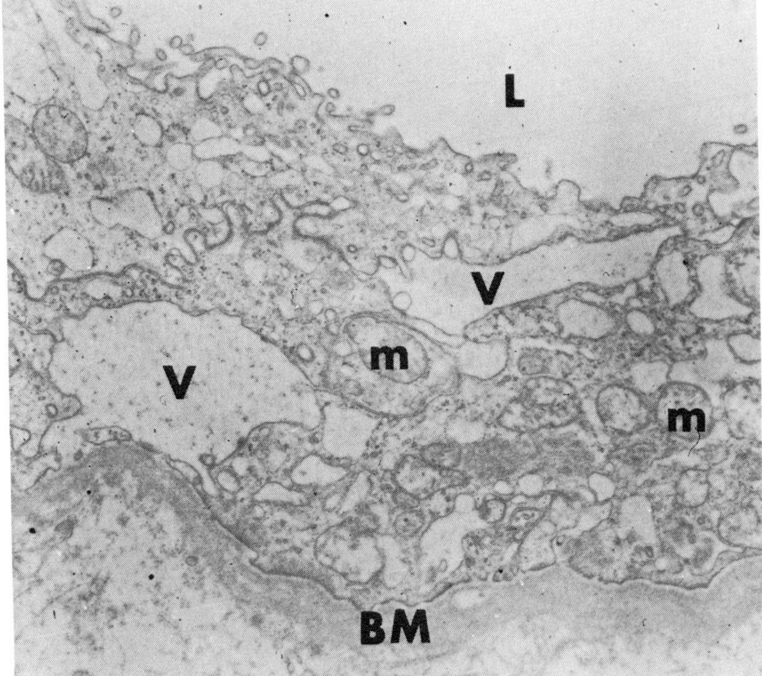

Fig. 2-21. Tubular regeneration after tubular necrosis. Electron microphotograph of renal biopsy taken during anuria from patient described in Fig. 2-14. Large vacuoles (V) were seen with the cortical tubules. The tubular lumen (L) was seen above. The tubular basement membrane (BM) was thickened. Several mitochondria (m) were seen in the cytoplasm. (×8,000.)

granular eosinophilic material mingled with erythrocytes and desquamated epithelial cells. By special stains, abundant hemoglobin could be demonstrated in this eosinophilic material. Hemosiderin was absent. In some of these tubules the lining cells showed obvious evidence of regeneration with clumps of epithelial cells projecting to the lumen. Henle's loops and the distal convolutions of tubules were often dilated with atrophic epithelium, and their lumina were filled by hyaline casts in which some hemoglobin could also be demonstrated. There was also a moderate degree of interstitial edema and minimal fibrosis with a few small clumps of lymphocytes. The small arteries were apparently normal.

The second renal biopsy study revealed that adequate cortex and medulla were present (Fig. 2-16). The glomeruli had a mild and irregular thickening of the capillary basement membrane more prominent near the vascular pole. All tubules appeared to be moderately atrophied. The convolutions of tubules were lined by relatively small cells that were often closely approximated and had hyperchromatic and irregular nuclei. Degeneration of these cells was minimal and necrosis was absent. These features suggested that these tubules were lined by a recently regenerated epithelium. Many tubules contained either granular or hyaline casts. Hemoglobin could be detected in most casts with the use of special hemoglobin stains. An occasional tubular cell contained hemosiderin granules. Some tubules had a slightly thickened basement membrane. The tubules were widely separated by an edematous and slightly fibrotic interstitial tissue in which a few small accumulations of lymphocytes were noted. The small arteries were slightly sclerotic. Several glomeruli had a prominent juxtaglomerular apparatus.

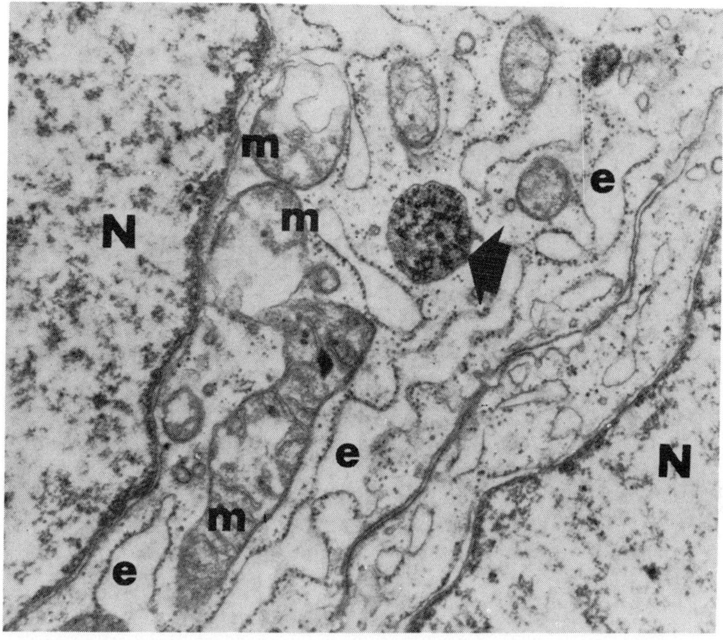

Fig. 2-22. Mitochondrial abnormalities in acute tubular necrosis. This electron microphotograph illustrates a portion of a tubular epithelial cell from patient described in Fig. 2-14. The biopsy study was made during complete anuria. A nucleus (N) was noted at left and a second nucleus at the right. Three small mitochondria were seen about a cytolysosome (arrow). The membranes of the endoplasmic reticulum (e) were separated. Coarsely granular ribosomes lined the membranes of the endoplasmic reticulum. Three degenerated mitochondria (m) were noted to the right of the left nucleus. The enclosing membranes of the mitochondria appeared invaginated. (×30,000.)

Electron microscopy findings revealed that no distinction could be made between the epithelial cells of the proximal, the distal, or collecting tubules. No brush border was seen. However, numerous short microvilli were seen projecting into the tubular lumen of some epithelial cells. The microvilli were more numerous in the crypts between cells (Fig. 2-20). The nuclei varied in size and shape. The mitochondria appeared swollen and contained a reduced number of cristae. Irregular clear vacuolar spaces were a common finding; they usually were present between the infolding of the cellular membrane (Fig. 2-21). Some of the spaces were large and apparently extracellular in location and were in direct contact with the tubular basement membrane.

In the cytoplasm a variety of round osmiophilic structures was seen. Many were the size of mitochondria and were outlined by a distinct membrane. Some of these contained indistinct residual cristae and often dense homogeneous osmiophilic granules and droplets. These structures were believed to represent mitochondria in various stages of degeneration (Fig. 2-22) or lysosomal (phagosomes) structures. In some of these structures the limiting membrane was incomplete or absent and the granular content appeared to be released in the adjacent cytoplasm. Huge osmiophilic inclusions were present within the tubular cytoplasm. They consisted of an irregular vacuolated homogeneous material limited by a dense membrane and were thought to represent erythrocytes in various stages of degeneration. Throughout the cytoplasm ribosomes could be identified along endoplasmic membrane as well as away from them. The grouping of ribosomes in small clumps in areas resembled ferritin (Fig. 2-23).

The tubular basement membranes were slightly and irregularly thickened with areas of varying density giving a laminated appearance. The interstitium had a loose appearance

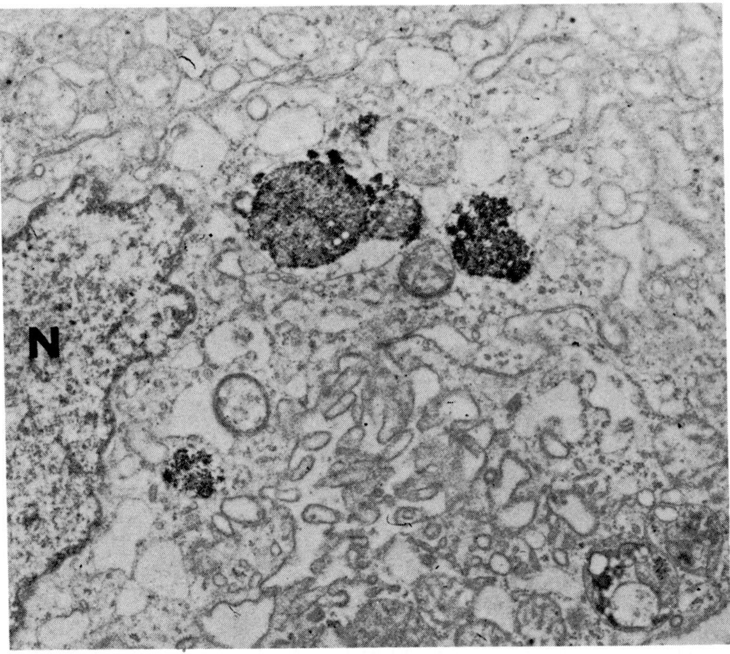

Fig. 2-23. Ferratin granules after severe hemolysis. This electron microphotograph illustrates a portion of a renal tubule studied during complete anuria associated with massive arsine-induced hemolysis. A nucleus (N) is seen to the left. Large oval bodies are noted containing small black granules. Ferratin granules were identified by high resolution electron microscopy. (×24,000.)

and contained numerous bundles of collagen fibers and a few polymorphonuclear leukocytes. Occasional large irregular cells with a large irregular nucleus and numerous cytoplasmic osmiophilic structures were noted. These osmiophilic bodies varied in density and were limited by a distinct membrane. They were believed to represent either degenerated mitochondria, reabsorption droplets, or lysosomes.

The third renal biopsy study revealed only renal cortex containing three glomeruli (Fig. 2-17). One glomerulus was completely fibrosed. There was a mild thickening of the glomerular capillary basement membrane with a slight axial hypercellularity. Bowman's capsule was moderately fibrotic. All tubules were moderately atrophic with increased atrophy when compared to the second biopsy. The tubules were lined by a low cuboidal cell with mild degenerative changes. Some tubule lumina contained granular casts. Hemoglobin could be demonstrated within the cortex by the use of special stains. Hemosiderin granules were found within a few tubular cells. The tubular basement membrane was slightly thickened. The abundant interstitial tissue was more fibrotic and less edematous than in the second biopsy. The interstitium contained scattered lymphocytes. Moderate arteriosclerosis and arteriolosclerosis were present.

Electron microscopic findings revealed, as in the previous biopsy, that the various types of cortical tubules could not be distinguished from each other. In general the appearances of the tubules were similar, as described in the second renal biopsy; however, the lining

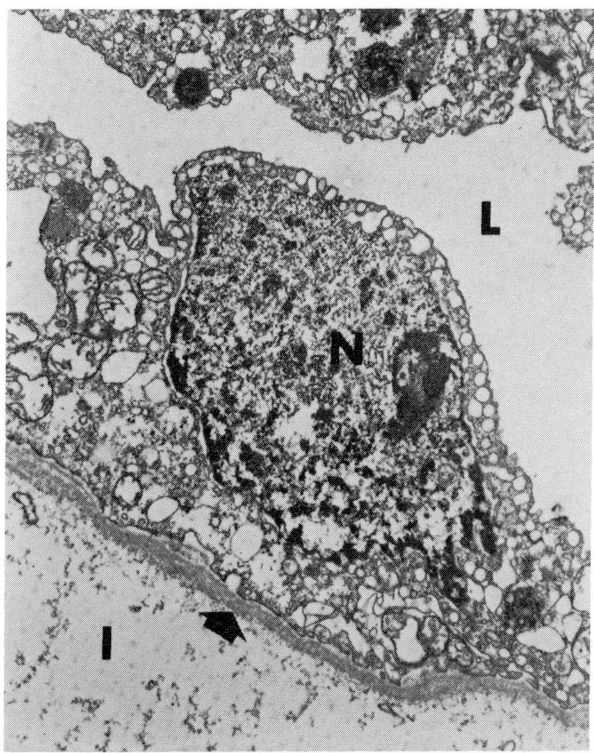

Fig. 2-24. Renal tubule at height of spontaneous diuresis. This electron microphotograph illustrates a renal tubule obtained by renal biopsy at the peak of a spontaneous diuresis. A large nucleus (N) fills much of the cell. The tubular lumen (L) separates the epithelial cells. Numerous small vacuoles are noted throughout the cytoplasm. The tubular basement membrane (arrow) is not thickened. The interstitial tissue (I) is edematous. (×12,000.)

tubular cells often appeared smoother and somewhat flat. Evidence of tubular cell proliferation was more pronounced. Within the cells numerous clear vacuoles were formed by membrane separation of the endoplasmic reticulum (Fig. 2-24), and numerous osmiophilic droplets of varying size were noted.

The tubular basement membrane of the cortical convolutions was often thickened. Some of the more severely degenerated and atrophic tubules were particularly denuded of living epithelium. The few remaining cells had a "ghost-like" appearance, usually without nuclei and often free in the tubular lumen. The mitochondria appeared vesicular and smaller with a reduction in the number of cristae within. The interstitium contained collagen fibers and many histiocytes and lymphocytes. In the glomeruli the capillary basement membrane was irregularly thickened in many areas. In general, the foot processes were well preserved, except for a few areas where they were found to be fused. The endothelial cells were swollen and the capillary lumen was considerably narrowed.

In brief, these findings indicated tubular cell atrophy and repair associated with more pronounced interstitial fibrosis and thickening of the tubular basement membrane. However, the collecting tubular basement membrane was not thickened.

The fourth renal biopsy study was conducted in two parts. After the fourth renal biopsy was taken, 25 gm of mannitol was given intravenously in a 20% solution. Thirty minutes later a repeat renal biopsy was taken. The first of these two biopsies consisted of a small fragment of renal tissue. No glomeruli were present. Few markedly atrophic tubules were recognized. These tubules had a thick basement membrane and were surrounded by an abundant dense fibrous connective tissue infiltrated by a small number of inflammatory cells. A few small arteries had considerable fibrosis of their wall.

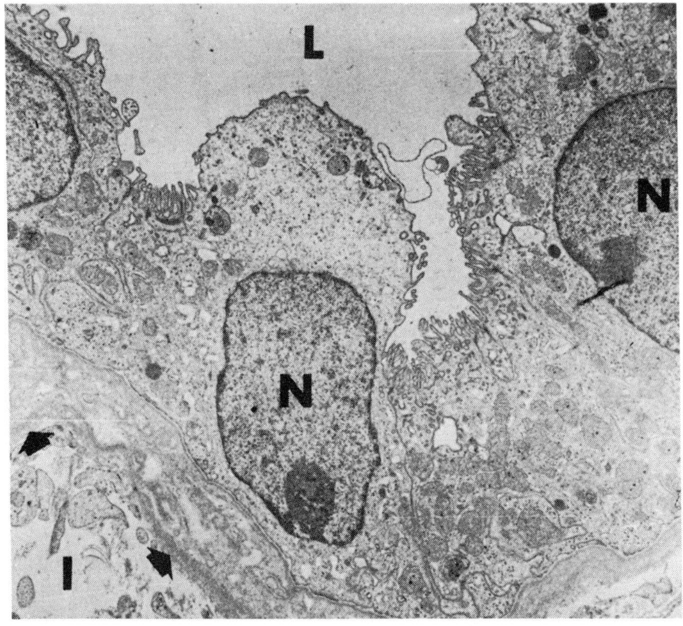

Fig. 2-25. Tubular regeneration 6 months after acute tubular necrosis. Six months following acute tubular necrosis the tubular epithelial cells were not normal. This photograph illustrates the fourth renal biopsy of patient described in Fig. 2-14. The nuclei (N) filled much of the cell. Short "crew-cut" brush borders were seen projecting into the lumen (L). The tubular basement membrane (arrows) was greatly thickened. The interstitium (I) was edematous. (×5,400.)

Study of the renal tissue taken 30 minutes after mannitol diuresis revealed renal cortex with six glomeruli with absence of medulla (Fig. 2-18). The glomerular capillary basement membrane was diffusely thickened. All tubules were markedly atrophied and were surrounded by a very thick and hyalinized basement membrane. Numerous vacuoles were noted within the cells. Few tubules contained hyaline and granular casts that contained traces of hemoglobin. No hemosiderin granules were detected in the tubular cells. The interstitial fibrous connective tissue was abundant and very dense. It contained small focal accumulations of inflammatory cells. The small arteries were moderately fibrotic. There was no apparent difference in the tubular cells before or after mannitol infusions.

Electron microscopic findings revealed that a distinction could not be made between the epithelial cells of the proximal, distal, and collecting tubules (Fig. 2-25). The cells were more regularly aligned but appeared to be incompletely differentiated. In the proximal convolutions of the tubules many of the lining cells were provided with a "crew-cut"–like brush border of closely approximated microvilli. The cytoplasm contained very few vacuoles and many mitochondria. In general, the mitochondria had few visible cristae and often some strongly osmiophilic granules. Larger inclusions were also noted in the cytoplasm. Some of these were in groups surrounded by a membrane that gave the appearance of lysosomes. Occasionally the portion of the epithelial cytoplasm projecting into the tubular lumen was not vacuolated and contained a few organelles. The basement membrane was greatly thickened and was in close contact with collagen fibers present in the interstitium (Fig. 2-26). This membrane had a laminated appearance and contained fine granules and small round structures that were possibly of cytoplasmic origin. In the distal tubules the

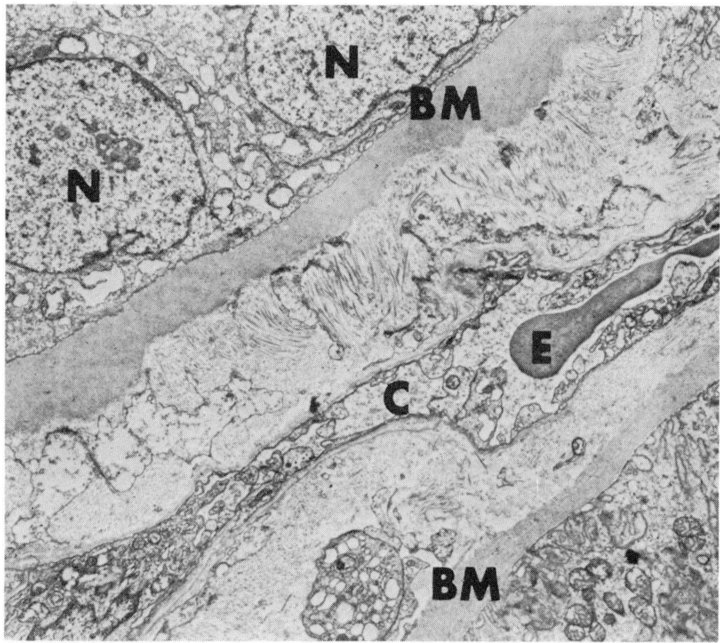

Fig. 2-26. Diffuse interstitial fibrosis following recovery from acute tubular necrosis. This electron microphotograph illustrates the diffuse interstitial fibrosis that followed healing of acute tubular necrosis. Mature bundles of collagen fibers were seen between thickened tubular basement membranes (BM) and the peritubular capillary (C) containing an erythrocyte (E). Two distal tubule cells are seen above containing nuclei (N). The renal biopsy study was done 3 years after recovery from acute tubular necrosis. (×6,000.)

mitochondria appeared well preserved and contained numerous cristae. Small clear vacuoles and lysosomes were present. The basement membrane of the distal convolutions of tubules was markedly thickened. The collecting ducts were lined by regularly aligned cells containing numerous osmiophilic inclusions, some of which were interpreted as degenerated erythrocytes. Polymorphonuclear leukocytes and erythrocytes were noted in the lumen. The basement membrane was not thickened. The glomeruli appeared similar to those of the third renal biopsy, but there was considerable thickening of the capillary basement membrane.

A renal biopsy taken 30 minutes after an intravenous injection of mannitol was similar to the previous biopsy except that an increased number of various-sized clear vacuoles was noted in the proximal and distal convolutions of tubules. The cytoplasm between the vacuole had a rarefied appearance suggestive of an increased content of water. The vacuoles were formed by a spreading apart of the endoplasmic reticular membrane.

The fifth renal biopsy study revealed adequate renal tissue containing seventeen glomeruli (Fig. 2-19). Thirteen of the seventeen were sclerosed and were closely approximated. Bowman's membrane of the remaining four glomeruli was thickened. In some areas the tubules appeared normal. In focal areas of interstitial fibrosis the tubules were atrophied.

Electron microscopic findings revealed that the glomerular basement membrane was focally thickened but in most capillary loops appeared essentially normal. The foot processes were focally fused. No osmiophilic deposits were seen adjacent to the capillary basement membrane.

The proximal convoluted tubules presented striking differences (Fig. 2-27). Many of the lining cells had a well-developed brush border that appeared to be essentially normal. However, other cells in the same tubules had only a few microvilli generally located within

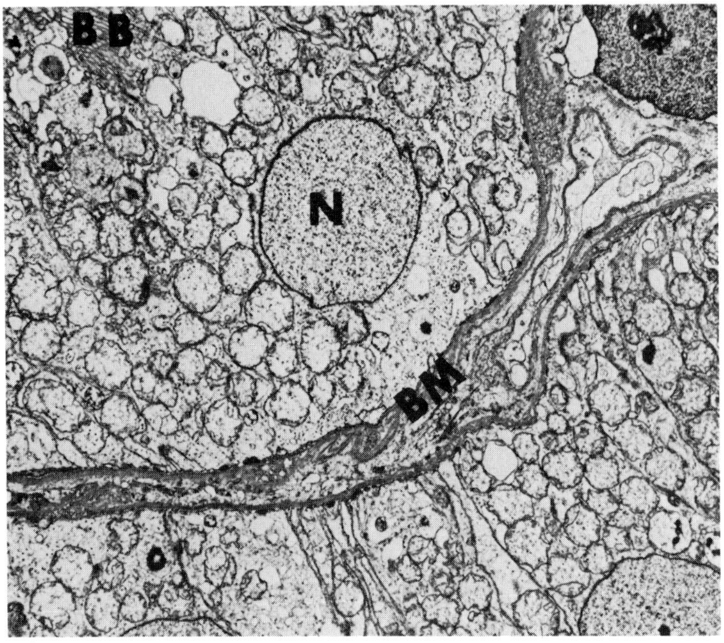

Fig. 2-27. Diffuse interstitial fibrosis becomes focal after recovery from acute tubular necrosis. This electron microphotograph is a renal biopsy taken 3 years after recovery from acute renal failure. The diffuse interstitial fibrosis noted in Fig. 2-18 became focal in distribution. The brush border (BB) is seen at the top. A proximal cell nucleus (N) is surrounded by numerous mitochondria. The tubular basement membrane (BM) is not thickened. There is no interstitial fibrosis separating the tubules. (×6,000.)

the crypts between the cells. In the cellular cytoplasm the mitochondria were quite numerous and were often smaller than normal. Some mitochondria had few or no cristae. In one area two entirely different types of mitochondria were seen side by side (Fig. 2-28). One type of mitochondria had the usual characteristics and was present in upper portions of the cell. The other type was in the basal portions of the cell, was surrounded by infolding basilar cellular membranes, and was somewhat more dense with numerous small and irregular cristae. Several mitochondria were noted to contain black granules or droplets of various sizes. Larger structures contained a variety of granules or lipids. Droplets were also present and were interpreted as lysosomes or phagosomes (Fig. 2-29).

In most cells the endoplasmic reticulum was poorly developed and few ribosomes were noted. In some cells the infolding membranes were poorly developed but in other cells they were closely approximated and appeared to be more numerous than normal.

The basement membrane of the proximal tubules was focally thickened and at times contained small granules. The cellular cytoplasm of the distal convolutions of tubules appeared in various forms and often contained black granules of various sizes. Some of the granules contained vacuolar structures and could have been lysosomes. The epithelial cells had what appeared to be a normal complement of mitochondria, some of which had abnormal cristae. The basement membrane was thickened and occasional fibers believed to be collagen were seen within it.

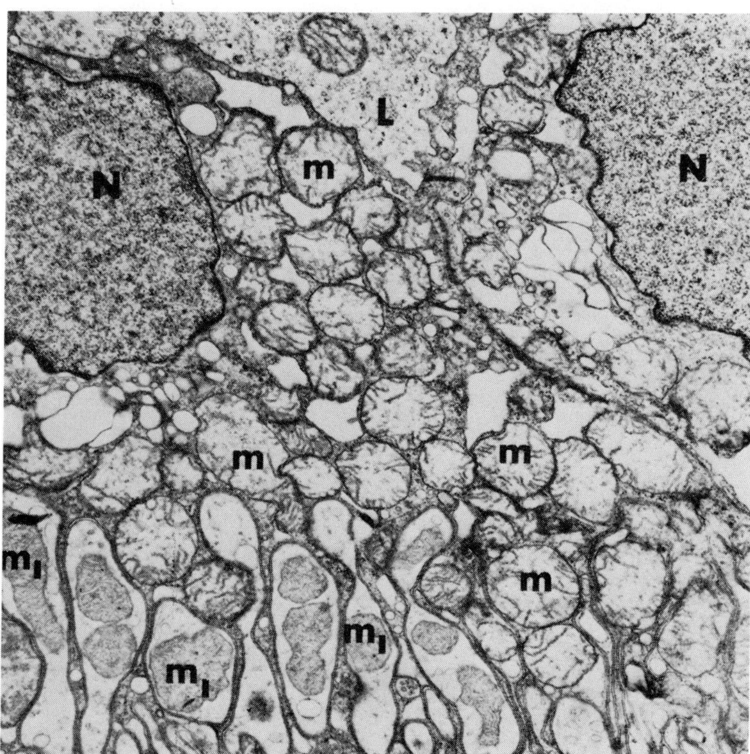

Fig. 2-28. Two types of mitochondria in healed acute tubular necrosis. This electron microphotograph illustrates a renal biopsy from patient described in Fig. 2-14. The biopsy study was done 3 years after the onset of acute tubular necrosis caused by arsine. Portions of two distal tubules are noted. The tubular lumen (L) is seen at the top. Portions of two nuclei (N) are present. Numerous mitochondria (m_1 and m) are seen within the infoldings of the cell membrane near the tubular basement membrane. ($\times$14,500.)

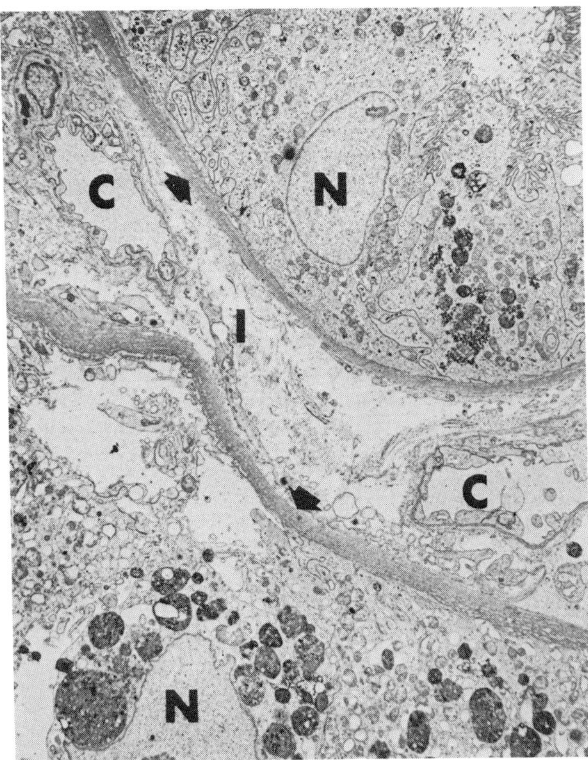

Fig. 2-29. Hemoglobin droplets in acute tubular necrosis. Renal biopsy taken from patient with acute anuria caused by severe intravascular hemolysis. A proximal tubule (upper right) contained numerous electron dense droplets to the right of the nucleus (N). The interstitium (I) was edematous and contained two peritubular capillaries (C). The tubules below appeared to be necrosed, and the tubular basement membrane (arrows) appears intact. Large electron dense bodies were seen surrounding the nucleus (N). Hemoglobin stains identified this material as hemoglobin pigment. ($\times$3,200.)

The interstitial cells, some of which were recognized as fibroblasts, contain numerous black granules of various sizes. The adjacent interstitial space was occupied by numerous bundles of collagen fibers. The intertubular capillaries had a normal appearance.

Comment. Correlations were made between the clinical and laboratory findings and the morphologic findings. The clinical and laboratory findings are summarized in Table 2-1. The morphologic analysis of serial light and electron microscopic renal changes are summarized in Table 2-2. The clinicopathologic observations were made on five renal biopsy specimens taken during complete anuria, early diuresis, the height of diuresis, the recovery period, and 23 months after recovery from acute renal failure.

Glomerular changes were not present in the first week of anuria. During early diuresis a progressive diffuse thickening of the glomerular basement membrane was evident. This was associated with slight axial hypercellularity. The glomerular changes resembled those seen in a diffuse vascular disease such as nephrosclerosis but differed in that the glomerular capillary membrane was more diffusely thickened and greater in proportion than the arteriolar changes. These glomerular changes are not clearly understood but appeared to be related to the progressive thickening of the tubular basement membrane and the interstitial fibrosis and not to the stage of acute renal failure.

Table 2-1. Serial clinical and laboratory observations made on patient with arsine-induced anuria

Days after arsine exposure	Blood pressure mm Hg	Urinalysis			BUN (mg %)	24-hour creatinine clearance (ml/min)	15 min excretion PSP (%)	Hematocrit (%)	Body weight (pounds)
		SG	Protein	Sediment					
2	120/68	—	—	—	135	—	—	17	—
7	118/70	—	—	—	—	—	—	—	—
31	110/68	—	—	—	—	Not done	0	—	—
66	118/75	1.011	2+	Few RBC casts; 10 to 20 RBC; several hyaline granular casts	79	10	0	24	—
74	130/78	1.010	1+	—	102	—	—	26	147
161	120/72	1.013	2.7 gm/24 hr	Several hyaline and hyaline granular casts	76	61	15	30	153
9 mos	120/78	—	—	—	39	—	—	33	165
13 mos	120/78	1.010	Trace	0	40	13.4	—	38	170
19 mos	108/65	1.010	1+	0	37	—	28	42	173
23 mos	110/68	1.010	88 mg/24 hr	Rare granular cast; 20 to 30 RBC	42	24	15.6	40	140

Table 2-2. Morphologic analysis of serial light and electron microscopic changes seen in renal biopsies from patient with arsine-induced anuria*

Biopsy	Time after arsine exposure	Glomeruli			Convoluted tubules					Interstitium			Arteriolar sclerosis
		Basement membrane	Cellularity	Sclerosis	Necrosis	Regeneration	Differentiation of regenerated cell	Basement membrane	Atrophy	Fibrosis	Edema	Cellular infiltrate	
1	7 days (Anuria)	0	0	0	4+	+	0	0	0	0	2+	+	0
2	33 days (Early diuresis)	+	0	0	4+	Complete	0	0	0	0	2+	+	+
3	66 days (Height of diuresis)	+	+	1+	0	Complete	2+	+	2+	2+ Diffuse	+	+	+
4	161 days (Recovery phase)	2+	+	1+ 2+	0	Complete	3+	4+	4+	4+ Diffuse	0	+	3+
5	23 months+	1+	+	3+	0	Complete	4+	2+	2+ Focal	3+ Focal	0	±	2+

*Severity of changes graded on semiquantitative scale; severity estimated on semiquantitative scale from 0 to 4+. Fourteen of seventeen glomeruli were completely hyalinized.

The greatest tubular damage occurred to the cortical convolutions of tubules—namely, the distal and proximal—and was characterized by marked tubular basement membrane thickening without alterations in the basement membrane of the collecting ducts. The severity of tubular lesions may have resulted in prolonged anuria. One week after arsine exposure and during complete anuria other tubules were lined by newly regenerated epithelium. The regenerated tubular cells could be differentiated from normal-appearing cells. In general, they had larger nuclei, a decreased size of cytoplasmic content, and a decreased number of mitochondria. The brush border was absent and the microvilli were decreased in number. Only a few microvilli were noted in the intercellular crypts. As the tubular cells underwent regeneration the mitochondria increased in number, the nuclei became normal in size, and the luminal villi became more numerous. However, 6 months after arsine exposure the patient was normotensive but had anemia and azotemia. The cells of the proximal convolutions of tubules were not yet normal. Mannitol diuresis was associated with morphologic changes in the cortical convoluted tubules. These changes, consisting of dilation of endoplasmic reticulum, were similar to changes in rats undergoing sucrose diuresis.

The most striking changes occurred in the interstitial tissue. Interstitial edema occurred early. Diffuse interstitial fibrosis was noted 66 days following arsine exposure, when the BUN was 79 mg per 100 ml. This fibrosis was uniform throughout the entire kidney. Twenty-three months following an apparent recovery from acute renal failure interstitial fibrosis was focal and severe nephrosclerosis was present. The blood pressure was normal, the BUN was 42 mg per 100 ml, and the hematocrit was 46%. The patient had chronic renal insufficiency.

Segmented tubular lesions

Although splitting the nephrons into specific sites for tubular necrosis is unrealistic, Sevitt has subdivided acute tubular necrosis into distal tubular necrosis, depending on the selected site of the main lesion.[995] He further divided distal tubular necrosis into diffuse and focal types, depending on the histologic damage.

These segmental tubular lesions can be explained by the maximal concentration of different nephrotoxic agents in specific portions of the nephron. Moreover, the tubular site of segmental tubular necrosis can be determined by the maximal concentration of any nephrotoxic agent. For example, specific nephrotoxic agents characteristically and reproducibly injure specific tubular areas. Segmented tubular necrosis of the proximal third is induced by mercury, carbon tetrachloride, *Amanita phalloides,* and serine. Necrosis of the middle and distal thirds of the proximal tubules results from diethylene glycol, tartrates, and chlorates. Arsine affects proximal and distal cortical tubules and spares cortical collecting tubules. The entire proximal tubule undergoes necrosis following arsenic and sulfonamides.

Histologic evolution of repair in acute tubular necrosis

Primary electron microscopic abnormalities are not seen to the same degree in all tubules.[256] The degree of tubular abnormalities depends on the severity of the initial insult. In such studies one must also consider the time relationship between onset of acute renal failure and the time the morphologic study is made. However, we have observed some tubules completely damaged and tubules in an adjacent nephron spared (Fig. 2-30). Uncomplicated tubular necrosis undergoes a rapid repair, and tubular lesions of mild necrosis may heal within days

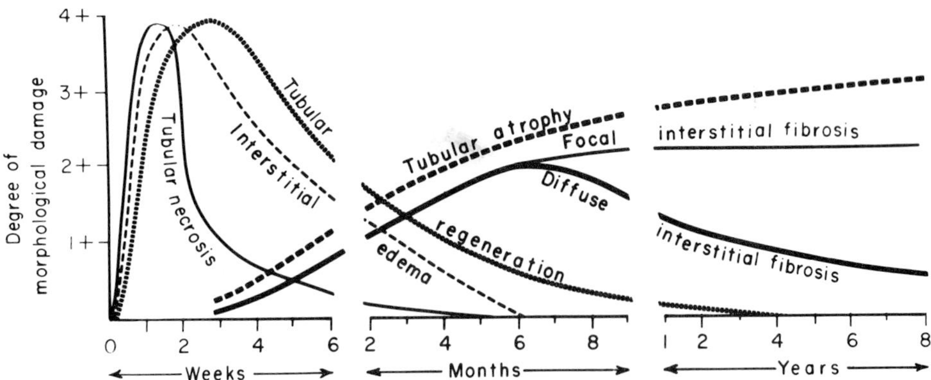

Fig. 2-30. Histologic evolution of acute tubular necrosis. This graph illustrates the evolution of renal changes that occurred during recovery from acute tubular necrosis. Tubular necrosis, tubular regeneration, tubular atrophy, interstitial edema, and interstitial fibrosis were analyzed on a semiquantitative scale from 0 to 4+ against time in weeks, months, and years. Tubular regeneration was rapid but covered a period of months. Healing was associated with interstitial edema. Diffuse interstitial fibrosis occurred and in time became focal.

after the initial insult. This may explain why necrotic lesions are not found if a renal biopsy is taken too late in the course of acute renal failure.

Serial renal biopsy study using an electron microscope reveals that tubular necrosis and tubular regeneration are extensive. In some patients it may be impossible to differentiate specific tubules as proximal, distal, or collecting. In severe acute tubular necrosis only remnants of the basement membrane may be found and spindles of fibrinoid may be seen in the epithelial cell debris. Cortical tubules can be identified when tubular necrosis is less severe. The proximal tubule may lose much of its brush border. In repair the epithelial cells have a simplified structure and mitosis is frequently seen.[257] The epithelial cells are low and cuboidal and they contain an enlarged round or oval-shaped nucleus. The mitochondria appear increased in numbers and have prominent cristae. Many months are required for epithelial cells of the cortical tubules to heal significantly for a possible differentiation of cell type. The histologic evolution of acute tubular necrosis is diagramed in Fig. 2-5.

If acute tubular necrosis is complicated by hemolysis, light osmiophilic inclusions are present within the tubular cytoplasm. They consist of irregular vacuolated homogeneous material of erythrocytes in various stages of degeneration. During diuresis the cortical tubule cells develop numerous small, clear vacuoles formed by spreading apart of the endoplasmic reticulum (Fig. 2-24). The proximal tubular brush border appears to regenerate by new villi developing in the intracellular crypts. Later the repairing brush border appears similar in the course of renal repair, and a diffuse interstitial fibrosis develops. In time this diffuse lesion becomes focal. The overall renal size decreases and the patient may progress to chronic renal failure with associated clinical and biochemical features.

It is difficult to explain how a diffuse process of interstitial fibrosis can subside and become focal in nature; nevertheless, this does occur. Associated with the evolution of interstitial fibrosis is death of nephrons with subsequent tubular atrophy and hyalinization of glomeruli.[482]

ACUTE BILATERAL RENAL CORTICAL NECROSIS

In 1896, Juhel-Renoy first described bilateral renal cortical necrosis at autopsy of a 16-year-old girl.[593] She developed anuria on the ninth day after developing scarlet fever, and she died on the fifteenth day. Ten years later Bradford and Lawrence described renal cortical necrosis associated with pregnancy.[142a] Since then numerous monographs have been written on this subject. The most well known are that by Sheehan and Moore[1004] and that by Duff and Murray.[321]

In general, bilateral renal cortical necrosis involves both kidneys with relatively the same severity.[419] It is a fulminant ischemic necrosis of the cortex involving glomeruli and tubules. On a single occasion the disease afflicted only one kidney; the opposite kidney had renal artery stenosis. Renal cortical necrosis can be suspected clinically, but the diagnosis can only be made by renal biopsy study or by postmortem examination.

Acute renal cortical necrosis produces the clinical setting of acute oliguric renal failure in 80% of the patients. It appears most frequently as a complication of pregnancy and occurs once in every one or two hundred patients with utero-placental asphyxia or obstetric hemorrhagic complications such as placenta abruptio and abortion. Other obstetric conditions include premature separation of the placenta and concealed retroplacental and massive accidental hemorrhage. These conditions are usually associated with afibrinogenemia. Rodriguez-Erdmann studied the pathogenesis of bilateral renal cortical necrosis induced by means of exogenous fibrin.[939] His studies have added greatly to our knowledge of this entity.

The degree and extent of renal involvement with cortical necrosis vary greatly. Cortical necrosis may involve a small foci of cortex including the columns of Bertini. The clinical course is directly related to the extent of the necrosis. The etiology of acute cortical necrosis is usually ischemic and results from massive uterine hemorrhage associated with pregnancy. The incidence of acute renal cortical necrosis is greater when the obstetric complications occur between the twenty-fifth to thirty-first week of gestation than towards the end of pregnancy. Infarctions of the anterior lobe of the pituitary gland and subsequent pituitary insufficiency may occur in association with the renal cortical necrosis of pregnancy.[214] The clinical syndrome produced by the infarction of the pituitary gland has been referred to as "Sheehan's syndrome."

Bilateral renal cortical necrosis has occurred in males, nonpregnant women, and children as a result of severe hemorrhage, trauma, severe infections, dehydration, diarrhea, vomiting, and burns.[674] When women with premature placental separation are excluded, the incidence of acute cortical necrosis is greater in men than in women. Gross hematuria and marked proteinuria occur and are followed by complete anuria or oliguria. Various numbers of leukocytes and granular and erythrocyte casts are noted. The oliguric stage is usually prolonged, and recovery from bilateral renal cortical necrosis is not common. The daily urinary output may reach a level of 400 ml but is never greater. Without long-term dialysis the patient would die. Acute cortical necrosis is more commonly seen in children. Using long-term dialysis, Alwall and colleagues kept two patients with renal cortical necrosis alive for 74 and 116 days, respectively.

The gross pathology of renal cortical necrosis is an increased kidney size within 2 weeks after the onset; later the size decreases. The kidneys involved with cortical necrosis are soft and enlarged for at least 2 weeks. The capsule strips easily from the yellow-mottled surface cortex. On cut surface the subcapsular

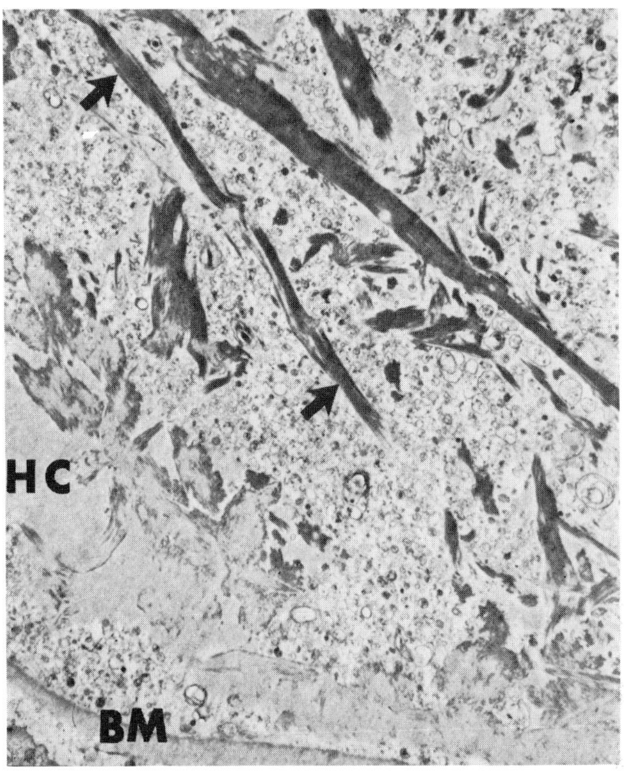

Fig. 2-31. Severe acute coagulative necrosis of cortical tubule. Extensive and severe acute tubular necrosis was found on light microscopic study of renal biopsy taken from a 43-year-old woman with fatal acute renal failure. This electron microphotograph reveals epithelial cell necrosis with cellular debris and spindles of fibroid material (arrows). Homogeneous coagular necrosis (HC) is seen below and around the fibroid material. The intact basement membrane (BM) is seen below. (×6,000.)

cortex is approximately 1 to 2 cm thick. It is usually intact, due to the collateral circulation to the subcapsular area. The remainder of the cortex is a yellowish gray necrotic zone. When necrosis is incomplete, multiple gray infarcted areas are seen within the cortex. The renal pyramids are dark purple. This gives the appearance that the medulla is congested with blood. Beyond the third week after onset the renal mass decreases in size and may become smaller than normal.

The histologic findings of acute renal cortical necrosis are best described in the time sequence reported by Sheehan and Moore. They studied the kidneys of a large group of women developing cortical necrosis following premature separation of placenta and concealed massive hemorrhage at 8 to 12 hours after onset. They found small fibrin thrombosis in the glomeruli, nuclear pyknosis of the tubular epithelial cell, and eosinophilic staining of the cytoplasm. At 14 to 18 hours after onset the glomeruli were dilated and there was nuclear pyknosis of tubular cells with reduced tubular necrosis. At 22 to 27 hours the glomerular capillaries were congested with erythrocytes, and the intertubular arteries and arterioles were dilated and had early necrotic changes in their media and intima. Erythrocytes within the glomerular capillaries underwent hemolysis by 36 to 72 hours; the histologic changes reached their fullest damage, without further change, for 2 to 3 weeks. When necrosis was complete there was death of all

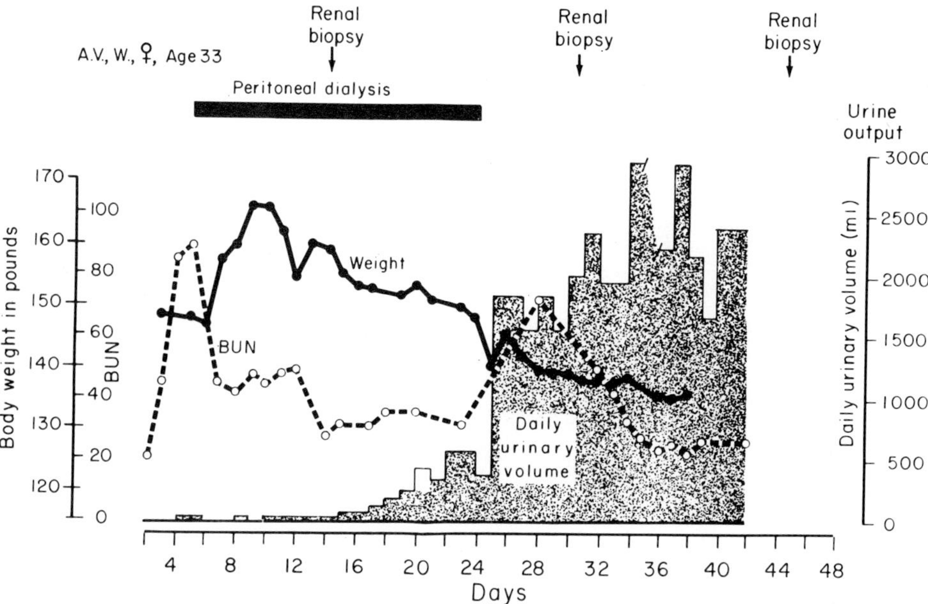

Fig. 2-32. Hospital course of patient with acute oliguric renal failure caused by partial acute renal cortical necrosis. This figure illustrates the hospital course of a 33-year-old Mexican woman who developed acute renal failure following a massive hemorrhage caused by premature separation of the placenta. When the BUN reached 158 mg per 100 ml, peritoneal dialysis was started and continued for 20 days. Renal biopsy studies were done on the thirteenth, twenty-ninth, and forty-third hospital days. A spontaneous diuresis occurred on the twenty-fifth day. Partial bilateral renal cortical necrosis was found on biopsy study.

types of cells. Glomeruli could still be recognized. There were various types of coagulation necrosis. The tubular epithelial cells stripped away from the tubular basement membrane into the capillary lumen (Fig. 2-31). This finding could not be attributed to a postmortem change, as it was observed in renal biopsy material.

The interstitium of the necrotic area was edematous without cellular infiltration. There was an abrupt change from necrotic area to the healthy tissue. However, the area adjacent to the necrotic area contained numerous interstitial cellular infiltrates of leukocytes, histocytes, and fibroblasts.

As the necrotic area underwent healing, interstitial fibrosis and cellular infiltration occurred. There was a revascularization of the necrotic cortex. Numerous small deposits of calcium occurred in necrotic glomeruli and tubules. The necrotic area shrank and became a fibrotic scar. The adjacent area underwent hypertrophy of nephrons and glomeruli. In some incidences cortical necrosis may be partial or focal and the clinical features of acute oliguric renal failure may be reversible.

Focal renal cortical necrosis

The three gradations of focal, partial, and gross acute renal cortical necrosis and their clinicopathologic correlations are discussed in the following three case presentations.

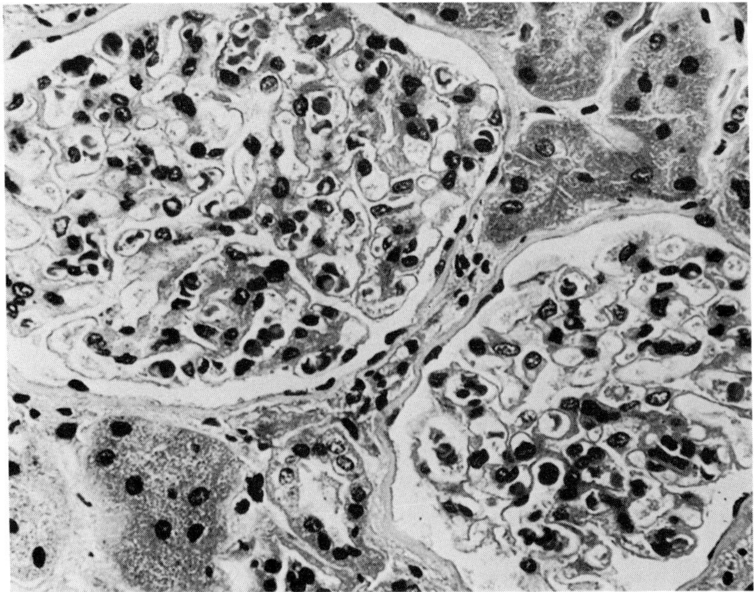

Fig. 2-33. Focal renal cortical necrosis associated with massive uterine hemorrhage. This microphotograph illustrates the first renal biopsy of patient described in Fig. 2-32. Tissue was obtained on the thirteenth day of oliguria. There was widespread acute tubular necrosis and only one glomerulus of eleven had morphologic changes of necrosis. The two glomeruli above appear normal. There is acute necrosis of the adjacent tubules. (H&E ×400.)

CASE PRESENTATION

A 33-year-old Mexican housewife, gravida IV, para III, was in her seventh month of pregnancy. On June 10, 1964, she developed massive vaginal bleeding and was admitted in shock to Gottlieb Memorial Hospital. She was given three transfusions of whole blood. Because bleeding continued the patient was taken to surgery; a Couvelaire uterus was found, and a Porro hysterectomy was done. The stillborn baby weighed 3 pounds, 10.5 ounces. An additional three units of whole blood raised her hematocrit to 38%. The BUN was 21.5 mg per 100 ml. The patient developed complete anuria, which did not respond to 25 gm of 20% mannitol solution infused rapidly intravenously.

The next day she was transferred to Presbyterian–St. Luke's Hospital for management of acute renal failure. (Her hospital course is plotted in Fig. 2-32.) On the fourth day of anuria the BUN was 92 mg per 100 ml. Peritoneal dialysis was started and was continued for 18 days. Over the first 14 days the daily urinary output remained below 65 ml, and most days was below 30 ml. On the twenty-first day the urinary output exceeded 500 ml, and diuresis ensued. A peak 24-hour urinary output of 2,935 ml was reached on the thirty-sixth day. On the forty-second day the BUN was stabilized at 31 mg per 100 ml. Two days later she was discharged.

On the second day of renal failure the hematocrit was 22% and the platelet count was 16,000/cu mm. The latter rose to 205,000/cu mm on the eleventh day. The total serum bilirubin was 4.2 mg per 100 ml (indirect bilirubin 3.1 mg). Hemoglobinuria was first looked for and was detected on the fourth day. It persisted to the sixth day. On the tenth day the direct and indirect Coombs tests were negative.

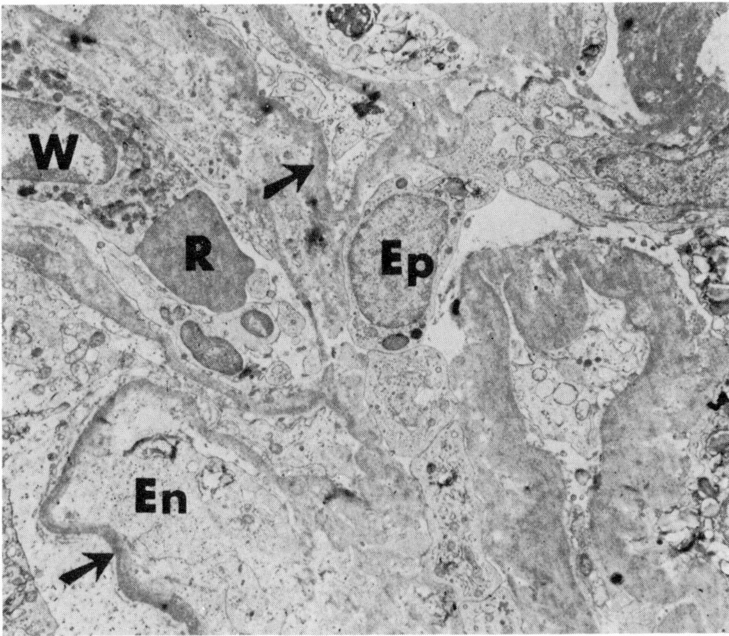

Fig. 2-34. Focal renal cortical necrosis. This electron microphotograph illustrates a necrotic glomerulus from a 33-year-old woman with acute renal failure. Renal biopsy was obtained on the fourteenth day of anuria. Seven days later the urinary output was 500 ml. The glomerular structure is disrupted. Epithelial cell foot processes are completely absent. The glomerular basement membrane (arrows) varies in thickness. The endothelial (En) and epithelial (Ep) cell membranes are disrupted. An erythrocyte (R) and a white blood cell (polymorphonucleocyte) (W) is seen within a glomerular capillary lumen. ($\times 6,000$.)

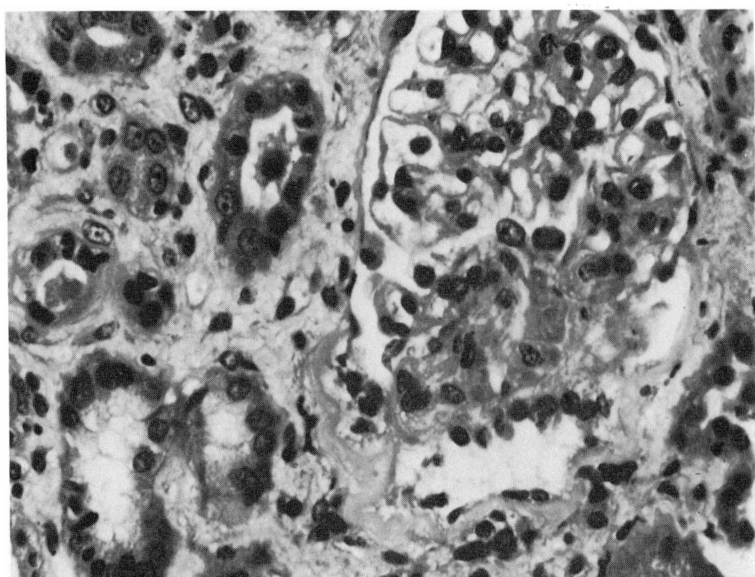

Fig. 2-35. Diffuse interstitial fibrosis following recovery from focal renal cortical necrosis. This microphotograph illustrates the second renal biopsy taken during early diuresis on the twenty-ninth day. There was focal necrosis of some glomeruli. Tubular regeneration was noted. The striking finding was in the interstitium. It was edematous and contained many collagen fibers, histocytes, and fibroblasts. Note the healed necrosis of the glomerular base. (H&E ×400.)

Three serial percutaneous renal biopsies were done during her hospitalization. The first biopsy was done on the fourteenth day while she was undergoing peritoneal dialysis—when the 24-hour urinary output was 29 ml and the BUN was 31 mg per 100 ml (Fig. 2-33). On the basis of one necrotic glomerulus acute renal cortical necrosis was diagnosed (Fig. 2-34). The second renal biopsy was done on the forty-fourth day when the BUN had "leveled" at 31 mg per 100 ml. Tubular regeneration appeared complete, and a diffuse interstitial fibrosis was present.

On December 13, 1964, she was readmitted to Presbyterian–St. Luke's Hospital for evaluation. Her blood pressure was 124/78 mm Hg, and the physical examination was essentially normal. The hematocrit was 39%. Urinalysis revealed proteinuria (1+) with a normal urinary sediment. The BUN was 18 mg per 100 ml and the 24-hour creatinine clearance was 76 ml per minute. A fourth renal biopsy was done 187 days after the onset of acute renal failure. Interstitial fibrosis was found as the only histologic abnormality (Fig. 2-35).

Comment. The prolonged oliguric phase that occurred in the patient is not unusual in postpartum women with acute oliguric renal failure. The histologic findings of one or more necrotic glomeruli would fit Sheehan's diagnostic criteria of acute cortical necrosis. The patient had this occasional necrotic glomerulus. The initial renal biopsy study revealed information that histologic recovery was possible, and time bore this forecast out. The finding of a subsequent diffuse interstitial fibrosis was probably the result of prolonged oliguria.

Partial renal cortical necrosis

Partial renal cortical necrosis involves scattered portions of the cortex. Recovery is still possible but depends on the extent of the necrotic lesion. This is discussed in the following case presentation.

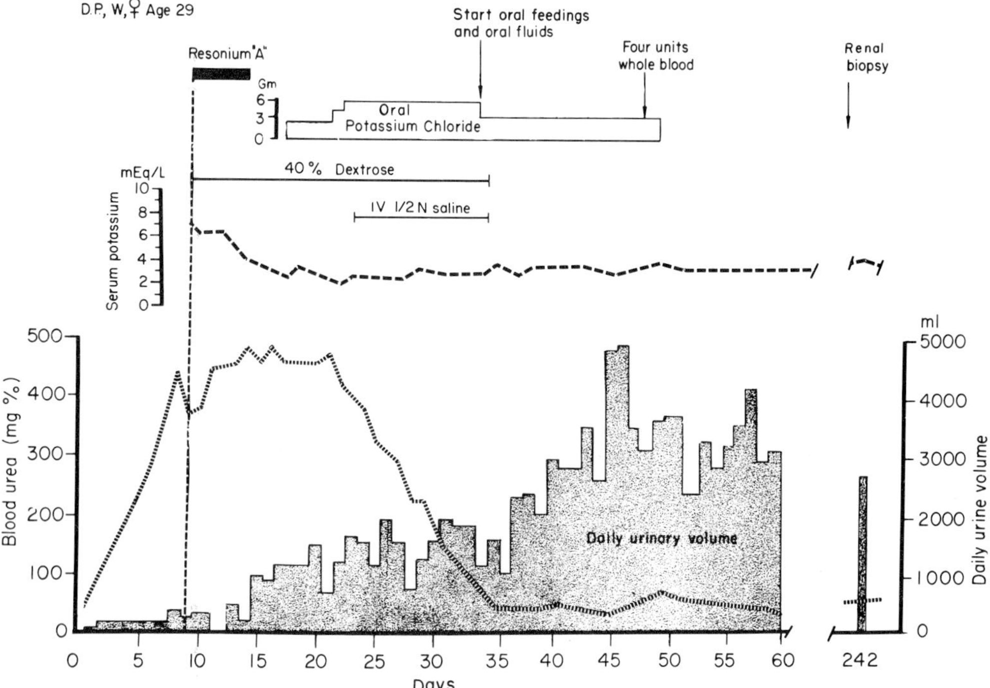

Fig. 2-36. Clinical findings of a patient with focal cortical necrosis. A 29-year-old woman developed a concealed intrauterine hemorrhage from premature separation of the placenta. She was treated conservatively. On the fourteenth day she entered the diuretic period and recovered. A renal biopsy study was done on the 242nd day after onset of renal failure.

CASE PRESENTATION

A 29-year-old white woman developed swelling of her ankles and fingers in the thirtieth week of her first pregnancy. Three weeks later, on February 14, 1955, she experienced a sudden onset of dull epigastric pain. This pain was intermittent and was followed by a vaginal hemorrhage of fresh blood estimated at 150 ml. The abdominal pain became severe. That evening, following a second vaginal hemorrhage of approximately one pint, she was hospitalized. On examination she was apprehensive, pale, and in pain. The blood pressure was normal (130/83 mm Hg). Because the uterus was tense, fetal parts were not palpable. No fetal heart tones were heard. Three pints of blood were given. Under light anesthetic the placental membranes were ruptured and a stillborn infant was delivered. A large retroplacental blood clot was expelled without excessive blood loss or fall in systolic blood pressure. The following day she had oliguria. Over the next 8 days the daily urinary output did not exceed 200 ml. Staphyloccocci, coagulase-positive, were cultured from the urine. There was gross proteinuria and microscopic hematuria associated with a low specific gravity. She was given a Bull-Borst dietary regimen and she developed nausea and vomiting.

On February 17 the hematocrit was 25%. She was transfused with three additional pints of blood. There was a steady rise in BUN, which was 440 mg per 100 ml on February 23. The following day she was transferred to Hammersmith Hospital. (Her hospital course over the next 51 days is plotted in Fig. 2-36.) She received conservative treatment of resins to remove potassium from the gut. Intravenous 40% glucose was given. On the eighteenth day oral potassium chloride was given. On the thirty-fourth day oral feedings were started. On the forty-eighth day four units of whole blood were given. She was discharged on the sixtieth day. A renal biopsy was done 241 days after the concealed hemorrhage. Study revealed areas of healed cortical necrosis (Fig. 2-37).

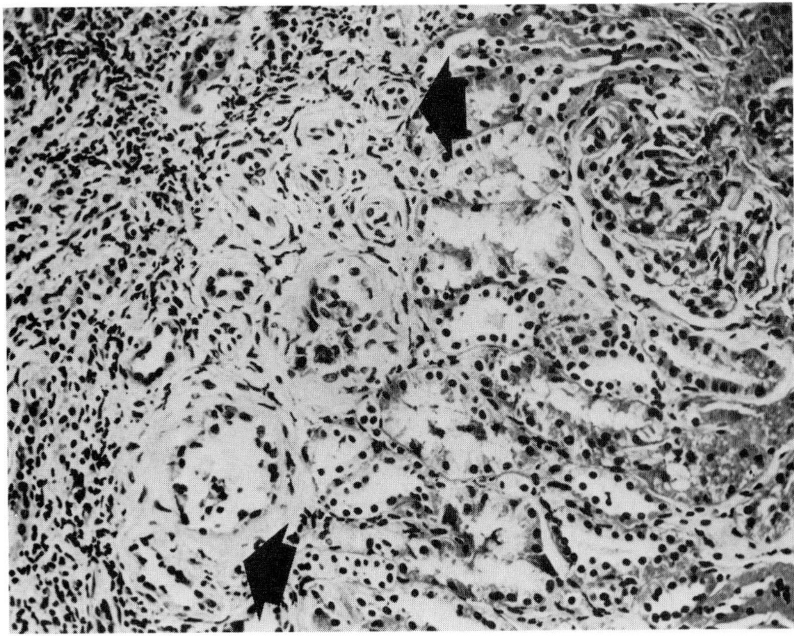

Fig. 2-37. Healed focal bilateral cortical necrosis. This microphotograph illustrates a renal biopsy from the patient described in Fig. 2-36. She had slightly impaired renal function. Eight months previously she had toxemia of pregnancy and premature placental separation followed by oliguria and diuresis on the fifteenth day. There is sharp demarcation (arrows) of scarring from healthy tissue. This finding confirmed the clinical diagnosis of focal bilateral cortical necrosis. (H&E ×375.)

Comment. The massive retroplacental hemorrhage following birth of a stillborn child resulted in a significant drop in glomerular blood flow and subsequently produced cortical ischemia. This ischemia resulted in renal cortical damage and subsequent acute oliguric renal failure. Conservative treatment was given. In time the kidneys gradually recovered. The diagnosis of renal cortical necrosis was made on the follow-up hospital visit when a renal biopsy revealed focal areas of healed scars. The degree of impaired renal function indicated the patchy and scattered involvement of scarred cortex.

Massive renal cortical necrosis

When massive renal cortical necrosis occurs the patient initially has anuria and later a prolonged oliguria, excreting less than 400 ml daily. The kidneys are more prone to infection with subsequent abscess formation. It is clinically very important to diagnose the underlying renal abnormality. Treatment by chronic dialysis and renal transplantation is based on this exact morphologic diagnosis. Renal biopsy is the only method during life to make this exact diagnosis.[450] Bilateral renal cortical necrosis can be diffuse and massive and can lead to irreversible and fatal acute renal failure.

The clinicopathologic correlations of massive renal cortical necrosis are discussed in the following case presentation.

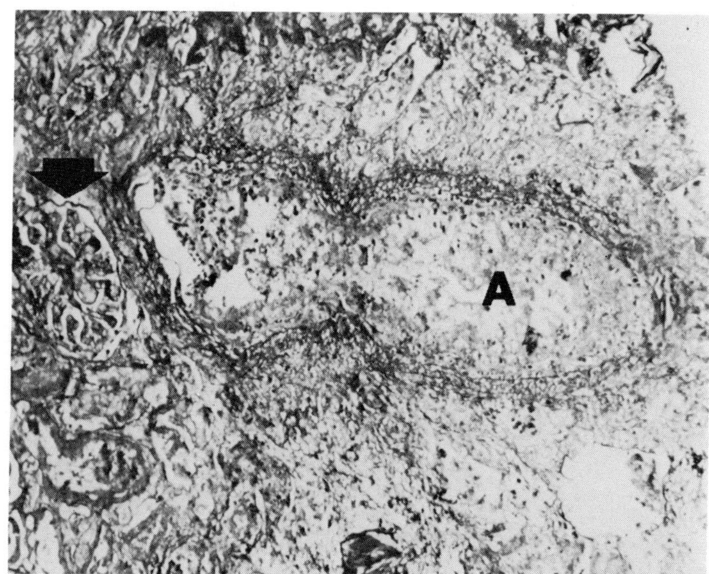

Fig. 2-38. Fatal acute renal cortical necrosis. A 40-year-old woman had a severe uterine hemorrhage during delivery of a stillbirth. She developed hematuria and acute oliguria. Peritoneal dialysis was started and a renal biopsy was obtained. Study of the tissue revealed massive cortical necrosis. A large necrotic artery (A) was seen. The adjacent tubules were pale. A degenerated glomerulus (arrow) was noted. The patient developed a superimposed acute pyelonephritis with septicemia and died. (H&E ×100.)

CASE PRESENTATION

A. S., a 41-year-old woman, had edema, hypertension, and proteinuria in her third pregnancy. Her first pregnancy occurred at age 13 years. Her second pregnancy occurred in January, 1960, and was complicated by weight gain, edema, hypertension, and proteinuria.

On May 22, 1961, she developed abdominal cramping and was admitted to Mary Thompson Hospital. The abdominal disturbance was followed by a massive vaginal hemorrhage. No fetal heart tones were heard. An emergency cesarean section was done. A placenta abruptio was found with approximately 1,000 ml of blood in utero. Immediately after surgery she developed acute oliguric renal failure. Five hours after surgery she had absolute anuria. She was treated with intravenous fluids. She became grossly overhydrated and developed congestive heart failure.

On May 24, 1961, she was transferred to Presbyterian–St. Luke's Hospital. Peritoneal dialysis was started. On July 28, 1961, a percutaneous renal biopsy was done to ascertain the need for future dialysis. Diffuse renal cortical necrosis was found (Fig. 2-38). Peritoneal dialysis was discontinued. She developed pyelonephritis and became comatose. She died in uremia on August 5, 1961.

Postmortem examination revealed bilateral renal abscesses with massive and complete bilateral renal cortical necrosis.

Comment. Renal biopsy study disclosed the massive cortical involvement of renal cortical necrosis. I wish to point out that it is rare for a patient with severe histologic involvement—such as just described—to recover from acute renal failure. The patient usually has severe chronic renal insufficiency and small kidneys. In general, the prognosis is grave once diffuse cortical necrosis occurs. The development of numerous small renal abscesses seen at autopsy is not unusual in kidneys involved with cortical necrosis.

RENAL VASCULAR LESIONS

Renal vascular lesions include bilateral occlusion of the renal artery and renal vein thrombosis. Renal artery occlusion follows dissection of aortic aneurysms, emboli, and traumatic thrombosis. Occlusion of the renal arteries leads to renal infarction and a clinical situation of acute oliguric renal failure.

BILATERAL RENAL ARTERY OCCLUSIONS

Renal destruction by ischemic infarction follows renal artery occlusions. The condition is considered grave because the time spent in making an exact diagnosis precludes prompt surgical treatment. Minor episodes of renal infarction may go undetected by both the patient and the physician. Unless anuria, oliguria, or hematuria develops the affliction usually goes undiagnosed. Renal artery infarction results from renal artery occlusions caused by a variety of conditions. These include emboli from bacterial endocarditis, aseptic valvular vegetation, mural thrombi from the left auricle in patients with atrial fibrillation, and mural thrombi from an aneurysm of the left ventricle. Renal artery occlusions can result from thrombosis following trauma, renal artery surgery, arteriosclerotic narrowing of the large renal vessels with thrombosis, polyarteritis nodosa, mural thrombi, aneurysm of the abdominal aorta, and dissection of the abdominal aorta into both renal arteries. Anuria follows renal infarction and in a few days the urinary output increases to between 300 and 400 ml daily. I observed two patients with bilateral renal artery obstruction caused by mural thrombi associated with "beer drinker's" cardiomyopathy[794] (Fig. 2-39, A).

Traumatic artery thrombosis

Traumatic renal artery thrombosis was first described by Von Recklinhausen in 1861.[1103] He described left renal artery thrombosis in a 13-year-old boy who died 8 days after a fall. In 1965 Steiness and Thaysen described bilateral traumatic renal artery thrombosis.[1042] They reported a previously healthy 18-year-old man who fell from his motorcycle while traveling at 50 miles per hour. The patient experienced bilateral back pain for 1 day. Except for 11 ml of bloody urine the patient had gross anuria. The diagnosis of renal artery thrombosis was made by renal aortography. A left nephrectomy was done. The right renal artery was resected and an end-to-end anastomosis was performed.

Bogaert and his colleagues reported two patients with acute renal failure caused by bilateral renal artery obstruction. They emphasized early diagnosis leading to surgical treatment or use of fibrinolytic drugs.

Collins and Jacobs hypothesized that the mobile kidney is suddenly moved by a direct blow or by sudden deceleration of the body from previous very great velocities.[228] The sudden movement the kidney creates overstretches the renal artery and subsequently damages the arterial wall. This occurs close to the junction between the aorta and the renal artery. The left renal artery is more

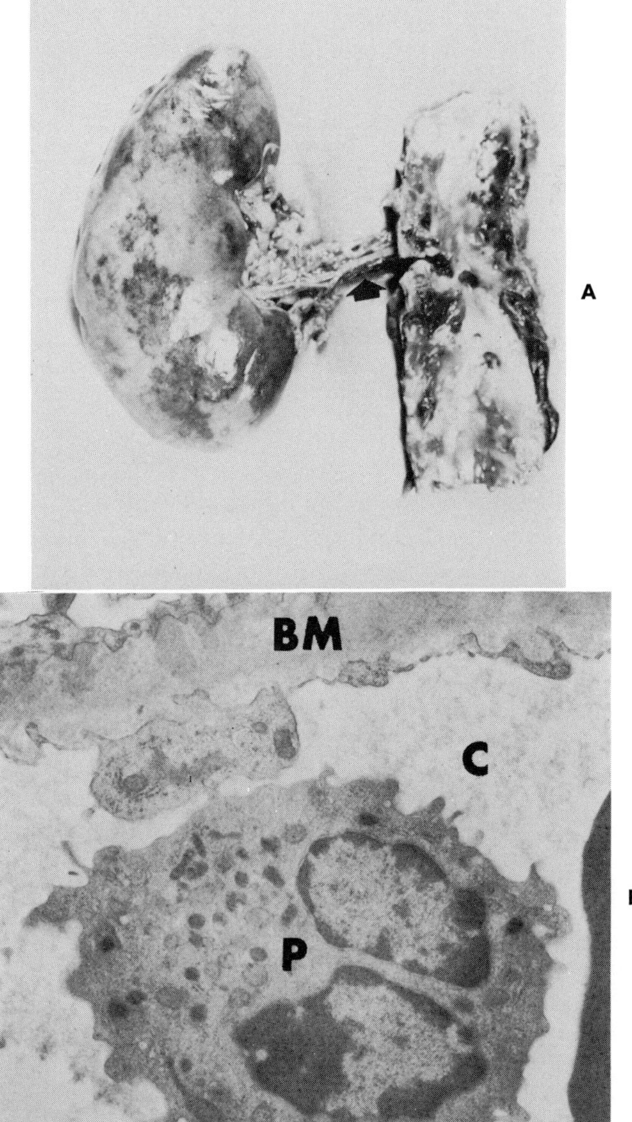

Fig. 2-39. **A,** Renal artery emboli from mural thrombi associated with alcoholic myocardiopathy. A 57-year-old man with a prolonged history of alcoholism was admitted to the hospital with congestive heart failure. After effective treatment the patient was ready for discharge; however, he suddenly developed gross hematuria and acute oliguria. He died of a cardiac dysrhythmia. At autopsy he was found to have alcoholic myocardiopathy with mural thrombi. The renal artery of a single kidney was occluded with a firm thrombus. This photograph illustrates the postmortem kidney. The thrombus (arrow) is noted in the renal artery. The kidney has several infarcted areas. **B,** Margination of leukocyte in renal vein thrombosis. This electron microphotograph illustrates a renal biopsy obtained from a patient with inferior vena cava thrombosis. A portion of a glomerular capillary loop is seen above. In the glomerular capillary lumen (C), a polymorphonucleocyte (P), is marginating (C) near the thickened glomerular basement membrane (BM). (×12,000.)

commonly involved. The overstretching of the renal artery may result in a complete convulsing of the artery.

Another mechanism is an intramural arterial lesion that does not completely interrupt the continuity of the renal artery. The arterial laceration extends from the intima to various depths down to but not including the adventitia. Rupturing of the arterial wall occurs and leads to artery occlusion. It is possible that local renal artery thrombosis also occurs. Management should be directed toward early diagnosis; renal aortography and prompt vascular surgical treatment should be used. All possible attempts should be made to reestablish renal blood flow. If a kidney is completely infarcted and destroyed it should be removed; otherwise, hypertension will follow.

Renal artery emboli

Renal artery embolic occlusion is the most common cause of renal infarction (Fig. 2-39, *A*). An episode of renal infarction has a self-limited course and cannot be recognized when it is in progress. The patient experiences a steady aching pain with tenderness over one or both kidneys. These findings are associated with fever, nausea, and vomiting. The kidney will be tender and may be enlarged. There is persistent pyelotubular backflow on retrograde pyelography. Surgical treatment should be prompt, before the small arterial branches are impervious to irrigation.

There is microscopic hematuria associated with leukocytosis, proteinuria, and renal epithelial cell casts. When both kidneys are infarcted, absolute anuria occurs and is followed by hypertension, which persists for approximately 4 to 8 days.

Renal vein thrombosis

Bilateral renal vein thrombosis occurs in children, usually infants. It can result in sudden oliguria or anuria.[605] The characteristic clinical feature is an acutely ill child with severe diarrhea and vomiting. Renal vein thrombosis usually develops in one kidney and then involves the other. Hemorrhagic infarction may occur.[638] In adults renal vein thrombosis produces oliguria or anuria when it is superimposed on kidneys that are involved by a chronic disease such as amyloid or diabetic glomerulosclerosis. Reversible acute renal failure caused by renal vein thrombosis was reported by Pollak and associates.[890] Their patient was a middle-aged woman who was treated with heparin and oral anticoagulants. She made a complete clinical and morphologic recovery.

On physical examination of the abdomen palpable masses in the kidney area are associated with gross or microscopic hematuria and increasing azotemia. Because of the renal masses the most frequently made diagnoses include hydronephrosis, renal tumor, and multicystic kidneys. A retrograde pyelogram will aid in establishing the correct diagnosis. In renal vein thrombosis there may be a cystic indentation of the renal pelvic veins resulting from a collateral circulation. Treatment should be directed toward improvement of the patient's general condition, correction of shock and dehydration, management of acute oliguric renal failure, and use of anticoagulants. Renal vein thrombosis in only one kidney can be successfully treated by nephrectomy and by removal of the propagated thrombosis from the inferior vena cava and the opposite renal vein.

The kidneys are large and appear to be congested with blood. Microscopic examination reveals prominent interstitial edema disproportionate to that seen in the kidneys of acute tubular necrosis. The tubules appear normal. The glomeruli are large and contain many erythrocytes. A prominent feature is margination of leukocytes in the glomerular capillaries (Fig. 2-39, *B*). If the process is prolonged, a membranous thickening of the glomerular capillary membrane occurs.

GLOMERULAR DISEASE

In the past, acute oliguric renal failure as a result of glomerular abnormalities was considered rare. More recently, acute oliguric renal failure has resulted from a number of diseases involving the glomeruli. These include acute poststreptococcal glomerulonephritis, lupus glomerulonephritis, glomerulonephritis caused by polyarteritis nodosa, drug-induced hypersensitivity glomerulonephritis, and necrotizing glomerulonephritis caused by Wegener's granulomatosis. In addition, thrombotic thrombocytopenic purpura (TTP) has produced acute renal failure caused by glomerular lesions.

The prominent clinical features of glomerular disease are hematuria and a rapidly decreasing urinary output ending in absolute anuria. There may be some degree of periorbital edema and hypertension. The urine is grossly bloody and contains erythrocyte casts and large quantities of heavy proteinuria. Unlike the fixed urinary specific gravity of acute tubular necrosis, the urinary specific gravity is usually high—for example, 1.025. In acute tubular necrosis the urinary sodium is above 30 mEq/L, while in acute glomerulonephritis the urinary sodium concentration during oliguria is usually below 30 mEq/L. Life should be sustained by repeated dialysis until a morphologic evaluation of the kidney is made. This provides an exact histologic diagnosis on which the physician can base his treatment and prognosis. In patients with acute oliguric renal failure caused by glomerular disease the use of adrenocortical steroids may be beneficial in resolving the glomerular abnormalities; otherwise, the prognosis is usually very poor and the patient does not recover.

Acute glomerulonephritis

In 1958, Brun and associates reported a clinicopathologic renal biopsy study of thirteen patients with acute glomerulonephritis.[163] Six of their patients died in uremia caused by acute oliguric renal failure. Death occurred within 22 to 24 days after onset. Diffuse glomerular changes were found; these included fibrinoid necrosis, cellular proliferation, and epithelial crescent formation. One patient died 10 months after onset of oliguria. A renal biopsy study earlier in the disease revealed a few intact capillary loops. Six patients recovered from acute oliguria. They had slight glomerular abnormalities but no fibrinoid necrosis or epithelial crescents. Persistent proteinuria was present for 1 to 2 years.

Alwall and his colleagues reported a clinicopathologic study of two adults with fatal glomerulonephritis and acute oliguric renal failure.[21] One patient remained uremic and had oliguria for 75 days. At autopsy diffuse glomerular abnormalities were found; these included thickening of the glomerular capillary basement membrane, hyalinization, crescent formation, and areas of fibrinoid necrosis.

In 1959, Bialestock and Tange described nine patients with fatal acute oliguria caused by acute glomerulonephritis.[105] They found a necrotizing glomerulonephritis characterized by amorphous eosinophilic material adherent to the capsule; a necrotic process appeared to have involved the afferent arteriole.

Harrison, Longhridge, and Milne reported twenty-one patients with acute oliguric renal failure caused by acute glomerulonephritis.[519] Eleven patients had a history of focal sepsis, such as a sore throat or otitis media, preceding the renal disease by a period of from 2 days to 5 weeks. Cultures from the throats of four of the eleven patients grew a hemolytic streptococcus. Two had elevated antistreptolysin O (ASO) titres.

The clinical findings in the remaining two patients were edema, hypertension, and cardiac failure. The urine was scanty and contained varying numbers of casts and erythrocytes. The diagnosis of acute glomerulonephritis was made by renal biopsy in seven patients and at autopsy in ten. On the bases of the clinical courses Harrison and associates divided their patients into three groups. Group I contained eight patients who had a diuresis with temporary or permanent recovery, Group II contained four patients who died following a partial diuresis, and Group III contained nine patients who died without diuresis from 14 to 91 days after onset.

The morphologic lesions were studied by renal biopsy from the fourteenth to the ninetieth day. Patients who recovered in Group I had mild renal lesions. In general, those with more advanced disease had epithelial crescents. They appeared as early as 14 days after onset. In some patients the glomerular lesion was fulminating and fibrinoid necrosis was seen.

Acute poststreptococcal glomerulonephritis

Acute poststreptococcal glomerulonephritis must be suspected when a previously healthy individual with a history of infection followed by a latent period subsequently develops hematuria, edema, and oliguria. One to two weeks following acute and severe inflammation of the upper respiratory system by a nephrogenic streptococcus, clinical features of acute glomerulonephritis become evident.[586] In particular, the patient experiences fatigue, anorexia, and generalized malaise, and he develops periorbital edema, gross hematuria, back pain, and

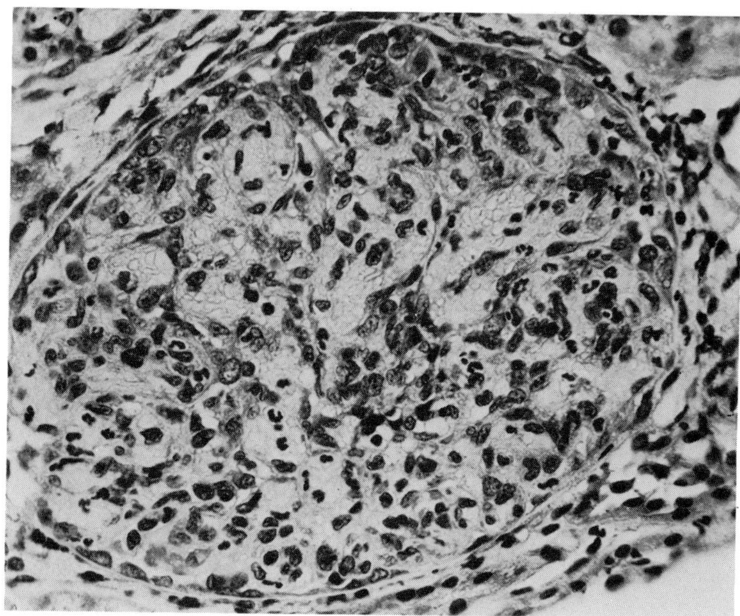

Fig. 2-40. Fatal acute renal failure caused by poststreptococcal glomerulonephritis. A 13-year-old high school student developed a streptococcal pharyngitis followed by gross hematuria and acute oliguric renal failure. This microphotograph illustrates a severe and fulminating poststreptococcal glomerulonephritis. The glomerulus was hypercellular and was ischemic in appearance. Numerous polymorphonucleocytes were noted. (H&E ×470.)

oliguria. Hypertension is prominent at the onset of oliguria. Retinopathy may or may not be present. Beta hemolytic streptococci are cultured from the nose or pharynx. The urinary specific gravity tends to be about 1.020, and the urine is strongly acid. The ASO titre is elevated. Diagnosis is uncertain if the illness is not carefully documented by bacteriologic studies or by immunologic proof such as the finding of streptococcal antibodies or reduced $beta_{1c}$ globulins. If attempts fail to identify a beta hemolytic streptococcal infection and if a streptococcal etiology is not documented, a percutaneous renal biopsy is helpful in establishing the diagnosis. Immunopathologic studies are most helpful (Fig. 2-40).

Extracorporeal hemodialysis is recommended to maintain the life of the severely uremic patient. By its use the clinical state of the patient improves and permits more definitive diagnostic studies such as renal biopsy or retrograde pyelography. Many patients may be brought through the critical period of acute oliguric renal failure by use of peritoneal or extracorporeal dialysis—the latter is preferred because a high incidence of peritonitis and other infections usually occurs with prolonged use of peritoneal dialysis. This is especially evident if the patient is receiving adrenocortical steroids and/or so-called immunosuppressive agents.[1057a]

Adrenocortical steroids have not been proved effective in arresting the progress of acute poststreptococcal glomerulonephritis. Recently, however, Kolff and associates found treatment with large doses of adrenocortical steroids (prednisone, 100 to 200 mg) over 6 weeks to be beneficial in promoting a diuresis.[826] Improvement occurred in approximately two-thirds of their patients. In addition, they found recovery more likely to occur when the brunt of the abnormalities was limited to the glomerular tufts rather than to Bowman's capsule. Diuresis occurred in approximately 25% of patients, and only 10% recovered.

Recovery was reported as being very uncommon in patients over 40 years old with acute oliguric renal failure caused by acute poststreptococcal glomerulonephritis. Severe or prolonged oliguria had a very dire prognosis. The most common cause of death in acute oliguric poststreptococcal glomerulonephritis was pulmonary edema and uremia. When peritoneal dialysis was used the common cause of death was infection such as pneumonia, septicemia, peritonitis, or pyelonephritis.

Grossly the kidneys are enlarged with thickened cortical area. The glomeruli may be hyalinized or completely necrosed. There is cellular proliferation along the mesangial area. Numerous leukocytes are seen in the capillary lumen. Epithelial crescents are noted (Fig. 2-41). The tubules appear relatively normal,

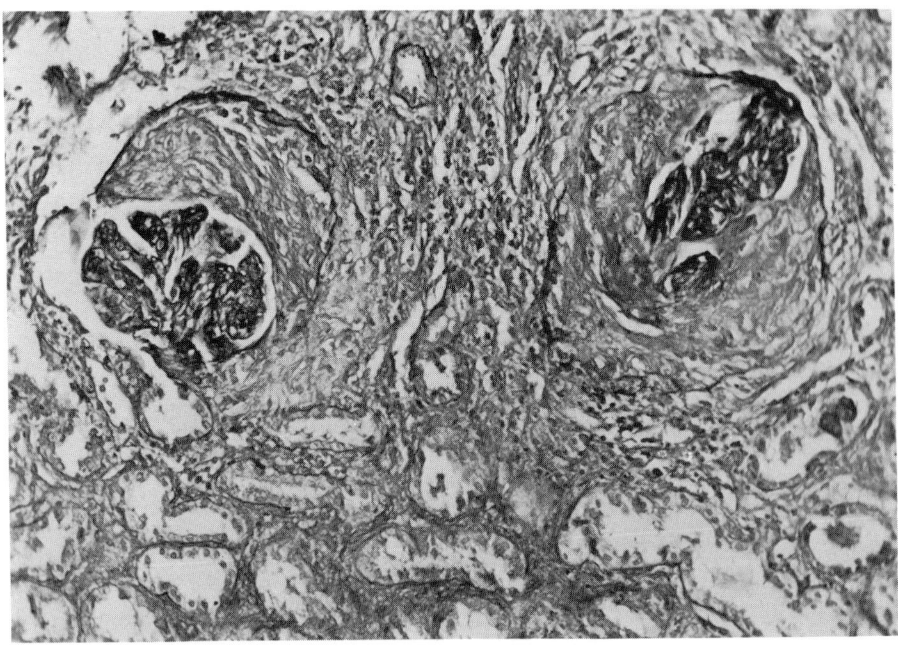

Fig. 2-41. Epithelial crescents. Renal biopsy study of a 24-year-old short-order cook with acute oliguric renal failure revealed poststreptococcal glomerulonephritis. Two glomeruli with prominent epithelial crescents are noted. There are diffuse interstitial edema and fibrosis. Eventually the patient made a gradual and complete recovery. (H&E ×350.)

and interstitial cellular infiltrates of lymphocytes and plasma cells are associated with interstitial edema. By means of electron microscopy numerous epithelial "humps" are seen in the capillary basement membrane. These humps were found by Jennings and Earle in patients with poststreptococcal glomerulonephritis,[586] and the humps have been found in luetic nephritis. Moreover, I have found such epithelial humps in an acute proliferative glomerulonephritis induced by high molecular weight dextran.

The clinicopathologic features of acute poststreptococcal glomerulonephritis described are discussed in the following case presentation.

CASE PRESENTATION

On October 3, 1966, M. S., a 13-year-old schoolgirl, was admitted to the pediatric wards of the University of Illinois College of Medicine Research and Educational Hospital. She had sickle cell anemia and had developed a severe pharyngitis in late September, 1966. Seven days later, on October 1, hematuria and periorbital edema occurred. Beta hemolytic

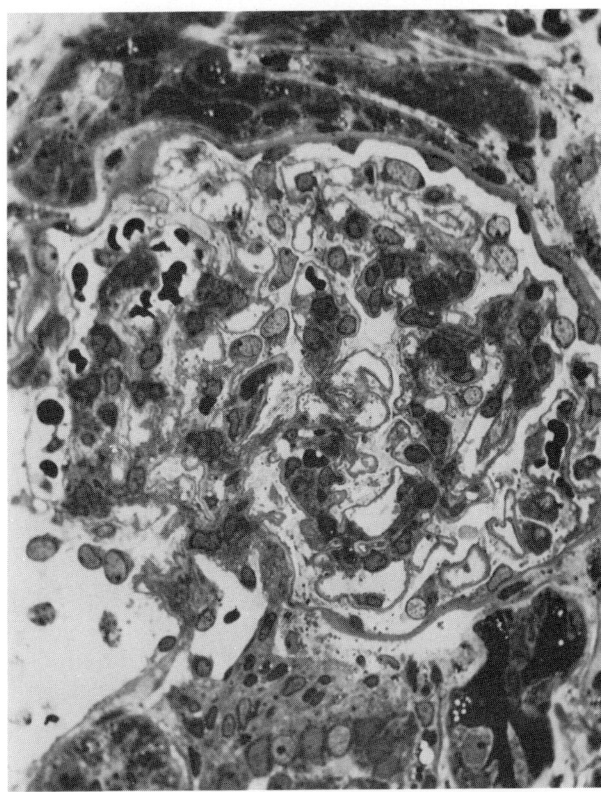

Fig. 2-42. Mesangial hypercellularity caused by poststreptococcal glomerulonephritis. This microphotograph illustrates the mesangial hypercellularity of acute poststreptococcal glomerulonephritis. A 10-year-old schoolgirl developed a beta-hemolytic streptococcal throat (infection followed by acute renal failure). Tissue was fixed in osmium and embedded in epoxy. The tissue was cut at 0.5μ and stained with methylene blue-Azure II. ($\times 670$.)

streptococci, group A, were cultured from the pharynx, and the ASO titre was 475 Todd units. Gross hematuria was present. The 24-hour proteinuria was 26 gm. The serum albumin was 1.4 gm per 100 ml. The serum cholesterol was 225 mg per 100 ml. Intramuscular injections of penicillin were started.

Oliguria occured on October 3. The next day a percutaneous renal biopsy was done. A severe acute poststreptococcal glomerulonephritis was found (Fig. 2-40). There was marked mesangial hypercellularity (Fig. 2-42) and marked polymorphonuclear cell infiltrates. Electron microscopic study revealed numerous epithelial osmiophilic humps and deposits on the glomerular basement membrane and extending into the urinary space (Fig. 2-43). The erythrocytes within the glomerular capillaries contained lysosomal bodies and vacuoles. They were identical to the erythrocyte vacuoles described by Kent and associates.[620] Although large doses of prednisone were started, the BUN continued to rise. Peritoneal dialysis was required twice. She developed a gram-negative septicemia and pneumonia. She died on November 10, 1966.

At autopsy the kidneys were found to be enlarged with a thickened and prominent cortex. The glomeruli were completely replaced by epithelial crescents and hypercellularity. The interstitial tissue had cellular infiltrates of plasma cells and polymorphonuclear leukocytes.

Comment. The morphologic lesions of a severe and active acute poststreptococcal glomerulonephritis followed a nephrogenic strectococcal pharyngeal infection. The electron microscopic findings of numerous epithelial osmophilic deposits were exceptional in number and degree. The characteristic clinical features were edema and oliguria. Initially the patient had all the laboratory findings of the nephrotic syndrome, except that her cholesterol was low. The

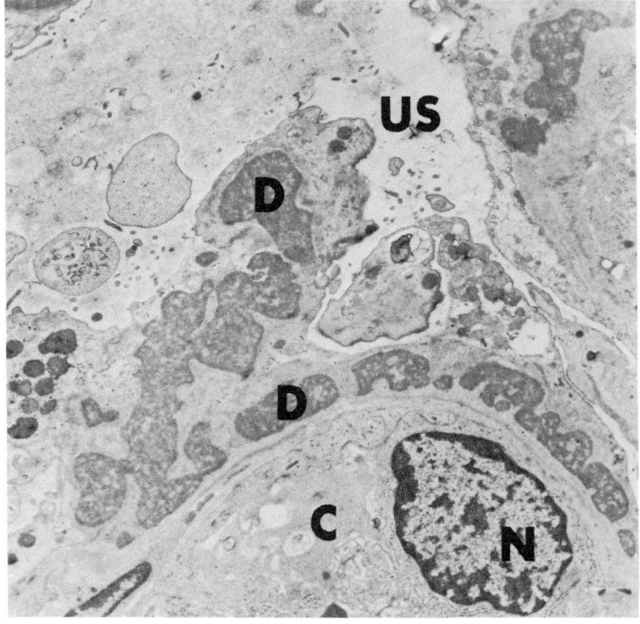

Fig. 2-43. Epithelial humps in poststreptococcal glomerulonephritis. This electron microphotograph illustrates the renal tissue described in Fig. 2-42. The biopsy was obtained during severe oliguria from a 13-year-old schoolgirl with fatal poststreptococcal glomerulonephritis. Dense epithelial humps or deposits (D) were seen on the epithelial side of the lamina densa and within the epithelial cells. The endothelial cells were swollen and contained large nuclei (N). The glomerular capillary lumen (C) was narrowed. The urinary space (US) contained proteinic material. (×7,000.)

clinical diagnosis of poststreptococcal glomerulonephritis was made when a beta hemolytic streptococcus grew from the throat culture and when a rising ASO titre was found.

Renal involvement with gross hematuria and the development of anuria is an unusual complication of a streptococcal infection. The fulminating acute and active nature of the glomerular disease was confirmed by renal biopsy study. The increase in daily urinary output occurred either spontaneously or in response to adrenocortical steroids. Peritonitis developed following use of 7.5% glucose dialysate fluid, and it progressed to a gram-negative septicemia and pneumonia. In spite of massive antibiotic treatment, she died. Study of the renal morphology at death indicated the severity and progressive features of the glomerular processes.

Lupus glomerulonephritis

Over half the patients with systemic lupus erythematosus develop renal disease. In approximately half of those, the renal disease is severe and progresses to chronic renal failure. In my experience acute oliguric renal failure caused by lupus glomerulonephritis has occurred in less than 4% of patients with systemic lupus erythematosus.

Since 1954, five patients with acute oliguric renal failure had "lupus sino lupo" nephritis. In all patients the diagnosis of systemic lupus erythematosus was

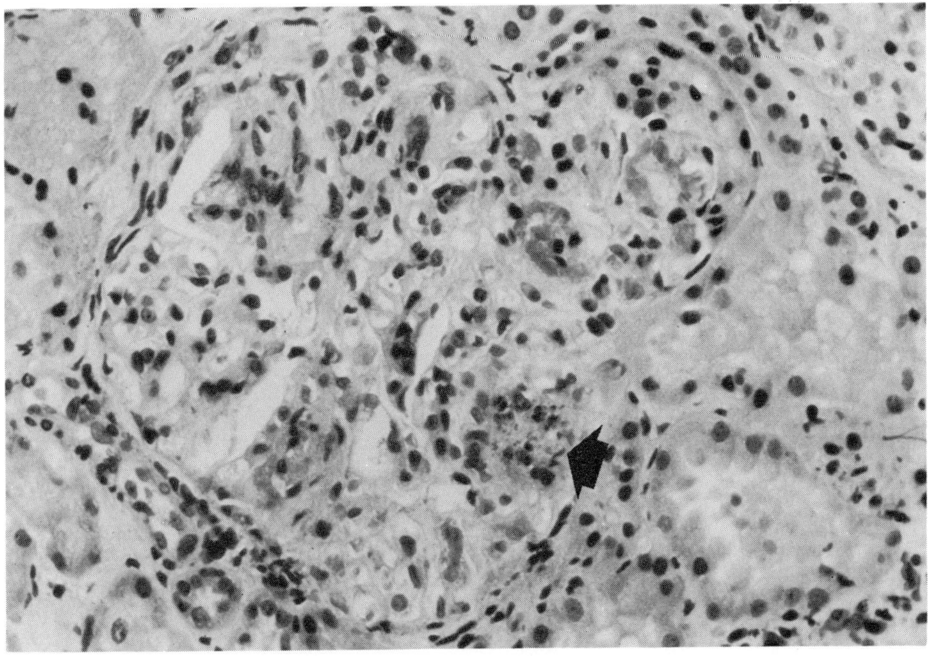

Fig. 2-44. Acute lupus glomerulonephritis. This microphotograph illustrates the renal biopsy findings in an 18-year-old schoolgirl with mixed proliferative and membranous glomerulonephritis. She had a positive LE cell test and a rapidly rising BUN with marked proteinuria. A marked glomerular hypercellularity was noted. Karyorrhexis (arrow) was noted. There was focal thickening of the glomerular capillary loop. The adjacent tubules appeared normal. (H&E ×525.)

made by finding LE cells. Lupus proliferative and membranous glomerulonephritis was found on renal biopsy study. In spite of intensive medical management and high doses of prednisone, all patients died. The clinical features were characterized by a sudden onset of hematuria, with decreasing urinary output to absolute anuria. On urinalysis all patients had a "telescoped" urinary sediment of erythrocytes, erythrocyte casts, leukocytes, hyaline and granular casts, fatty and waxy casts, and numerous renal broad casts.

Treatment consisted of high doses of prednisone, and in some patients repeated peritoneal dialysis was done. Immunosuppressive agents were used in one patient. A fulminating infection followed. In spite of massive antibiotic treatment, the patient died.

Grossly, the kidneys of patients with lupus glomerulonephritis are enlarged. On cut surface the kidneys are dark red with yellow swelling. They are not as pale or yellow as the kidneys seen in patients with acute poststreptococcal glomerulonephritis. The cortical thickness is usually increased. Histologically, an acute active mixed proliferative and membranous lupus glomerulonephritis is seen. There is a proliferation of endothelial and mesangial cells in the glomeruli (Fig. 2-44). The glomerular capillary wall is irregularly thickened. Acute lesions

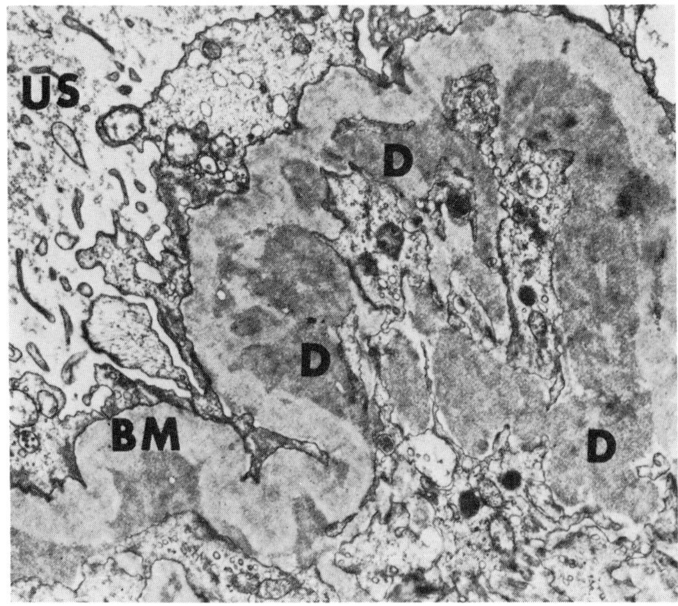

Fig. 2-45. Lupus glomerulonephritis. This electron microphotograph illustrates a small portion of a glomerular capillary loop from the patient with acute renal failure described in Fig. 2-46. The glomerular basement membrane (BM) appears collapsed. The capillary lumen is difficult to identify. Large amounts of electron dense material or deposits (D) are noted on the endothelial side of the basement membrane. Proteinic material fills the urinary space (US). (×11,000.)

consist of fibrinoid changes, hyaline thrombi, hematoxylin bodies, karyorrhexis, and wire loop formations. Hyaline thrombi may be obliterating the glomerular capillary loops. These lesions involve all glomeruli in a diffuse manner. The tubules usually reflect few if any abnormalities By means of electron microscopic study, osmiophilic deposits are usually seen on the endothelial side of the basement membrane (Fig. 2-45). The endothelial cells are swollen and almost occlude the capillary lumen. Necrotizing glomerular capillary changes have not been seen by electron microscopy.

The clinical and pathologic features of acute oliguric renal failure caused by lupus glomerulonephritis are discussed in the following case presentation.

CASE PRESENTATION

On September 2, 1964, K. R., an 18-year-old college student, was transferred to Presbyterian–St. Luke's Hospital for evaluation of proteinuria, hematuria, and progressive azotemia. Four weeks prior to admission proteinuria was found during a routine college entrance physical

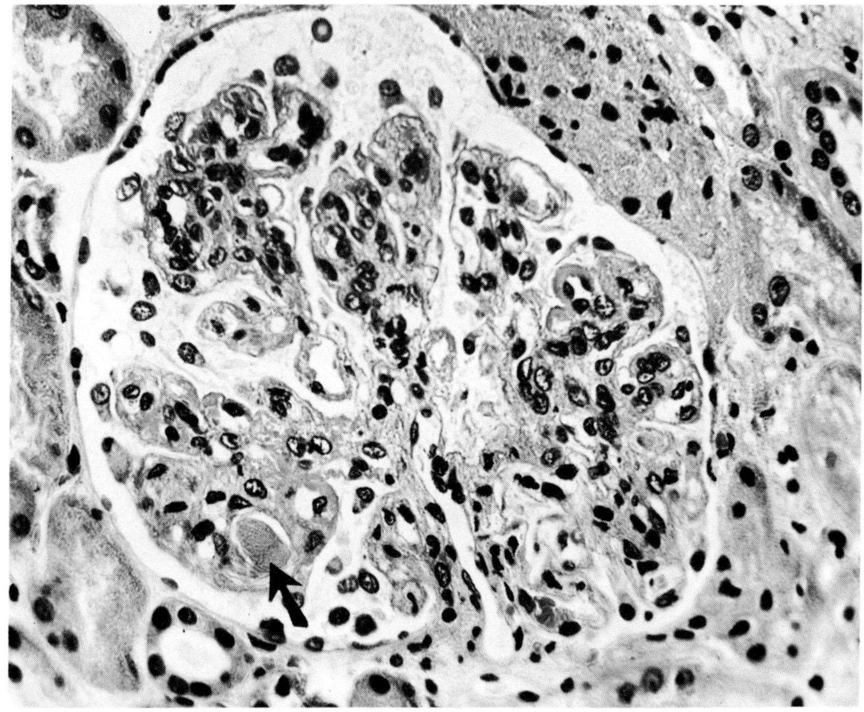

Fig. 2-46. Fatal acute renal failure caused by lupus nephritis. An 18-year-old college student developed rapidly progressing oliguria associated with azotemia and hematuria. The LE cell preparation was positive. Peritoneal dialysis was done. A renal biopsy was obtained on the twelfth day of oliguria. Adrenal corticosteroids in large doses were given with immunosuppressive agents. The patient died on the nineteenth day of his illness. An active proliferative and membranous lupus glomerulonephritis was diagnosed. Numerous wire loop lesions were noted. A large hyaline thrombus was seen (arrow). (H&E ×470.)

examination. In early August, 1964, he developed eyelid edema, later ankle swelling, and a weight gain of 10 to 12 pounds. There was no history of sore throats, joint pains, or face rash.

On August 26, 1964, he entered Highland Park Hospital. His blood pressure was 140/86 mm Hg, and his BUN rose from 108 to 125 mg per 100 ml. His total serum protein was 3.65 gm per 100 ml. The serum albumin was 2.6 gm per 100 ml, and the serum cholesterol was 272 mg per 100 ml.

Physical examination revealed an alert, husky male in no acute distress. There was moderate periorbital edema and pitting edema (2+). There was no lymphadenopathy. Findings from funduscopic examination were normal. There was no hepatosplenomegaly.

Admission urinalysis revealed a specific gravity of 1.011. There was proteinuria (2+), 20 to 30 leukocytes, and 150 to 200 erythrocytes per hpf. The hematocrit was 30%. The leukocyte count was 2,800/cu mm, the platelet count was 75,000/cu mm, and the serum potassium was 6 mEq/L. The CO_2 combining power was 20.9 mM/L. The BUN was 138 mg per 100 ml, and the LE cell test was positive. The ASO titre was 12 Todd units. The total serum proteins were 3.3 gm per 100 ml, and the serum albumin was 1.2 gm per 100 ml. The 24-hour proteinuria was 2.7 gm, and the 24-hour creatinine clearance was 5 ml per minute. Oliguria persisted from the time of admission.

On September 4, 1964, a daily intravenous dose of 3 gm Solu-cortef was begun. Ten days later peritoneal dialysis was started. The platelet count rose to 220,000/cu mm. On September 13, 1964, peritoneal dialysis was stopped. The next day a percutaneous right renal biopsy was done with the patient sitting upright. Severe active lupus glomerulonephritis was found. The tubules, vessels, and interstitium appeared normal. There was a marked proliferation of cells throughout the glomerular tuft. Marked focal thickening of the glomerular capillary membranes was noted (Fig. 2-46).

Electron microscopic study of renal tissue revealed marked mesangial cell proliferation,

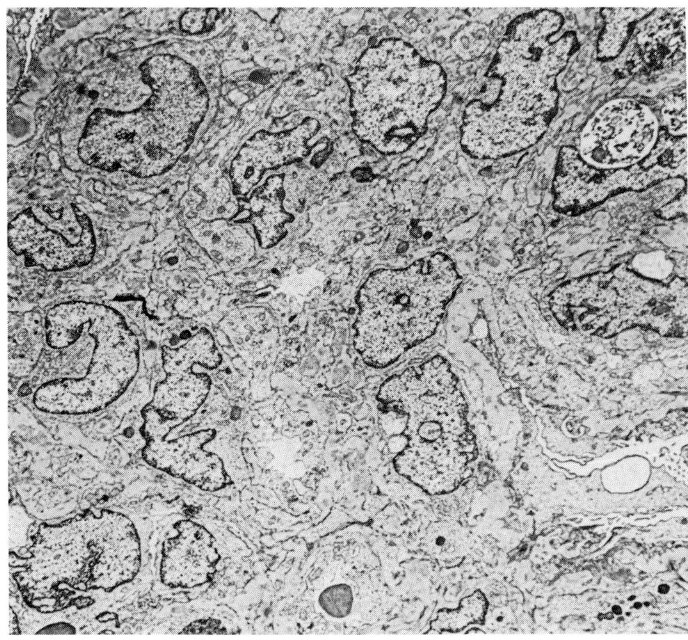

Fig. 2-47. Lupus glomerulonephritis. This electron microphotograph illustrates an active proliferative and membranous lupus nephritis. There is great difficulty in detecting either the urinary space or the glomerular capillary lumen. (×3,100.)

epithelial cell proliferation, and prominent osmiophilic deposits on the endothelial cell side of the glomerular basement membrane (Fig. 2-47). The glomerular capillary loops appeared to be occluded by endothelial cell proliferation and were relatively free of erythrocytes. The cortical tubules appeared normal, but there was a small amount of interstitial edema separating the tubules.

The patient continued to have gross hematuria and progressed to complete anuria. Peritoneal dialysis was restarted on September 19, 1964. A pseudonomas peritonitis developed. A dose of 500 mg of ampicillin was given four times daily, and 5 mg of Coly-mycin was added to each of the peritoneal dialysis exchanges. A total dose of 4 mg/kg of nitrogen mustard was given intravenously, and azathioprine (Imuran) was started. There was no clinical response to the therapy, and the patient developed a severe peritonitis. He died on September 21, 1964.

Comment. This young man developed a sudden, severe, active, and rapidly progressive lupus glomerulonephritis. Initially there was no clinical finding to suggest lupus erythematosus such as face rash, joint pains, fever, splenomegaly, or lymphadenopathy. On a clinical basis lupus erythematosus without these physical findings has been referred to as "lupus sino lupo." Initially the patient appeared to have the nephrotic syndrome, except that the serum cholesterol was normal. Gross hematuria and progressive decrease of urinary output to anuria was suggestive of a glomerular lesion.

The diagnosis of systemic lupus erythematosus was confirmed by the positive LE cell test. The renal basis of lupus glomerulonephritis was established by biopsy study. This morphologic study, by means of light and electron microscopy, revealed the diagnosis of lupus proliferative and membranous glomerulonephritis. Moreover, it revealed an active, acute, and progressive lesion, one that was possibly irreversible.

Intensive treatment was given in very high doses of adrenocortical steroids and immunosuppressive agents. Unfortunately, an incurable pseudomonas infection developed; in the presence of a leukopenia, this infection resulted in the death of the patient.

Hypersensitivity glomerulonephritis

Drug-induced hypersensitivity glomerulonephritis has resulted in acute oliguric renal failure following treatment with dextran, sulfonamides, trichloroethylene, and bunamiodyl. The clinical features are similar to those of acute poststreptococcal glomerulonephritis. The patient develops fatigue, low back pain, periorbital edema, and hematuria. Later there is hypertension associated with absolute anuria. When the urine is examined, erythrocytes and erythrocyte casts are found in association with a relatively high specific gravity—for example, 1.020— and an acid urine. It is most important to establish the diagnosis of glomerular involvement that is caused by drug sensitivity. Effective treatment with high doses of adrenocortical steroids may reverse the glomerular abnormalities. Hypersensitivity glomerulonephritis caused by bunamiodyl is discussed in the following case presentation.

CASE PRESENTATION

M. B., a 36-year-old mother of five children, developed nausea and pain in the right upper quadrant. A cholecystogram was ordered by her physician. On May 8, 1961, bunamiodyl (Orabilex) was given. Because there was no gallbladder filling, the next day a double dose of bunamiodyl was given. She developed loin pain, absolute anuria, fever, and a leukocytosis. Hemodialysis was done on the eleventh day of anuria when the BUN was 202 mg per 100 ml. (Her clinical course is plotted in Fig. 2-48.) Intravenous Solu-cortef, 2 gm daily, was given for 5 days. Later, prednisone, 200 mg daily, was given. She entered the diuretic stage on the seventeenth day, and the BUN began to fall.

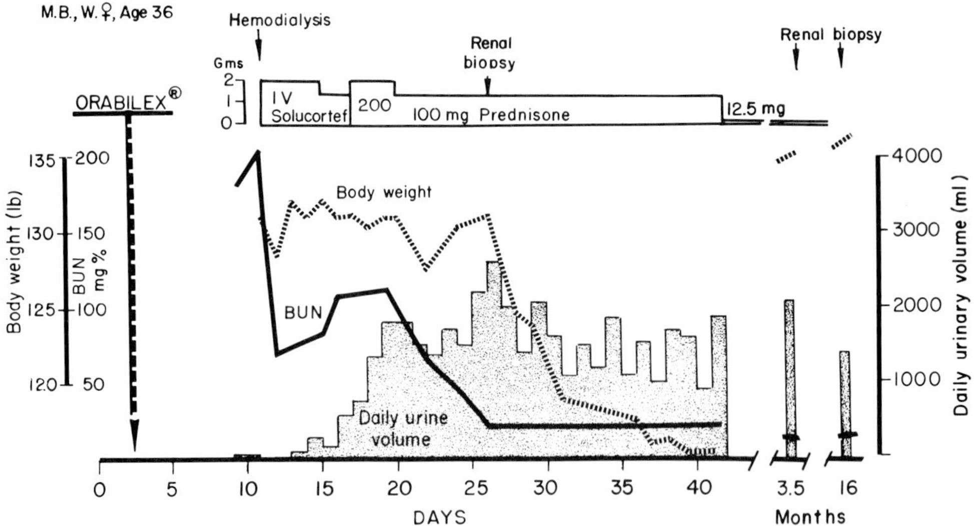

Fig. 2-48. Clinical course of patient with acute renal failure from bunamiodyl. A 36-year-old mother of five children developed acute oliguric renal failure following a double oral dose of bunamiodyl. Oliguria lasted for 17 days. Hemodialysis was done on the eleventh day. Intravenous Solu-Cortef and later prednisone were given. A percutaneous renal biopsy was done on the twenty-fifth day when diuresis was greatest and the BUN was near normal. Serial renal biopsies were done at 3½ and 16 months.

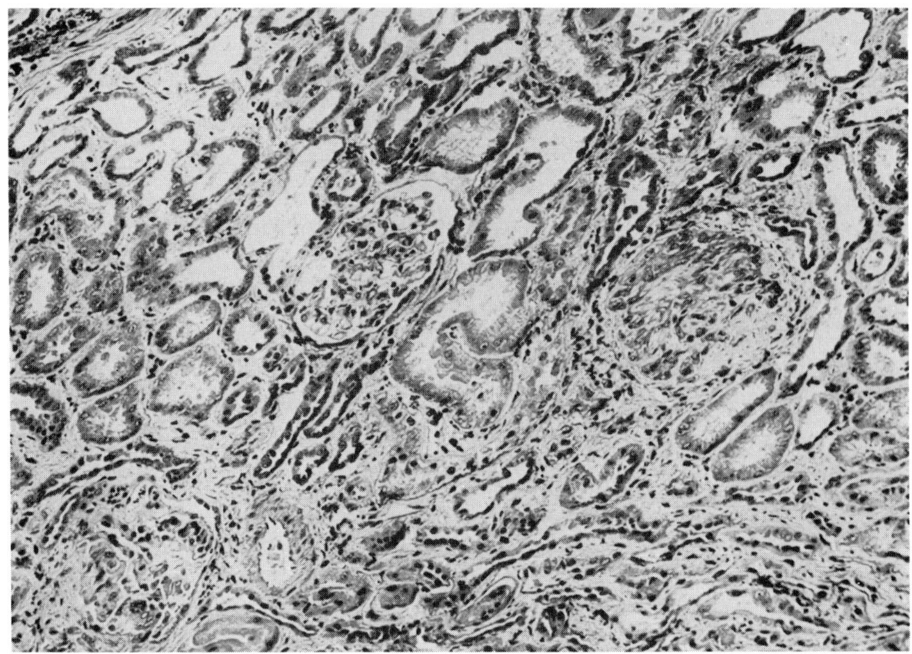

Fig. 2-49. Hypersensitivity glomerulonephritis from bunamiodyl. This microphotograph illustrates the first renal biopsy taken from the patient described in Fig. 2-48. A proliferative glomerulonephritis was found. The tubular regeneration was noted. There were interstitial edema and fibrosis. (H&E ×300.)

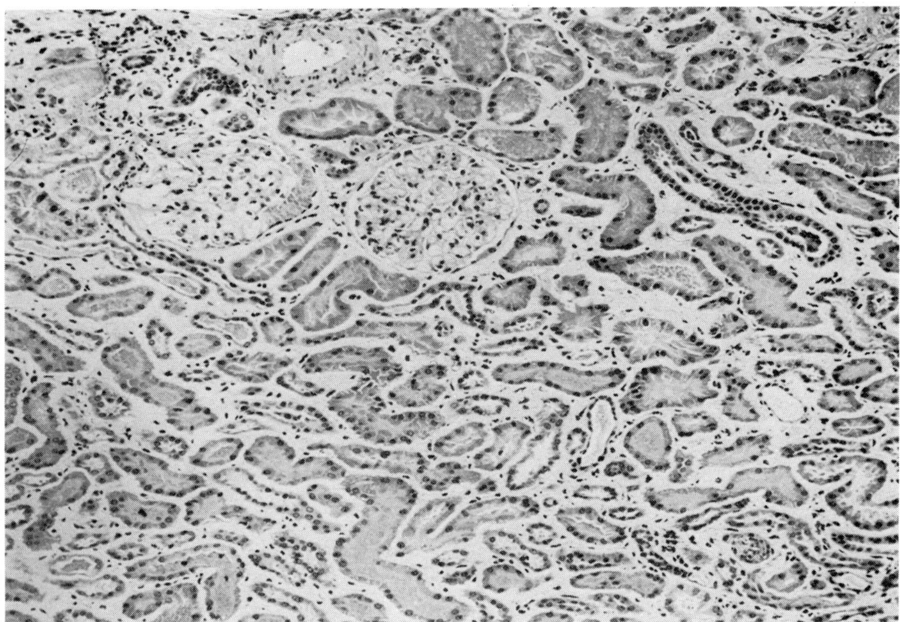

Fig. 2-50. Resolving hypersensitivity glomerulonephritis. This microphotograph illustrates the second renal biopsy of the patient described in Figs. 2-48 and 2-49. It was taken 3½ months after bunamiodyl ingestion. The glomeruli appeared normal. Tubular cell repair was still active. There was a striking diffuse interstitial fibrosis. (H&E ×300.)

A percutaneous renal biopsy was done on the twenty-fifth day (Fig. 2-49). The renal biopsy study revealed a severe proliferative hypersensitivity glomerulonephritis with associated tubular necrosis, tubular regeneration, and interstitial edema. Serial renal biopsies were performed following recovery of acute renal failure at 3½ months (Fig. 2-50) and at 16 months (Fig. 2-51). These serial biopsy studies indicate the complete healing of the glomeruli and tubules. The only abnormality at 16 months was a diffuse interstitial fibrosis.

Comment. The morphologic lesions of hypersensitivity glomerulonephritis justify the use of high doses of adrenocortical steroids. Without steroid treatment it was believed that recovery may not have occurred. The exact immunologic reaction is not known, but it may well be a cytotoxic mechanism. This can be explained as follows: iodine within the bunamiodyl molecule drew the molecules to protein of the glomerular basement membrane and produced a hypersensitivity glomerular reaction. Although the patient recovered from acute oliguric renal failure and the glomeruli returned to normal, she developed mild interstitial fibrosis.

During the past 5 years twenty-six patients were reported to have developed acute oliguric renal failure following administration of bunamiodyl.[734] Most of these patients received a double dose; in some it was fatal. On morphologic study the common lesion was acute tubular necrosis. Bunamiodyl has since been removed from the market by the manufacturer.

Thrombotic thrombocytopenic purpura

Renal involvement in thrombotic thrombocytopenic purpura (TTP) is common but is usually not severe. Moderate azotemia may occur in the terminal stages, but death from uremia is rare. The clinical picture is usually dominated by fever, purpura, hemolysis, and various neurologic manifestations.

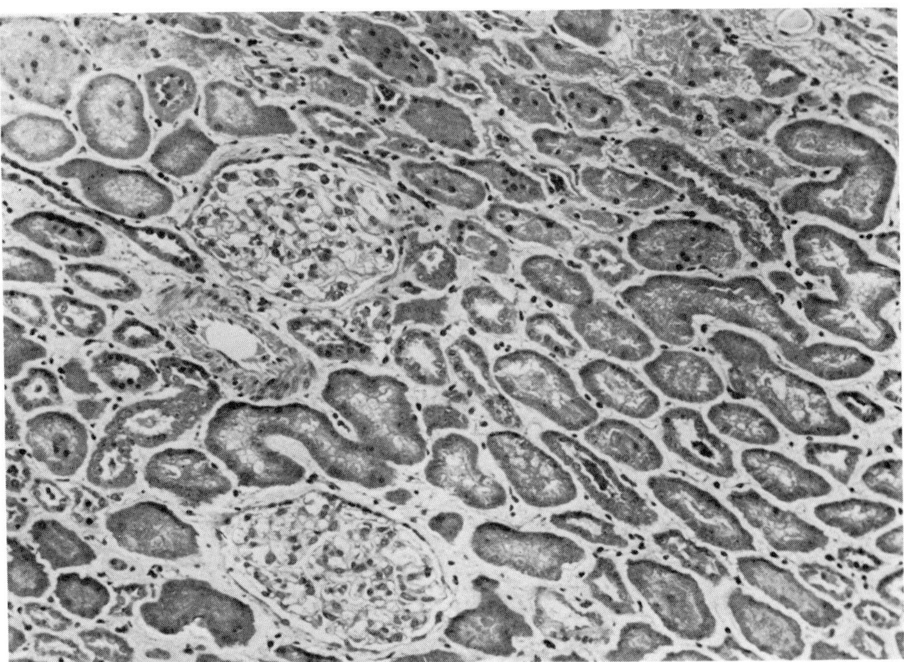

Fig. 2-51. Complete healing of hypersensitivity glomerulonephritis. This microphotograph illustrates the third renal biopsy from the patient described in Figs. 2-48, 2-49, and 2-50. Urinalysis revealed a trace of protein. The 24-hour creatinine clearance was reduced. The glomeruli were normal. Although the tubules appeared normal, a diffuse interstitial fibrosis was present. (H&E ×300.)

The renal lesion of TTP was first described by Moschcowitz in 1925.[798] It was characterized by the incorporation of erythrocytes into an eosinophilic amorphous material to form a hyaline thrombotic occlusion. In 1952, Orbison demonstrated a significant vascular dilatation into an aneurysm of capillary and arterioles.[851] The clinicopathologic features of acute oliguric renal failure in TTP are discussed in the following case presentation.

CASE PRESENTATION

E. B., a 44-year-old white female, was admitted to Presbyterian–St. Luke's Hospital in April, 1965, with acute oliguric renal failure and jaundice. Hypothyroidism had been diagnosed in 1959, and she had been maintained on thyroid extract. She had suffered from migratory and generalized joint pains associated with occasional joint swelling since 1961. Her shoulders, knees, wrists, fingers, and occasionally other joints were involved. There was morning stiffness but no deformity. No lupus erythematosus cells were found. Fixation tests were latex positive (1:5,120) and a diagnosis of rheumatoid arthritis had been made. She had received occasional courses of chloroquine, gold salts, and adrenocortical steroids. Some relief of her symptoms occurred.

Recently her joint pains had become progressively more severe; on April 22, 1965, phenylbutazone (600 mg daily) was prescribed. On April 24 she developed an acute illness with severe chills and fever, vomiting, diarrhea, and colicky abdominal pain. The following day

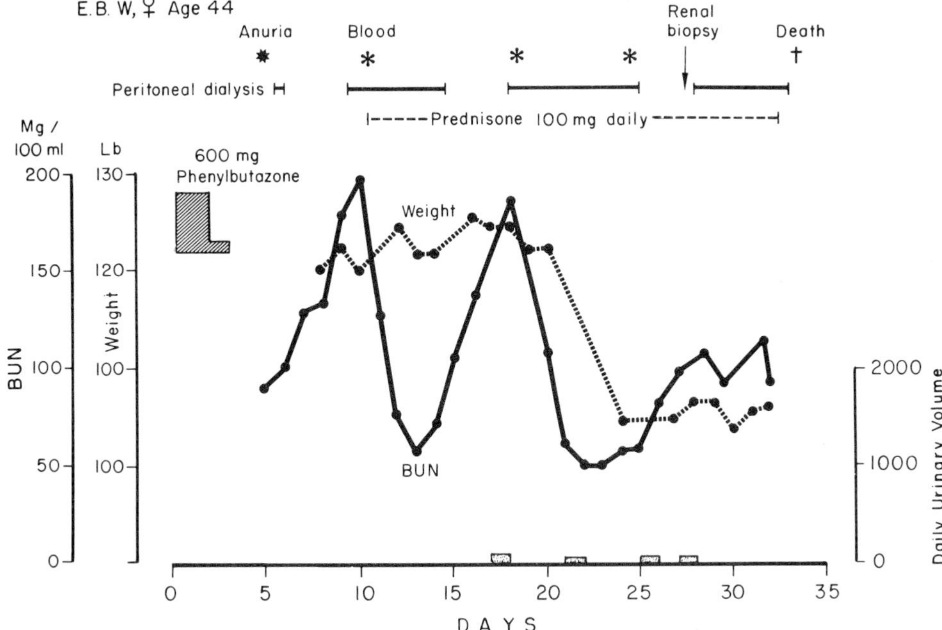

Fig. 2-52. Clinical features of patient with thrombotic thrombocytopenic purpura (TTP). Phenylbutazone was given for 3 days. Acute anuria developed. The patient had four peritoneal dialyses, and three whole blood transfusions were given. An open renal biopsy was done on the twenty-eighth day. Prednisone and heparine were given. The patient died on the thirty-third day.

she had anuria and was jaundiced. She was admitted to another hospital, where peritoneal dialysis was begun on April 27. Two days later she was transferred to Presbyterian–St. Luke's Hospital. Since January, 1964, a number of short episodes of fever and chills lasting for several days had occurred. No definite cause was ever found. (Her clinical course is plotted in Fig. 2-52.)

Physical examination on admission revealed an acutely ill, drowsy white female complaining of severe generalized abdominal pain. Marked jaundice was noted, but neither purpura nor petechia was seen. There was palmar erythema. Blood pressure was 110/88 mm Hg, and the optic fundi were normal. The thyroid gland was not palpable. Findings of examination of the heart and lungs were normal. The abdomen was moderately distended with fluid, and generalized tenderness with rebound was noted. The liver and spleen were not enlarged and no masses were palpable. There was marked tenderness over both kidneys. Neurologic examination revealed a course "flapping" tremor, frequent twitching, generalized hypertonia, and hyperreflexia. Plantar responses were extensor.

The peripheral blood smear revealed marked poikilocytosis and anisocytosis; numerous burr cells, helmet cells, schistocytes, and occasional spherocytes were seen. The findings were as follows: BUN–132 mg per 100 ml; serum creatinine–11 mg per 100 ml; total serum bilirubin–34 mg per 100 ml (direct–16 mg per 100 ml); alkaline phosphatase–11.4 units (Bessey-Lowry); serum glutamic oxalacetic transaminase (SGOT)–225 IU; serum glutamic pyruvic transaminase (SGPT–77 IU; LDH–2,250 IU; prothrombin time–20%; blood ammonia–66 μg/100 ml. Numerous lupus erythematosus preparations were negative. The Coombs tests (direct and indirect) initially were positive, later became negative, and were again positive after incubation of erythrocytes with phenylbutazone. The chrominum[51] red cell half-life was 2½ days. The bone marrow study revealed slight erythroid hyperplasia.

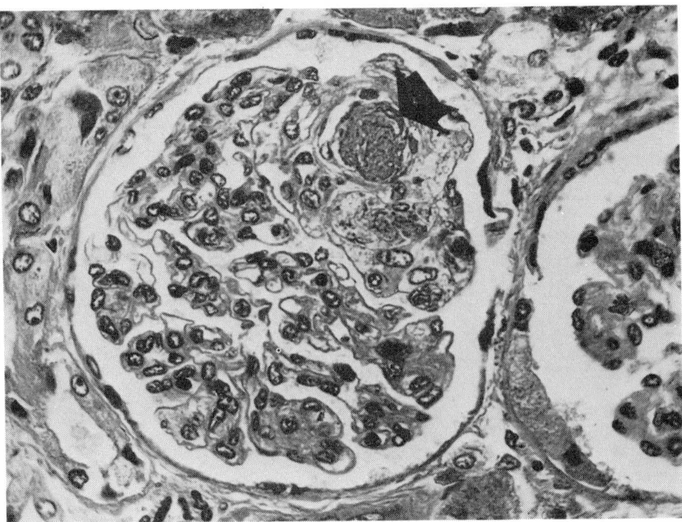

Fig. 2-53. Drug-induced TTP. Microphotograph of kidney from patient with phenylbutazone-induced TTP. Renal biopsy was taken on the twenty-eighth day of anuria. A large eosinophilic hyaline thrombus is seen at upper right (arrow). Adjacent renal tubules appear normal. (H&E ×630.)

Complete anuria persisted throughout her hospitalization. Peritoneal dialysis was reinstituted periodically. Fluctuating neurologic signs were observed for the first 2 weeks while she continued to show signs of liver disease and hemolysis. Prednisone, 120 mg per day, was started on May 1. After 14 days her general condition gradually improved. Neurologic signs subsided. She became more lucid and jaundice subsided. Because of her critical condition renal biopsy was delayed until an open biopsy was done on May 18. By the end of the fourth week her clinical condition had improved but renal function had not been restored. Heparin was administered in an attempt to alleviate intravascular thrombosis, but bleeding occurred within the first 16 hours of treatment with that drug. She died quietly on May 24, 1965.

The morphologic finding within the kidneys was characteristic of TTP. The lesions were usually located near the base of the glomeruli and extended to the peripheral glomerular capillary loops (Fig. 2-53). In addition to a conglomeration of platelets, fibrin, and erythrocytes within an amorphous matrix, the thrombi contained lipoid material. The separation of the capillary basement membrane and epithelial cells from the endothelial layer gave the appearance of aneurysmal dilatation of the capillary loop (Fig. 2-54). This electron microscopic finding could be similar to the aneurysmal dilatation reported by Orbison.[851] The amorphous material seen between the basement membrane and endothelial layer appeared to originate from the mesangial cells.

Comment. The phenylbutazone-induced hemolytic anemia, thrombocytopenia, and glomerular capillary changes can be best explained by a cytotoxic immunologic reaction. The proof of this reaction was that the initial negative Coombs test became positive when phenylbutazone was added to the test tube.

In spite of large doses of adrenocortical steroids and intravenous heparin, the lesions of thrombotic thrombocytopenia were progressive and ended in a fatal anuria.

The morphologic renal lesion bears no resemblance to the granular lesions induced in rabbits by the Shwartzman reaction.[1011] In an electron microscopic study by Pappan and associates, dense fibrinous material was seen to occlude most capillary loops.[859] In addition, balloon-like vesicles were originating from endothelial cells. The renal lesion in TTP can be differentiated

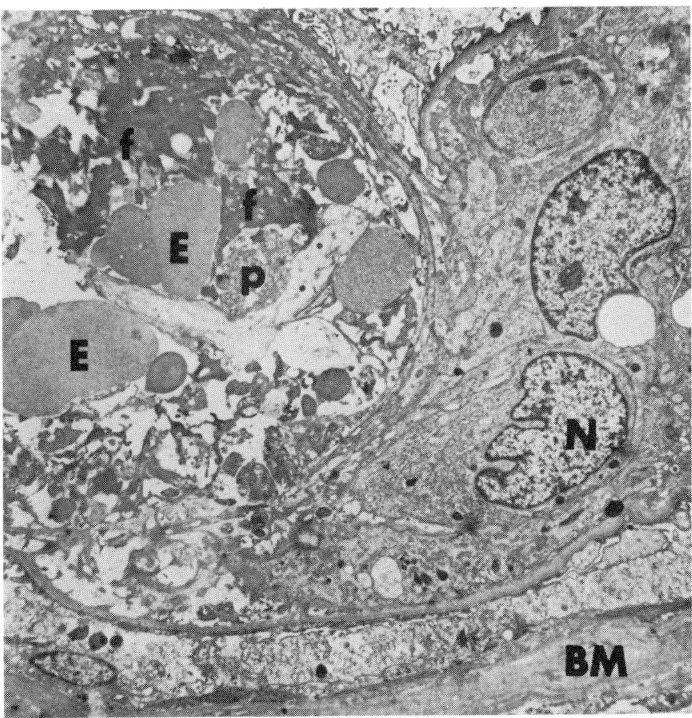

Fig. 2-54. Glomerular capillary thrombosis in TTP. This electron microphotograph illustrates a glomerular capillary thrombosis in the patient with TTP described in Fig. 2-52. The peripheral glomerular capillary was dilated and contained a hyaline thrombus. The thrombus contained erythrocytes (E), fragments of platelets (P), and fibrinoid material (f). Bowman's membrane (BM) was seen below. Three mesangial cell nuclei (N) were noted (×3,078.)

from that of other conditions that also contain fibrin within the glomeruli. These lesions include renal cortical necrosis, eclampsia, and lupus nephritis. In TTP the presence of platelets and fibrin within the tubular lumen is distinct from the presence of fibrinoid material seen incorporated into the glomerular capillary membrane in cortical necrosis or eclampsia of pregnancy. Moreover, acute tubular necrosis is usually present in cortical necrosis and may be present in toxemia of pregnancy or eclampsia. In TTP, as occurred in this patient, the renal tubules are quite normal.

Wegener's granulomatosis

Wegener's granulomatosis is a syndrome associated with angiitis and focal necrosis and with granulomatous lesions beginning in the respiratory tract. It spreads to other organs and terminates in a focal necrotizing glomerulonephritis.

In 1951, Goodman and Churg established the histologic criteria for the diagnosis of Wegener's granulomatosis.[438] Although Klinger described the granulomatosis process in 1931, it was Wegener who clearly characterized the disease that bears his name.[1117] Wegener's granulomatosis has an insidious onset and a fulminating febrile course. The disease starts with a necrotizing hemorrhagic upper

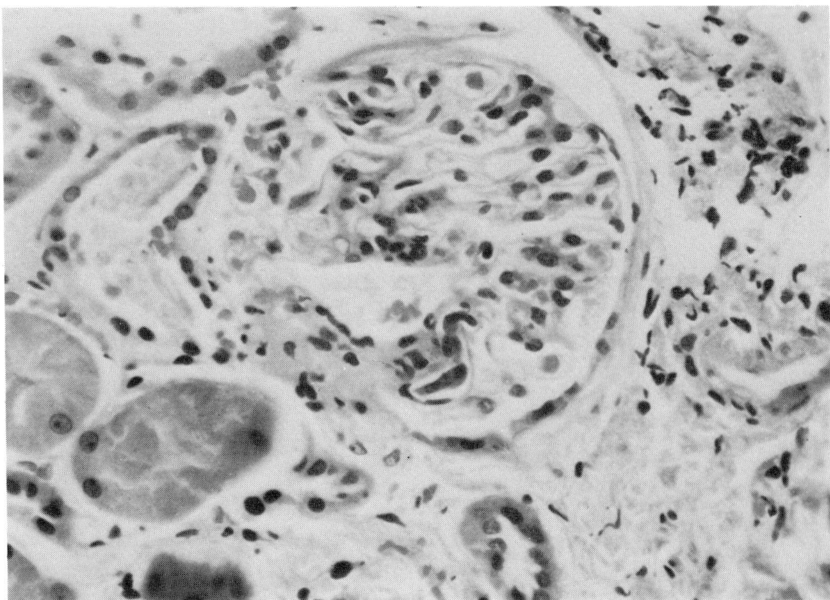

Fig. 2-55. Wegener's granulomatosis. A 54-year-old farmer developed a hemorrhagic sinusitis followed by acute oliguria. A renal biopsy study revealed Wegener's granulomatosis. A proliferative and necrotizing glomerulonephritis was found. Although large dosages of adrenal corticosteroids were given, the patient died in uremia. (H&E ×425.)

respiratory lesion and should be differentiated from Goodpasture's syndrome[815] and associated respiratory infections.[864] The lesion varies from a necrotizing sinusitis to a necrotizing bronchitis. Acute oliguric renal failure with progressive uremia and death within weeks is not unusual. Administration of adrenocortical steroids has produced remission in some patients, but only for a brief period. The effect of large doses of adrenocortical steroids on Wegener's granulomatosis has not been satisfactory. The early diagnosis of Wegener's granulomatosis can be established by renal biopsy. Such early diagnosis would permit the physician to commit his patient to high doses of adrenocortical steroids or so-called immunosuppressive agents.[564,1057a]

The striking characteristic lesion is a local necrotizing glomerulonephritis. This morphologic lesion may resemble a severe active and proliferative lupus glomerulonephritis. The necrotizing process may extend to and involve Bowman's membrane (Fig. 2-55). Initially fibrinoid material is found to be lining the capillary wall. Later there is an occlusion of the glomerular capillary wall, followed by necrosis. There is usually a proliferative and membranous glomerulonephritis with formation of epithelial crescents. In addition, granulomatous lesions are seen in the periglomerular areas.[630]

The cortical arteries, arterioles, veins, and, in some patients, capillaries become involved with necrotizing lesions with fibrinoid deposition within the subendothelial layers. A necrotizing arteriolitis occurred in approximately 77% of cases reported by Walton.[1112] This lesion must be differentiated from the allergic granulomatous angiitis and the hypersensitivity form of polyarteritis nodosa. The renal interstitium becomes involved with a granulomatous inflammatory reaction. The vascular lesions are usually prominent in and closely peripheral to the margins of the granulomas. They may be apart from the granuloma. Foci of necrosis are enveloped by a granulomatous lesion consisting of giant cells, polymorphonuclear cells, plasma cells, and lymphocytes.

Henoch-Schönlein purpura

Henoch-Schönlein purpura, a clinical syndrome, usually occurs in children or young adults.[969a] It is characterized by purpura, abdominal pain, and gastrointestinal tract symptoms of nausea, vomiting, and diarrhea. In addition, the joints may be tender and painful. Renal disease is always present. Hemorrhage can usually be found in the skin, mucosal areas, conjunctiva, joints, and viscera.

Hematuria is the outstanding feature of renal involvement. In addition, there is proteinuria and the presence of numerous casts including red blood cell casts. The microscopic findings may represent a telescoped urinary sediment. Acute oliguric renal failure is unusual and occurs in 5 to 8% of the patients with an active renal lesion. If acute oliguric renal failure develops, the disorder is fatal.

The striking morphologic renal abnormality was found in the glomeruli; in some patients with acute oliguric renal failure renal biopsy study revealed a severe acute proliferative to a necrotizing glomerulonephritis. Fibrin thrombi and fibrinoid material have been observed in the glomerular capillaries (Fig. 2-56, A). The necrotizing glomerulonephritis may be indistinguishable from a lupus necrotizing glomerulonephritis or that seen in Goodpasture's disease[721] and Wegener's granulomatosis. The arteriole lesions of Henoch-Schönlein purpura are similar to those classified as a hypersensitivity angiitis by Zeek.[1151] In addition, there is a focal interstitial nephritis with mild tubular degeneration.

INTRARENAL ARTERY AND ARTERIOLE DISEASE

Diseases of the renal arcuate and segmental arteries and arterioles can cause acute oliguric renal failure. These intrarenal artery and arteriole diseases include acute necrotizing arteriolitis, malignant nephrosclerosis, polyarteritis nodosa, and progressive systemic sclerosis. The clinical features are hypertension with papilledema, hematuria, erythrocyte casts, and proteinuria. Although at a great risk to the patient, the histologic diagnosis can be made by renal biopsy. The clinical course is a rapid deterioration that ends in death.

Acute necrotizing arteriolitis

Acute necrotizing arteriolitis can result from a variety of drugs, chemicals, and biologic products. These include sulfonamides,[1157] alpha naphthalene, chlorothiazide,[345] and pertussis vaccine.[110] Acute oliguric renal failure develops and,

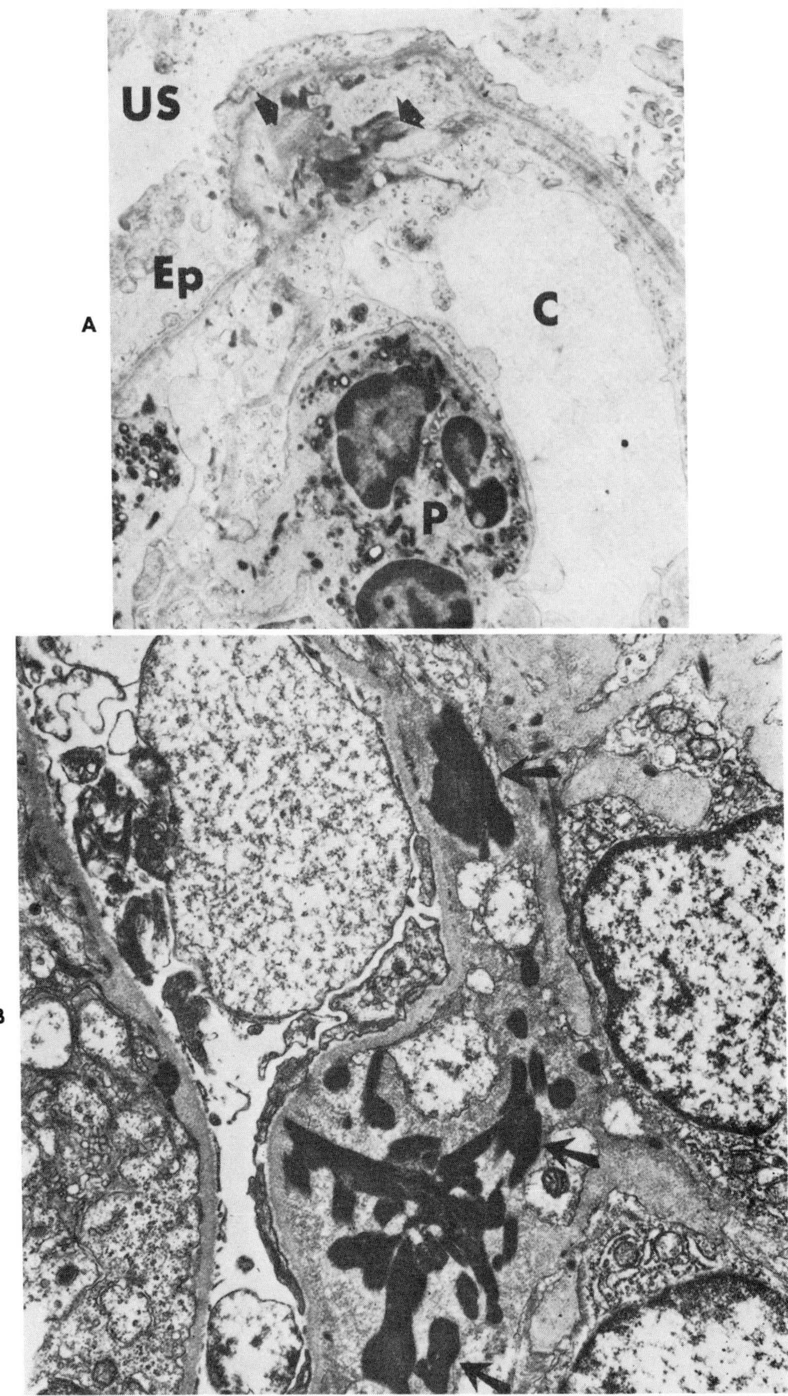

Fig. 2-56. For legend see opposite page.

in spite of adrenocortical steroids in high doses, the patient dies. In some patients the etiology of necrotizing arteriolitis is unknown. The prominent clinical features are gross hematuria, malignant hypertension, and rapidly progressing fatal renal disease.

Acute necrotizing arteriolitis with acute oliguric renal failure has developed in women immediately postpartum. The onset is delayed from 1 to 3 weeks postpartum and usually occurs in women with uncomplicated deliveries. Initially the blood pressure is normal. Later in the course of acute oliguric renal failure the blood pressure may become elevated. The retinal arterioles are narrowed and gross hematuria is common. Hemoglobin and erythrocyte casts are found in the urine. The daily proteinuria may reach 3 or more gm. Despite intensive management that includes high doses of adrenocortical steroids and hemodialysis, the lesion is fatal.

The most striking morphologic abnormalities are found in the intralobular arteries and afferent arterioles. These findings include marked intimal fibrosis and fibrinoid necrosis (Fig. 2-57, *B*). The interstitium is edematous and contains cellular infiltrates of polymorphonuclear cells and fibroblasts. Scattered glomeruli may be infarcted.

Fatal acute necrotizing arteriolitis has followed inoculations with pertussis vaccine.[110] Sulfonamides are drugs that can produce granulomatous and necrotizing arteriolitis.[1157] The larger vessels may be involved with an acute hypersensitivity arteriolitis that resembles polyarteritis nodosa. In addition, there may be granulomatous interstitial nephritis.

An acute granulomatous necrotizing arteriolitis was possibly induced by hydrochlorothiazide in a 62-year-old woman. She had fever, kidney pain, and gross hematuria. The renal biopsy changes were different from those of an allergic granulomatous vasculitis in that there was an absence of fibrinoid-type necrosis, giant cells, significant eosinophils, leukocytes, and glomerular abnormalities.

Acute necrotizing ateriolitis was observed in a middle-aged chemist with an exposure to para naphthalene. This is discussed in the following case presentation.

Fig. 2-56. **A,** Fibrinoid material within glomerulus of patient with acute oliguric renal failure. This electron microphotograph illustrates a renal biopsy from a 5-year-old girl with acute oliguric renal failure. Fibrinoid material (arrows) was seen on the endothelial side of the glomerular basement membrane. Polymorphonucleocytes (P) were noted within the capillary lumen (C). The urinary space (US) contained proteinic material. The epithelial cell (EP) foot processes were either fused or absent. (×7,000) **B,** Fibrin material in glomerulus. A 14-year-old schoolboy with Henoch-Schönlein purpura had rapidly progressing acute renal failure. A renal biopsy study revealed severe acute proliferative glomerulonephritis. On electron microscopy large quantities of fibrin material (arrows) were found in the glomerular capillary loop. (×13,233.)

CASE PRESENTATION

On August 27, 1963, R. R., a 46-year-old chemical engineer in acute oliguric renal failure, was transferred to Presbyterian–St. Luke's Hospital from Elkhart General Hospital. In 1962, the patient was known to have a normal blood pressure and normal renal function. During 1962 and 1963, he worked with para naphthalene. By August 14, 1963, he had developed generalized fatigue and breathlessness. The next day he had dark urine.

On August 16, 1963, he consulted his physician and 4 days later was admitted to Elkhart General Hospital. There he was found to have proteinuria, hematuria, a BUN of 140 mg per 100 ml, and a hemoglobin of 10.6 gm/100 cc. The serum potassium rose from 4.2 mEq/L on August 21 to 6.2 mEq/L on August 26, 1963. He was then transferred to Presbyterian–St. Luke's Hospital.

On August 27, 1963, physical examination revealed the patient to be alert; his blood pressure was 150/76 mm Hg. There was mild periorbital edema. Findings from funduscopic examination were normal. Urinalysis revealed a specific gravity of 1.012, proteinuria (3+), numerous erythrocytes, and hyaline, granular, and erythrocyte casts. The urine was examined for naphtols, and 243 mμ of absorbing substance (alpha naphtol) was found.

Throughout his hospital course his urinary output remained below 400 ml daily. The BUN rose to 184 mg per 100 ml. On August 31, 1963, peritoneal dialysis was started and continued intermittently. On September 5 the blood pressure was 190/98 mm Hg. The pulse was 112 per minute. Retinal hemorrhages were noted. Numerous petechiae were noted over the entire body. The platelet count was 57,000/cu mm and remained low. The patient developed mental confusion, marked lethargy, and generalized convulsions.

On September 12, *Staphylococcus aureus,* coagulase-positive, was grown from the peritoneal

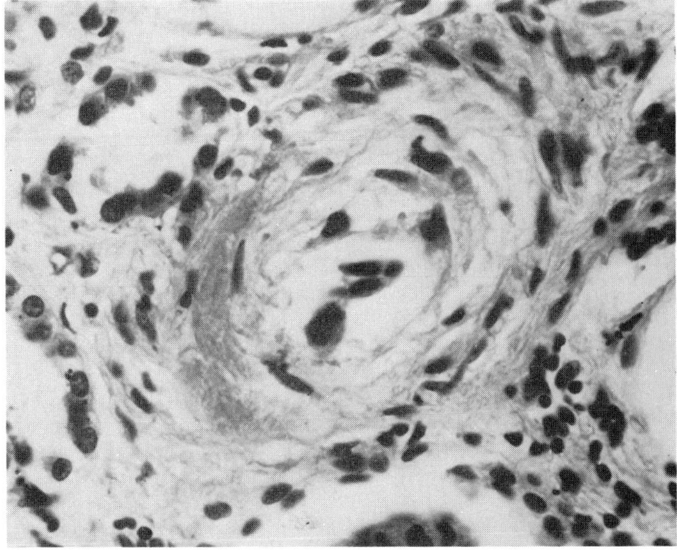

Fig. 2-57. Necrotizing arteriolitis following prolonged exposure to para-naphthalene. This microphotograph illustrates the kidney at autopsy taken from a 46-year-old chemist who was exposed to para-napthalene for 1 year. He developed generalized fatigue, dyspnea, and hematuria. He had hypertension, a hemolytic anemia, thrombocytopenia, and acute oliguric renal failure. Morphologic study revealed a proliferative glomerulonephritis caused by a necrotizing arteriolitis. This vascular abnormality is seen above. In addition, there were interstitial edema and fibrosis associated with tubular degeneration. (×750.)

2-60). The lesion was usually a cellular one with a matrix composed of acid mucopolysaccharide. The matrix was supported by a fine reticulum, which stains positively to Alcian blue, is metachromatic to toluidine blue, and stains slightly positive with periodic acid-Schiff. The mucoid lesion occurred more frequently in older individuals than in younger ones. The second lesion was found in patients with chronic progressive systemic sclerosis. There was a marked fibrotic thickening of the intima and it contained many fibers. The morphologic abnormalities of intimal fibroelastosis usually occurred in younger patients and were seldom associated with hypertension.

Afferent arteriolar thrombosis (hemolytic uremic syndrome)

In 1955, Gasser and associates described a syndrome of unknown etiology that occurs in children and that is characterized by anemia with irregularly contracted erythrocytes (burr cells), thrombocytopenia, and acute oliguric renal failure.[420] They named this syndrome the "hemolytic uremic syndrome." Since then, numerous case reports have extended our knowledge into the natural history of this illness. Moreover, clinicopathologic studies, especially those of Desmit and associates, have clarified the morphologic evaluation of the renal lesions.[296] Most of the children are younger than 1 year of age. However, the illness can afflict children up to the age of 5 years.

"Hemolytic uremic syndrome" is a poor descriptive term, for neither hemolysis nor uremia is the prominent clinical feature of the disease.[1120] The outstanding features of the disease are related to gastrointestinal symptoms—anemia with irregularly contracted erythrocytes, massive proteinuria, hematuria, and acute oliguric renal failure. The severity and clinical features of the illness vary considerably. In some patients the disease is so relatively mild that it is often overlooked. In other patients the illness is rapidly progressive and eventually fatal. In over half the patients reported to have the hemolytic uremic syndrome the diagnosis was made retrospectively.

The clinical features of the syndrome may begin with coryza, nausea, anorexia, and malaise. Gastrointestinal symptoms of abdominal pain, vomiting, and diarrhea may be present for at least 3 weeks. Some patients have frequent and watery stools that contain gross blood. This bloody diarrhea adds to the severity of the anemia and dehydration. Oliguria, edema, and hypertension are prominent later in the course of the disease. Ecchymosis or petechia is present in approximately 50% of the children but is not a striking finding. Although jaundice is uncommon, hepatomegaly is present in approximately 50% of the reported cases.

In the past, the prognosis of a child with the hemolytic syndrome was usually poorer than that of a child with acute renal failure caused by poststreptococcal glomerulonephritis.[200] The use of heparin in the treatment of the hemolytic uremic syndrome may reduce the mortality rate and may give rise to an improved prognosis.[296] Further investigative studies on the use and effectiveness of heparin are needed.

All patients have massive proteinuria and hematuria. In some the hematuria is gross and hemoglobinuria may be found. The urinary specific gravity during oliguria varies from 1.010 to 1.014. All patients have a moderate anemia with severe structural alterations of the erythrocytes. On examination of the peripheral blood smear one may find anisocytosis, fragmentation, poikilocytosis, burr cells, helmet cells, or polychromasia. The burr cells are characterized by dense staining of smaller than normal erythrocytes with irregular outline and small projections or burrs. The survival time of the erythrocyte is reduced. Brain, Dacie, and Hourihane suggested the term "microangiopathic hemolytic anemia" to describe the anemia associated with disease processes of the small'blood vessels.[147] Thrombocytopenia is usually present at some phase of the illness and, unless looked for, may be missed. The reticulocyte count is always increased, usually more than 10%. In all patients, the sedimentation rate is elevated, the Coombs test is negative, and the BUN is moderately elevated. The total serum bilirubin is slightly elevated (not over 5.6 mg per 100 ml) in less than 50% of the patients. The LE cell preparation is negative and the ASO titre is not elevated.

The hemolytic uremic syndrome must be differentiated clinically and pathologically from acute inflammatory diseases involving the glomeruli. These include poststreptococcal glomerulonephritis, TTP, Schönlein-Henoch purpura, bilateral renal cortical necrosis, lupus glomerulonephritis, and drug-induced acute renal failure. For example, features common to the hemolytic uremic syndrome are seen in patients with acute poststreptococcal glomerulonephritis. These findings are anemia, oliguria, and progressive azotemia.

Although other diseases such as TTP, lupus glomerulonephritis, and polyarteritis nodosa have in common both clinical and morphologic features with the hemolytic uremic syndrome, the latter has characteristic clinicopathologic features to classify it as a distinct clinical entity.

The clinicopathologic correlations made by renal biopsy have delineated the histologic evaluation of the renal lesion. Grossly the kidneys become enlarged and their capsules strip easily. Numerous small petechiae dot the renal surface. The renal cortex is edematous and thickened. The columns of Bertini are prominent.

The kidneys have a distinctive histologic lesion characterized by a hyaline thrombosis within the lumen of the renal afferent arterioles. This lesion is referred to in the French literature as a "microangiopathic thrombotique." The intralobular and afferent glomerular arterioles have their lumina obliterated by the thickening of the intimal cells with subendothelial hyaline deposits. The prominent feature is a fibrinoid necrosis and hyaline thrombosis within the arteriolar lumen extending as microthrombi into the glomerular capillary tuft. Although the lesions are not pathognomonic, they are repetitive and easily recognized. A patchy to almost complete renal cortical necrosis may occur. In glomeruli less involved there is a centrilobular hypercellularity that appears similar to poststreptococcal glomerulonephritis. The hypercellularity varies from a focal glomerulitis to a proliferative glomerulonephritis with epithelial crescents.

Interstitial changes consist of a slight periglomerular edema and focal infiltrates of mononuclear cells. Round cells can be seen around an occasional afferent arteriole. In general, the cortical tubules are normal. Erythrocytes, erythrocyte casts, hemoglobin, and hyaline casts are prominent within the tubular lumen. In children who recover from acute renal failure a few hyalinized glomeruli, tubular atrophy, and focal interstitial fibrosis are found.

Involvement of various areas and levels of the colon ranges from simple edema to intense inflammatory lesions. For example, vascular lesions similar though less prominent than those observed in the renal afferent arteriole are seen in the submucosal arterioles of the colon. More intense lesions of acute fibrinoid necrosis of arterioles are seen in the serosa and muscle layers. These inflammatory lesions in the gut may explain the gastrointestinal symptoms that occur in patients with the hemolytic uremic syndrome. Of interest to note is the self-limiting nature of the arteriolar lesions and their ability to undergo healing and repair with almost complete resolution in renal function.

The problem of differentiating the clinical and pathologic features common to the hemolytic uremic syndrome and acute post streptococcal glomerulonephritis is discussed in the following case presentation.

CASE PRESENTATION

On December 24, 1966, B. H., a 5-year-old girl, was admitted to West Suburban Hospital because of vomiting and diarrhea of 3 days' duration. Puffiness of the eyelids and mild swelling of the legs had been present since December 22, 1966. The next day she had oliguria.

On Noverber 25, 1966, she had a low-grade fever and complained of a sore throat. Her family consulted her pediatrician. He cultured her throat, and beta hemolytic streptococcus grew on the blood agar plate. She received 600,000 units of penicillin intramuscularly for 2 days (November 25 and 26) and oral penicillin in a dosage of 250 mg three times daily for 10 days. On December 12 her father had a sore throat. On December 14 she developed a mild erythematous rash on her arms. This rash lasted 1 day.

On admission she weighed 48 pounds. Her blood pressure was 140/90 mm Hg. There was periorbital edema and pitting edema (2+) of the legs. Purpura and petechia were not seen. The throat was hyperemic and cervical adenopathy was present. There was diffuse abdominal tenderness but no renal tenderness. The liver and spleen were not enlarged.

Admission urinalysis revealed proteinuria (4+), microscopic hematuria, a specific gravity of 1.014, erythrocyte casts, and numerous granular and hyaline casts. The hematocrit was 28%. On a peripheral blood smear there were poikilocytosis, polychromasia, and anisocytosis. There was a reticulocytosis of 6.4%. The leukocyte count was 7,500/cu mm, and the platelet count was 135,000/cu mm. The serum bilirubin was normal. The Coombs test, ASO titre, and LE cell preparation were normal. The serum $beta_{1c}$ component of complement was reduced. The admission BUN was 66 mg per 100 ml, the serum potassium was 6.9 mEq/L, and the CO_2 combining power was 13 mM/L. Nasopharyngeal culture failed to grow beta hemolytic streptococci. The total serum protein was 5.2 gm per 100 ml (albumin 2.23 gm per 100 ml and globulin 2.97 gm per 100 ml). The serum cholesterol was 270 mg per 100 ml. The ASO titre was normal.

On January 12, 1967, the $beta_{1c}$ component of complement was 35 units (normal 35 to 50), the antihyaluronidase titre was 1,024 (abnormally high), and the bactericidal test for Type

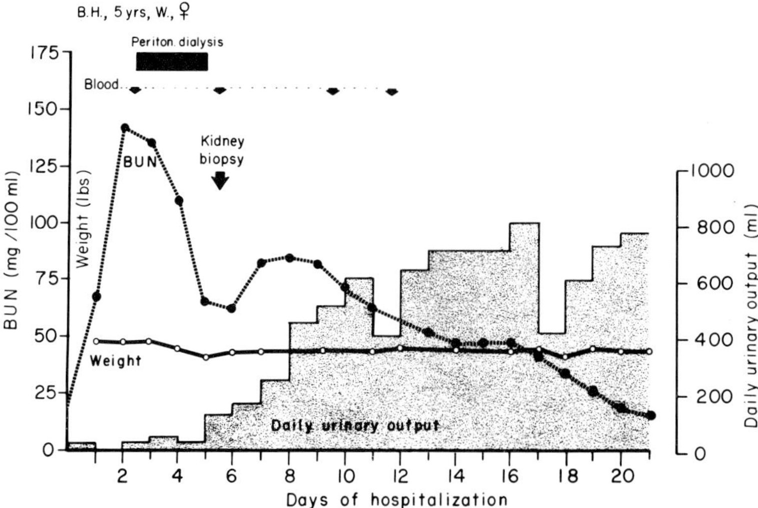

Fig. 2-61. Hospital course of child with acute renal failure caused by a proliferative glomerulonephritis. A 5-year-old girl developed oliguria 1 month after a beta-hemolytic streptococcal pharyngitis. Although she was treated with penicillin injections she developed gross hematuria and oliguria. Her BUN rose to 147 mg per 100 ml. Peritoneal dialysis was done on the third to fifth day. Four whole blood transfusions were given during her course. Her urinary output increased step-wise. On the fifth day a renal biopsy was done. On the twenty-third day the BUN was normal.

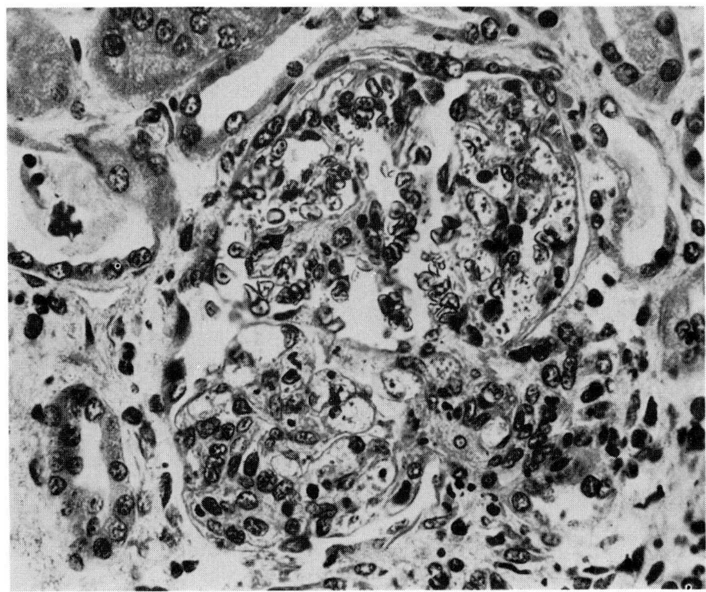

Fig. 2-62. Proliferative glomerulonephritis. This microphotograph illustrates a renal biopsy taken from the patient described in Fig. 2-61. The glomerular capillaries appeared dilated and contained numerous erythrocytes and leukocytes. There was increased cellularity of the epithelial and endothelial cells. The afferent arterial was thickened. The interstitium was normal. (H&E ×470.)

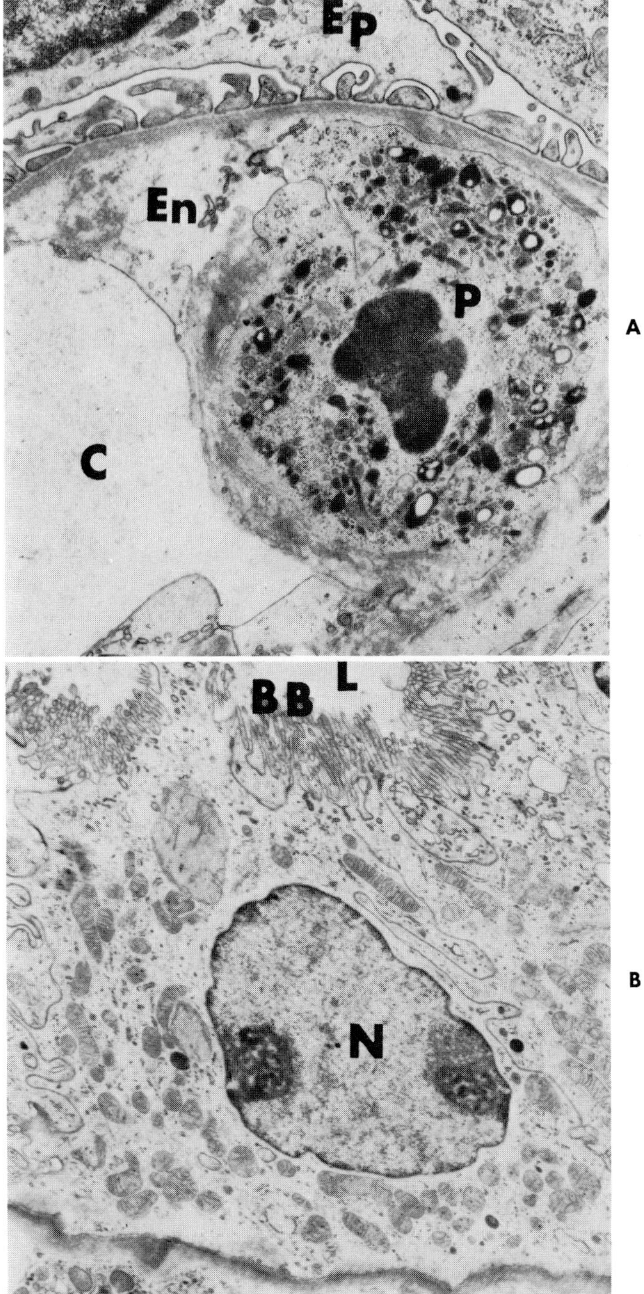

Fig. 2-63. Ultrastructural study of proliferative glomerulonephritis. A renal biopsy was obtained on the fifth day from the patient described in Fig. 2-62. Tissue was studied by light and electron microscopy. **A,** A portion of a glomerular capillary loop is seen. The capillary lumen (C) contains a polymorphonucleocyte (P) that is directly up against the lamina densa and an endothelial cell (En). The foot processes appear normal. An epithelial cell (Ep) is seen above. No epithelial humps were noted. (×12,000.) **B,** A proximal tubule is seen. The brush border (BB) projects into the tubular lumen (L). A large nucleus (N) contains two accumulations of chromatin. (×6,500.)

XII antibodies was positive. The long chain test showed poor growth and was negative, suggesting the presence of antibodies in the serum. (Tetracycline was given for an upper respiratory infection from January 8 to January 13, 1967.) (The clinical course is plotted in Fig. 2-61.)

Enemas containing sodium polysulfonated resins were started. The total fluid intake containing sodium bicarbonate 44 mEq was limited to 350 ml daily. Although the serum potassium dropped to 6.5 mEq/L, the CO_2 combining power rose to 20 mM/L. The BUN rose to 141 mg per 100 ml. Complete anuria occurred. Peritoneal dialysis was started on December 26 and was discontinued 2 days later after thirty-nine exchanges of 750 ml each of 1.5% glucose dialyzing fluid. Her weight dropped to 41 pounds and the BUN to 64 mg per 100 ml. Packed erythrocytes of 100 ml were given on December 25 and December 29.

On December 29 a percutaneous renal biopsy was done. A proliferative glomerulonephritis was found (Fig. 2-62). No apparent arteriolar thrombosis was seen. Following renal biopsy the patient gradually recovered.

Comment. Initially poststreptococcal glomerulonephritis was suspected as the cause of acute oliguric renal failure. It was highly unlikely that poststreptococcal renal disease would occur 1 month after a beta hemolytic streptococcal infection. In addition, the admission laboratory findings of a negative ASO titre and "negative" throat culture failed to confirm the diagnosis.

Although the hemolytic uremic syndrome usually occurs in infants, it was included in the differential diagnosis because of the clinical features of vomiting, diarrhea, and anemia associated with variation in the shapes of erythrocytes. The morphologic finding of a proliferative glomerulonephritis would favor a clinical diagnosis of either poststreptococcal glomerulonephritis or the hemolytic uremic syndrome.

The glomerular hyperemia and glomerular infiltrates of polymorphonuclear leukocytes could be part of the histologic finding of a poststreptococcal glomerulonephritis. Electron microscopic study revealed glomerular hypercellularity and in some areas a sublamina densa deposit of fibrin-like material. This was more readily seen on a tangential cut of the glomerular capillary (Fig. 2-63). No epithelial humps were noted. Although the humps are not pathognomonic of poststreptococcal glomerulonephritis, their presence would aid in a morphologic diagnosis of poststreptococcal glomerulonephritis.[802]

Normal ASO titres can be found in approximately 15% of patients with proved streptococcal infections. In this patient the diagnosis of poststreptococcal glomerulonephritis was finalized on the laboratory findings of an initially low $beta_{1c}$ component of complement, the return of $beta_{1c}$ component to normal, and the elevated antihyaluronidase titres.

Chapter 3

Clinical features of acute oliguric renal failure

In Chapter 2 acute oliguric renal failure was described as an omnibus syndrome that is an acute result of innumerable causes[642] stemming from major and minor renal artery involvement, the renal veins, glomeruli, interstitium, renal tubules, and obstructive uropathy.[384,394,1048] The primary illness precipitating acute renal failure can greatly modify the natural history of the disorders.[510,974] Thus, clinical courses and prognoses of patients with acute oliguric renal failure may be extremely variable.*

Today, the most common underlying pathologic abnormality of acute oliguric renal failure has been attributed to "acute tubular necrosis." Although electron microscopic studies of renal tissue obtained early in oliguria have revealed normal or minimal tubular changes, the term "acute tubular necrosis" will be used in relation to the wide spectrum of these tubular abnormalities. This spectrum of tubular findings extends from morphologically normal tubules seen by electron microscopy to severe tubular necrosis with dissolution of the tubular basement membrane.

When acute oliguric renal failure caused by acute tubular necrosis is uncomplicated by high catabolic conditions such as infection or fever or by surgical trauma or associated injuries, the clinical course and natural history with its biochemical abnormalities and clinical complications are quite predictable[243,858] With proper treatment the patient has an excellent chance of survival, and recovery may be relatively complete. In general, the ability of the patient to recover depends on the primary illness and associated complications. For example, in patients with uncomplicated acute renal failure due to medical or obstetric causes, the mortality rate is approximately 25%. On the other hand, when the acute renal failure is complicated by surgical and accidental infection and trauma, the mortality rate is over 70%.

---

*See references 473, 842, 875, and 1056.

STAGES OF ACUTE OLIGURIC RENAL FAILURE

The course of the illness may be short or long and the disorder may be mild or severe.[125] In general, the clinical course of patients with acute renal failure follows similar basic stages regardless of difference in etiology or pathogenesis. The clinical course was divided by Bull, Joekes, and Lowe into five distinct stages.[173] These stages were more precisely adapted for clinical use by Lough-bridge and associates and were related to patients with uncomplicated acute tubular necrosis[708] (Fig. 3-1). The first is the onset stage, which is followed by the oliguric-anuric stage. Following oliguria is the early diuretic stage, then comes the late diuretic or recovery stage. During this phase, the recovery of renal function and tubular healing take place. Finally the convalescent stage occurs, in which the patient is rehabilitated and is returned to productivity and usefulness as a member of society. The clinical course of acute renal failure can often be forecast if the type of precipitating disorder is known; in at least 25 to 30% of cases, however, no exact diagnosis can be made because the precipitating factor is not known.

Onset stage

The onset stage in acute tubular necrosis is that short period between the acute precipitating event and the subsequent development of oliguria or anuria. The onset stage ends when the daily urinary output is less than 400 ml in the

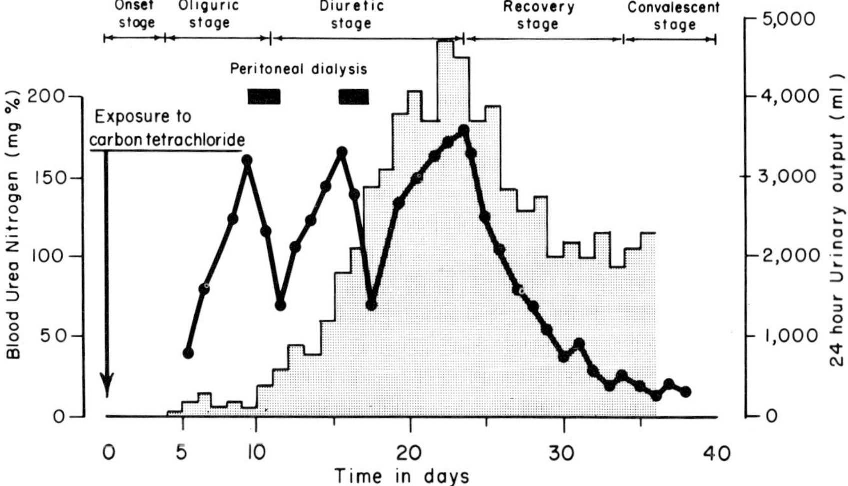

Fig. 3-1. Five distinct clinical stages of acute oliguric renal failure. The onset stage starts with the patient's exposure to the precipitating factor and extends to the occurrence of oliguria. The oliguric stage begins the first day the daily urinary output is less than 400 ml and extends to the onset of the diuretic stage. The diuretic stage starts with the first day the daily urinary output exceeds 400 ml and extends to the day the BUN starts to fall. The recovery stage begins the day the BUN falls and extends to the day it becomes stabilized or returns to normal. The convalescent stage follows and ends when the patient returns to normal life.

adult and 50 ml in the child.[206] The precipitating factors include accidental or surgical trauma, nephrotoxins, shock, hypovolemia, hemolysis, peripheral vaso-constriction, and any condition producing obstructive uropathy.

In patients with shock or bilateral renal artery thrombosis, the onset stage is very brief. In patients exposed to carbon tetrachloride or patients developing periureteral fibrosis because of methysergide maleate (Sansert) administration, the onset stage may be quite prolonged. I have managed two patients with carbon tetrachloride-induced acute tubular necrosis with an onset stage of 7 and 9 days, respectively. Another patient with periureteral fibrosis progressed to acute renal failure 9 weeks after stopping methysergide.

Oliguric-anuric stage

The oliguric-anuric stage begins when the daily urinary output drops below 400 ml in adults and below 50 ml in children. Although oliguria or anuria is the outstanding feature by which to recognize acute renal failure, the condition has been temporarily overlooked by some physicians, especially if they are occupied with a severe primary illness.

Although oliguria is common in uncomplicated acute tubular necrosis, anuria is extremely rare and unusual. The mean duration of this stage is 12.5 days,[708] and it usually lasts from 8 to 15 days. The duration of the oliguric-anuric stage is related to the precipitating factors of the primary illness and the underlying renal lesion. In a rare case of renal cortical necrosis or severe acute tubular necrosis, the oliguric stage has lasted for long periods.[930]

Absolute anuria of more than 2 weeks' duration has a poor prognosis. When complete anuria occurs, glomerulonephritis (poststreptococcal, hypersensitivity, lupus, and so on), large renal artery lesions, renal cortical necrosis, or obstructive uropathy must be suspected. Diagnostic procedures such as retrograde pyelography, renal biopsy, and renal angiography are of great clinical value. With information from these procedures the physician can more exactly base his treatment and management of the individual patient; with adequate and repeated dialysis the physician can maintain the patient alive for relatively indefinite periods.

Because acute renal failure occurs infrequently, the patient and his physician may be completely unaware of oliguria for days until symptoms of azotemia develop. This condition is more likely to be undiagnosed if serious illness pre-occupies the physician. Prominent symptoms of hiccups, nausea, and vomiting occur, usually in the morning. Unless the patient undergoes dialysis or spontaneous diuresis, additional symptoms and findings of uremia follow such as infection, pericarditis, congestive heart failure, gastrointestinal hemorrhage, and neurologic complications. The patient becomes confused, has somnolence, develops lethargy, and progresses into coma.

Biochemical changes of metabolic acidosis and hyperkalemia intensify this stage. The patient is unable to combat infections; in approximately 50% of cases surgical wounds may rupture. The common complication of the oliguric-anuric stage is overhydration. The patient with acute oliguric renal failure is very susceptible to excessive amounts of water. Overhydration leads to congestive heart failure, pulmonary edema, and death. This usually results from unrecognized acute renal failure and the forcing of excessive intravenous fluids. Cardiac arrest can result from severe hyperkalemia. I have obtained frequent monitored traces of patients with acute oliguric renal failure and have observed numerous types of cardiac dysrythmias. These include atrial fibrillation, sinus tachycardia, complete heart blocks, and ventricular tachycardia (Fig. 3-2).

During the first 2 days of the oliguric stage, the rise in BUN level is usually greater than in the following days. In uncomplicated acute tubular necrosis, the daily rise of BUN is approximately 25 to 30 mg per 100 ml. This represents a low endogenous protein breakdown of 40 gm per day. This breakdown is much

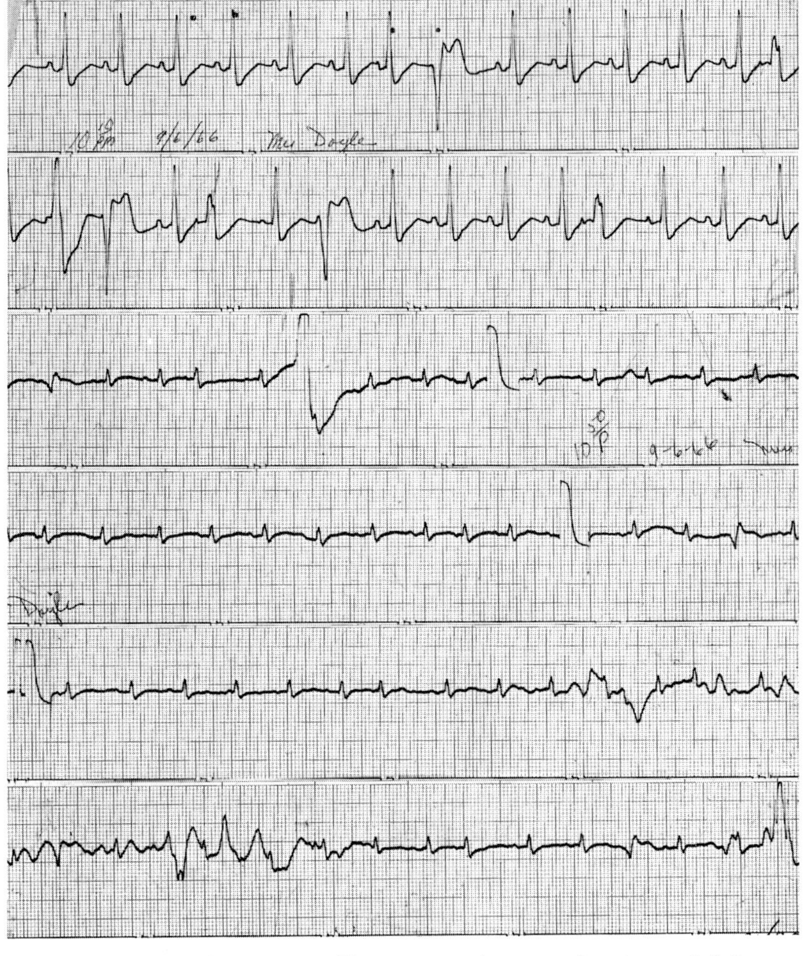

Fig. 3-2. Cardiac rhythm of a 70-year-old woman with acute oliguric renal failure resulting from acute tubular necrosis. During peritoneal dialysis she developed ventricular tachycardia, numerous extra ventricular contractions, and atrial fibrillation.

greater when acute tubular necrosis is complicated by a hypercatabolic condition such as infection, burns, fever, and trauma.

Cameron and associates reported a hypercatabolic rate of BUN rise of 108 mg per 100 ml per 24 hours.[198] This was considerably greater than the rate found by Silva and associates and indicates the need for early and frequent dialysis.[1014] Hypercatabolic patients have a mortality rate of 80 to 90%. If fluid balance is adequately controlled the patient loses approximately 1 to 1.5 lbs daily. This weight loss results from tissue breakdown and use of tissue stores for metabolic needs. The rate of urea lost in the decreased daily urine in sweat, gastric juice, and feces is directly in proportion to the urea concentration in the blood.[1014] During the oliguric-anuric stage, the daily urinary output increases stepwise until it exceeds 400 to 500 ml.

Meroney and Rubini studied urinary sodium/potassium (Na/K) ratios during acute oliguric renal failure in patients with acute tubular necrosis.[771] In their study, urinary sodium decreased and urinary potassium increased with each succeeding day of oliguria-anuria. This Na/K ratio suggests gradual improvement of tubular function in the nephrons that produce urine. The kidney is able to secrete urine with a pH of 5.5 or lower, which suggests an intact acidifying mechanism.

Early diuretic stage

The early diuretic stage is the first indication of recovery from acute renal failure. It begins when the daily urinary output persistently exceeds 400 ml and ends when the serum urea nitrogen fails to rise. Return of tubular function is rapid in most patients but very slow in others. The daily urinary volume gradually increases stepwise in amounts of 100 to 500 ml. The magnitude of diuresis reflects the degree of overhydration during the oliguric-anuric stage. The state of hydration at the beginning of the early diuretic stage is the important factor in determining the amount of water and electrolytes to be replaced. Daily urinary output varies between 1,500 ml and 4,000 ml for 4 to 8 days. The patient may lose as much as 30% of his body weight, which is usually the result of water loss. Marked sodium wasting occurs and may last for 1 to 2 days. During the diuretic stage death may occur from water depletion and/or electrolyte depletion if those substances are not replaced. The occurrence of diuresis may mislead the physician and the nursing staff into a false sense of relief. Approximately 25 to 50% of the deaths occur in this stage, usually as a result of cardiovascular complications, electrolyte deficiencies, and infections.

Complications occurring during the oliguric stage are carried over to the diuretic stage and may be intensified in the latter stage. These include infections, pulmonary edema, bleeding, and convulsions, especially when acute renal failure is associated with severe trauma or primary infection during a prolonged and complicated oliguric stage. In addition, delayed wound healing and pulmonary emboli may occur during diuresis, when water or electrolytes are not replaced in sufficient amounts.[288]

It is rare that a patient who is comatose requires intravenous fluids to replace electrolytes and water. The urine is hypotonic to blood early in this stage; therefore, a daily urinary output of at least 1,500 ml with a specific gravity of 1.010 is required before the serum urea nitrogen starts to fall. The serum uric acid will start to fall at the end of this stage. After the physician makes the correction of acidosis, he may unmask a hidden potassium deficiency.

Late diuretic or recovery stage

The late diuretic or recovery stage is that period between the first day the BUN falls and the first day it is stabilized or is within the normal range. In some patients the BUN remains elevated and permanent irreversible renal disease is present.[286] In this stage urea excretion exceeds urea production and there is a concommitant increase in the renal blood flow. However, the clearance of creatinine, inulin, and para-aminohippuric acid (PAH) may not reach normal values for months. The patient is unable to concentrate his urine. The overall effects of tubular repair are found whenever urea-urine/plasma ratios reach 10, creatinine-urine/plasma ratios reach 20, and sodium-urine/plasma ratios reach 5.

The patient is bedridden with severe nutritional depletion and has metabolic exhaustion. The serum electrolytes depend upon a balance between urinary losses and replacement of electrolytes.[292]

Convalescent stage

The convalescent stage follows the recovery stage and ends when the patient is able to return to employment or other productive activities. After urine volumes and urea levels return to normal, renal function gradually continues to return to normal. In the weeks following the diuretic stage, clearance of inulin, mannitol, creatinine, Diodrast, and para-aminohippurate increases rapidly.

A period of several months is needed before renal function returns to normal.[215] Some patients may recover from the acute renal failure, only to develop persistent renal damage, chronic renal damage, and chronic renal insufficiency, especially if diffuse interstitial nephritis develops to complicate acute tubular necrosis. The duration of this stage varies from one country to another. Because of medicolegal situations, it is usually more prolonged in the United States.

A marked anemia persists for weeks and even months following recovery from acute renal failure. Some physicians use whole blood transfusions to correct the anemia prior to the patient's discharge from the hospital. However, the patient continues to gain strength and energy gradually returns. Ankle edema may be present for several weeks; it is controlled by a salt-restricted diet and oral diuretic agents such as chlorothiazide.

Acute nonoliguric (high output) renal failure

Although oliguria and/or anuria are the classic clinical features of most patients with acute renal failure, some patients with acute renal failure will have neither oliguria nor anuria but will have a normal or a high urinary output. The frequency with which this occurs is not known, and the condition of many patients with nonoliguria will go unrecognized. It is possible that acute non-oliguric renal failure occurs in a similar if not a greater incidence as does acute oliguric renal failure. Moreover, patients with acute nonoliguric renal failure often do well without dialysis and are not referred to renal dialysis centers if they are diagnosed by their physician.

Acute renal failure without oliguria or anuria can result from the same numerous causes that produce oliguria.[76a] This type of acute renal failure was emphasized by Grabe and Sevitt in patients who develop a high urinary output associated with a rapidly increasing BUN and an impaired creatinine clearance.[458] In this condition, the kidneys have an inability to excrete a large urea load.

Acute nonoliguric renal failure can be induced by nephrotoxic drugs and chemicals, eclampsia, burns, shock,[76a] and hemorrhage. Why the same nephrotoxic agent produces severe oliguria in one patient and massive urinary output in others is not known. For example, I observed that severe tubular necrosis with oliguria occurred in a woman following treatment with aristolochic acid, and that the same agent in another patient produced a high urinary output failure of 16 liters daily.

The ratio of acute nonoliguric renal failure to oliguric renal failure varies from one reported series to another. For example, Vertel and Knochel reported a nonoliguric ratio of 11 to 14,[1100] Swann and Merrill reported a ratio of 3 to 82,[1056] and Handa and Lazor reported a ratio of 2 to 42.[514]

The clinical course of the patient with acute nonoliguric renal failure is quantitatively similar to that of the patient with acute oliguric renal failure. Acute oliguric renal failure is usually mild and should require conservative medical management. Hyperkalemia in the patient with nonoliguric renal failure usually does not require dialysis treatment. However, if the physician does not diagnose nonoliguric renal failure serious problems of overhydration may occur.

Patients with acute nonoliguric renal failure have urine sodium concentration ranging from 0.9 mEq/L to 11 mEq/L. This is in contrast to the patients with acute oliguric renal failure, in whom the sodium concentration ranges from 20 mEq/L to 77 mEq/L. Graber and Sevitt believe that the major functional defect in patients with nonoliguric renal failure is glomerular and not tubular.[458] On the other hand, Finckh and colleages conclude that acute nonoliguric renal failure has a functional defect rather than a structural one.[367] Renal biopsy studies usually reveal apparently normal glomeruli and tubules by light and electron microscopy. Thus, clinicopathologic studies in patients with nonoliguric renal failure are impossible to correlate. When tubular damage is found in non-oliguric renal failure it is usually very mild and undergoes rapid repair.

Teschner and associates reported acute nonoliguric renal failure in eight wounded soldiers who were in the Korean War.[1073] They emphasized that, under unusual combat conditions, battle casualties without obvious clinical symptoms of uremia may go undiagnosed through the regular chain of evacuation.

No doubt many patients have acute renal failure without reduction in urinary output. In fact, they may go unnoticed and spontaneously recover. Atlas and Gaberman's statement is most appropriate in this regard: "There is no substitute for repeated non-protein nitrogen or blood urea nitrogen determinations to evaluate renal failure."[41] I would like to add that observations should be made on the daily urinary output. This is especially true if nephrotoxic drugs are used.

The following case presentation describes high output renal failure in an obstetric patient.

CASE PRESENTATION

On July 13, 1964, L. P., a 29-year-old Caucasian, para VIII, gravida VII, was first seen in the Presbyterian–St. Luke's Hospital Obstetrical Clinic, 2 months prior to her expected date of confinement (Fig. 3-3).

Physical examination was not remarkable except for an asymptomatic ostium primum defect diagnosed 10 years previously. The blood pressure was 154/82 mm Hg. The hemoglobin was 13.8 gm per 100 ml, and the urinalysis was negative for protein, blood cells, and casts. She was seen 2 weeks later. The blood pressure was 170/74 mm. Hg, and another urinalysis was normal.

On August 4, 1964, at 7 AM, she was admitted in early labor with a 4 cm dilated cervix. Abnormal physical findings included a blood pressure of 180/118 to 190/120 mm Hg, distended neck veins, cardiac enlargement, a prominent apical Grade III systolic murmur, and

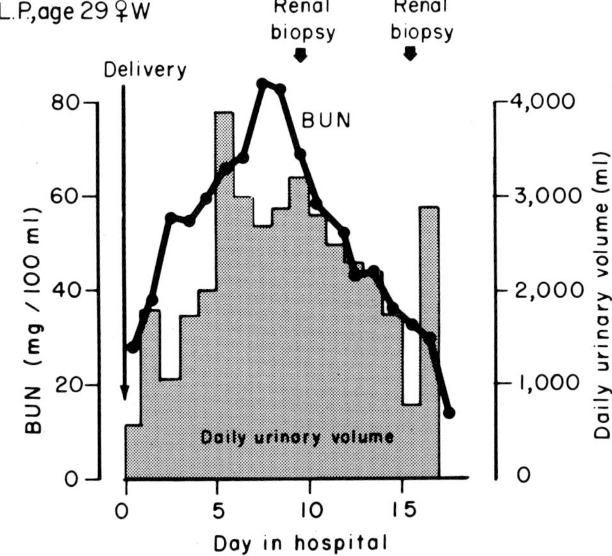

Fig. 3-3. Hospital course of a 29-year-old postpartum woman with acute nonoliguric renal failure. A 29-year-old woman developed severe hypertension prior to an uncomplicated delivery. Postpartum, she developed a so-called high output renal failure. The daily urinary output exceeded 700 ml and ranged up to 4,100 ml. On the ninth postpartum day the BUN was 85 mg per 100 ml. On the seventeenth day the BUN was normal. Renal biopsy was done on the ninth and fifteenth days.

a retinal sheen that was most marked in the perimacular area with absence of nicking, spasm, hemorrhages, or exudates. Admission hematocrit was 46%, with a leukocyte count of 12,050/cu mm. Urinalysis revealed a specific gravity of 1.025, a pH of 7, proteinuria (4+), and 50 leukocytes and an occasional erythrocyte per hpf. No casts were seen.

An hour after admission she began to complain of backache, which increased in intensity for the next few hours. Four hours after admission she passed brown urine, which was inadventently lost to examination. A catheterized urine specimen had a specific gravity of 1.015, a pH of 5, protein (4+), and 10 to 20 leukocytes and many erythrocytes per hpf. No casts were present. A few hours later she was jaundiced. Serum bilirubin was found to be elevated (total 4.0 mg per 100 ml, direct 1.5 mg per 100 ml); a urine urobilinogen on the following morning was a low normal.

The bilirubin fell rapidly to within normal range over the next 12 hours. On the morning of August 5, 1964, 24 hours after admission, petechiae were not present but a platelet count was 13,500/cu mm. Urinalysis at this time revealed only a few erythrocytes per hpf and persistent proteinuria. The spleen was easily palpable 3 cm below the left costal margin. Papain screening was negative. A 24-hour creatinine clearance was recorded as 10.5 ml per minute. Bleeding, clotting, and prothrombin times and prothrombin consumption were normal. Blood pressure remained between 120 to 130 systolic and 90 to 100 diastolic.

Forty-eight hours after admission she delivered a 4 lb 3 oz viable son. Her platelet count 3 hours later was 18,500/cu mm. Her course was one of slow recovery of renal function. Seven days after admission, despite daily urine volume exceeding 1,550 ml, the BUN rose to 84 mg per 100 ml. Twenty-four hours postpartum the platelet count was normal; the hematocrit, however, dropped to a low of 27% within 6 days before a reticulocytosis occurred.

On August 11, 1964, the 24-hour creatinine clearance was 11 ml per minute. Ten days later the excretion of intravenous injected phenolsulfonphthalein was 13% in 2 hours; 9 days later it rose to 29%. Glucose-6-phosphate dehydrogenase and 6-phosphogluconic acid levels were normal, as were the results of autohemolysis studies.

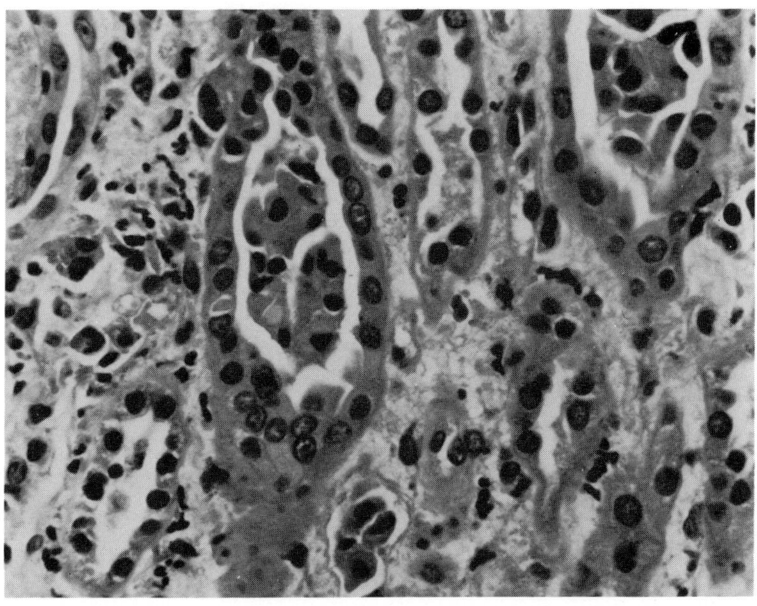

Fig. 3-4. Acute nonoliguric (high output) renal failure. Renal biopsy study was done at the height of BUN elevation when the urinary output was 4,725 ml. Tubular damage was associated with interstitial edema. Numerous casts were noted within the tubular lumen. The tubular epithelium was flattened and appeared to be undergoing repair. (H & E X 425.)

During the hemolytic episode on August 6, a bone marrow study revealed a reactive marrow with erythroid hyperplasia, reduced stainable iron, slight eosinophilia, and adequate to increased numbers of megakaryocytes. Other laboratory tests included lupus erythematosus cell preparations (3−), alkaline phosphates of 3.9 units, cholesterol of 179 mg per 100 ml, eight sterile blood cultures, and absent cold agglutinins. The blood type was O-positive with a negative panocell. The blood type of the infant was A-positive with a negative direct Coombs test.

A renal biopsy was done on August 13, 1964, and was repeated 6 days later because of an inadequate specimen (medulla only). The patient was discharged on August 23, 1964.

Renal biopsy findings. The first biopsy contained only medulla and was therefore considered inadequate for histologic evaluation. However, hyaline and erythrocyte casts were noted in medullary tubules.

Light microscopic study of the second renal biopsy revealed adequate cortex (six glomeruli). There was a mild focal increase in mesangial cellularity, and the matrix appeared normal except for minor focal basement membrane thickening and wrinkling. In some glomeruli, the mesangial matrix appeared to be slightly increased. The convoluted tubules, ascending limbs of Henle, and collecting ducts were unremarkable except for focal basement membrane thickening and scattered osmiophilic inclusions. In one area the interstitial tissue was infiltrated by cells believed to be of leukocytic origin, one of which was an eosinophil (Fig. 3-4).

Comment. Acute nonoliguric renal failure occurred postpartum in a young woman with eclampsia. She developed a hemolytic uremic syndrome with a thrombocytopenia. Fibrin thromboses were not found in the renal biopsy. The exact pathogenesis of acute renal failure in this patient remains obscure. However, it was quite possible that mild renal tubular necrosis occurred and rapidly underwent healing prior to the renal biopsy study. Unfortunately, it was necessary to delay the taking of renal tissue because of the low platelet count.

In spite of an excellent urinary output, proper medical management was required to ensure a healthy outcome. This management consisted of blood pressure control, administration of supportive measures, and adequate but not excessive fluids and electrolytes.

Acute oliguric renal failure in newborns and infants

Acute oliguric renal failure is commonly seen in children under 1 year of age.[206] It occurs in newborns and infants who have infectious diarrhea, bronchopneumonia, pyelonephritis, and septicemia. It uncommonly occurs associated with drug intoxication, water intoxication, hemolytic uremic syndrome, renal vein thrombosis, and central nervous system disease.[449]

Excluding the hemolytic uremic syndrome, the oliguric stage lasts approximately 5 days. The BUN increases rapidly and acidosis with hyperkalemia are present. Most deaths occur during oliguria and anuria. The diuretic stage is shorter than that of adults and usually lasts 3 to 5 days. Complete recovery in function occurs.[600]

The exception to this is the occurrence of acute bilateral cortical necrosis and renal infarction following septicemia, diarrhea with and without renal vein thrombosis, and the hemolytic uremic syndrome. In the latter, glomerular hyalinization and arteriolar thrombosis were associated with cortical infarctions.

The mortality rate varies from 35 to 55%.[71] Most deaths occur within 12 hours; the incidence of death increases with the duration of oliguria until effective treatment is started. The mortality rate in nondialyzed infants is approximately 90%, and in dialyzed infants it is 49%. Once the diagnosis of acute oliguric renal failure is made the treatment of choice is peritoneal dialysis. In the newborn the maternal precipitating factors include eclampsia, diabetes mellitus, and pyelonephritis. In many infants acute oliguric renal failure is associated with prematurity, neonatal apnea, urologic defects, cardiac defects, and gastrointestinal defects.

PROGNOSIS

The ability of physicians to forecast the outcome of patients with acute oliguric renal failure is an art at which only a few excel. After a careful analysis of the prime factors influencing the outcome of patients with acute renal failure, however, one can more accurately make exacting predictions through an appropriate clinicopathologic appraisal of the patient.

In 1955, Strauss and Raisz stated: "The mortality in acute tubular necrosis itself can be reduced by the combination of physiologic measures and external dialysis to nearly zero."[1049] Unfortunately, the results of treatment for acute renal failure in renal centers throughout the world have been uniformly discouraging.

The prognosis of patients with acute renal failure depends on several prime factors—the precipitating factors of acute oliguric renal failure and their relationship to mortality statistics, the common complications causing death in acute renal failure, the clinical and biochemical complications resulting from acute renal failure, and the severity and irreversibility of pathophysiologic damage sustained by the kidney once recovery is made from acute renal failure.[219]

Mortality rate

The overall mortality rate of patients with acute oliguric renal failure reported by several renal dialysis centers varies from 34 to 65%.* In an extensive analysis of 1,350 patients, the overall mortality rate was 42% (Table 3-1). The mortality rate in the group above age 51 years is approximately 58% and is similar in both sexes.[632,732] The mortality rate in the group below age 50 years is approximately 31% and is twice as high for men as for women. This sex difference is due to the large group of obstetric patients. When they are excluded, the sex ratio in the group below age 50 years is quite similar. It can be seen from this analysis that the mortality rate of acute oliguric renal failure is greatly dependent upon the following factors: the nature and severity of the primary illness, the precipitating factors producing acute renal failure, the site and severity of the renal lesion, the clinical condition of the patient on arrival at a renal dialysis center, and the promptness and effectiveness of the medical team in utilizing adequate facilities and knowledge in the management of the patient.

Nature and severity of primary illness

During the Korean campaign, Teschan and his colleagues found that patients with acute renal failure associated with severe injury to voluntary muscle had a

---

*See references 24, 52, 71, and 624.

Table 3-1. Mortality rates in 1,350 patients with acute oliguric renal failure in relation to the precipitating factors

Authors	Following obstetric complications			Hemolysis			Nephrotoxins and other intoxications			Postoperative			Posttrauma		
	Number	Dead	Mortality rate (%)	Number	Dead	Mortality rate (%)	Number	Dead	Mortality rate (%)	Number	Dead	Mortality rate (%)	Number	Dead	Mortality rate (%)
Alwall	8	1	13	6	1	17	—	—	—	33	17	51	—	—	—
Balslov and Jorgensen	16	3	19	3	1	33	64	28	44	177	111	63	7	6	86
Bluemle and others	16	4	25	24	7	29	9	5	55	32	23	72	6	5	83
Guild and others	—	—	—	—	—	—	20	5	25	—	—	—	—	—	—
Kiley and others	10	0	0	4	0	0	9	2	22	28	17	61	17	9	53
Legrain and others	216	21	10	64	16	25	42	8	19	71	46	64	38	26	68
Loughridge and others	20	4	20	—	—	—	7	2	29	—	—	—	—	—	—
Lunding and others	20	2	10	3	0	0	13	2	15	105	58	53	15	7	42
Palmer and Henry	—	—	—	—	—	—	16	6	38	—	—	—	—	—	—
Parsons and McCracken	25	2	8	—	—	—	—	—	—	18	14	78	7	4	57
Russel	34	8	24	—	—	—	—	—	—	—	—	—	—	—	—
Salisbury	—	—	—	17	9	53	—	—	—	—	—	—	—	—	—
Shackman and others	—	—	—	—	—	—	—	—	—	50	42	84	29	22	76
Smith and others	—	—	—	—	—	—	—	—	—	—	—	—	51	27	53
Totals	365	45	12	121	34	28	180	58	31	514	328	63	170	106	62

much more fulminating course than the average civilian patient without such complication.[1073] Parsons and McCracken,[866,867] as well as Bluemle and associates,[126] found that patients with acute tubular necrosis caused by medical and obstetric illness had a mortality rate of less than 25%. When severe injuries such as battle trauma or surgical operations produced acute tubular necrosis, the mortality rate was greater than 70%.

The mortality rate was high in patients with acute renal failure associated with a systemic condition, such as fibrin thrombin formation within renal arterioles caused by eclampsia. The mortality rate was extremely high in patients with lupus glomerulonephritis, polyarteritis nodosa,[519] TTP, or the generalized Shwartzman reaction. This was true in spite of treatment with high dosages of adrenocortical steroids, heparin, or a combination of both. The mortality rate was high in patients in endotoxemic shock caused by gram-negative septicemia. The mortality rate is especially high in jaundiced patients following peptic ulcer perforation. Patients with massive body burns and septicemia have a mortality rate near 100%. Moreover, any burned patient who develops uremia from acute oliguric renal failure usually dies.

Other primary conditions that lead to an absolute mortality rate and that produce acute renal failure are hemorrhagic pancreatitis, severe cerebral lesions such as cerebral hemorrhage, vascular trauma with hemorrhage, massive myocardial infarction, severe barbiturate intoxication, advanced cirrhosis of the liver with hydroperitoneum, and exposure to large and excessive quantities of a protoplasmic nephrotoxic agent such as arsine, mercuric chloride, and ethylene glycol.

Lunding, Steiness, and Thaysen analyzed their patients with acute renal failure regarding the nature and severity of the primary illness.[716] They divided their patients into three risk groups according to the nature of the primary disease. Patients in risk group I were "good risks"; their acute renal failure followed obstetric conditions, intravascular hemolysis, and nephrotoxic agents. The primary disease of this group was potentially reversible and was usually under control by the physicians.

Risk group II contained patients with a "dubious risk." In this group the renal failure followed an often very severe primary disease such as acute surgical emergencies, prolonged surgery, or trauma. The primary illness was sometimes irreversible and generally dominated the overall condition.

Patients in risk group III were very "poor risks." Their acute renal failure followed extensive myocardial infarction with shock, marked hepatocellular failure, septicemia, burns, tetanus, and so on. The primary disease was very severe and the illness was prominent throughout the course of the disease.

Precipitating factors

The precipitating factors have a great influence on the mortality rate of acute renal failure. For example, patients with obstetric complications have the best prognosis. In a group of 365 women the mortality rate was 12%. In women with renal cortical necrosis or severe eclamptic lesions of fibrin thrombosis, however, the mortality rate was much greater and approached 80%.

In patients with acute renal failure caused by a variety of conditions that produce intravascular hemolysis, the mortality rate is 28%. In patients with hemolysis caused by arsine vapors or falciparum malaria, the mortality rate may approach 60%; in patients with arsine-induced anuria, the mortality rate may approach 100%.

Patients with acute renal failure caused by nephrotoxic agents have an overall mortality rate of approximately 31%. The mortality rate was greater in patients with other organ damage such as acute yellow atrophy of the liver induced by carbon tetrachloride. In these patients the mortality rate approached 100%.

In some patients with drug-induced acute renal failure a hypersensitivity reaction may involve the arteries by a hypersensitivity polyarteritis nodosa or necrotizing angiitis, may involve the glomeruli by a hypersensitivity glomerulonephritis, or may involve the interstitium by a Councilman interstitial nephritis. In these patients, the use of adrenocortical steroids has remarkably improved recovery.

The greatest overall mortality rate (63%) occurred in a group of patients who developed acute renal failure following either surgery or extensive accidental trauma. In patients with trauma-induced acute renal failure, the greatest single mortality rate occurred in patients with severe body burns, especially if more than 50% of the body was burned. In some reports the mortality rate in severely burned patients approached 100%. It has been my experience that, when patients have 50 to 90% of their body surface burned, they develop renal failure and die.

Severity and extent of renal lesions

The degree of renal damage is directly related to the occurrence of oliguria or high output failure and to the duration of the oliguric-anuric stage. The physician feels reassured if the urinary output is adequate, and he feels discouraged if the patient has oliguria for a prolonged period. In general, the greater the renal damage the more prolonged the oliguric-anuric stage of acute renal failure. This is not a hard or steadfast rule of thumb, as minor tubular changes are sometimes found in some patients with prolonged oliguria. If exposure to the precipitating factor is intense or prolonged, oliguria is also prolonged and the mortality rate sharply increases. The mortality rate is high for patients with acute renal failure caused by either renal artery occlusion or a dissecting abdominal aortic aneurysm. This grave complication usually results in renal infarction and death.

Patients with extensive bilateral renal cortical necrosis or acute proliferative glomerulonephritis have a prolonged course of renal failure and usually die.[284] The urinary output remains below 400 ml for weeks or even months. Patients with renal cortical necrosis are more prone to develop pyelonephritis and,

in patients with burns, surgical trauma, or accidental trauma such as crushing muscle injuries and open fractures.

The bacterial infection appears more virulent. In uremic patients treated conventionally the infection progresses rapidly. When patients undergo frequent and prophylactic dialysis the infection is more easily treated, improves, and resolves.[588] Meroney stressed that infection in patients with acute renal failure may be completely overlooked by the physician because he is confused by the clinical symptoms of uremia.[768] In patients with acute renal failure the occult infections are usually pneumonia, bacterial endocarditis, pyelonephritis, and renal abscesses.

The prophylactic use of antibiotics or chemotherapeutic agents is definitely contraindicated. The foremost prophylactic treatment is reverse isolation, which decreases the chances of the patient's developing an infection. The antibiotics of choice are selected on the basis of laboratory in vitro sensitivity tests. Once bacterial invasion occurs in the uremic patient with acute renal failure, the infection is usually extremely difficult to control.

The dosages of antibiotics are greatly reduced for oliguria or anuria; antibiotics are given in a so-called stat dose.[773] During peritoneal dialysis, however, drugs are given in the usual parenteral dose. The dosage of antibiotics metabolized by the liver given to patients with oliguria or anuria is almost the same as that given to patients with normal renal function. These antibiotics include erythromycin and chloramphenicol. However, other antibiotics that are largely excreted by the kidneys must be given in greatly reduced dosages; otherwise, severe toxic effects may result. These include streptomycin, colistin, and kanamycin.

Treatment with antibiotics should be prompt, vigorous, and aggressive; they should be given at the first indication of infection, but only after appropriate cultures are taken. Table 3-2, modified from Kunin, is most helpful to the physician.[650] It contains data on the usage and particularly on the specific dose levels of a large group of antibiotics and chemotherapeutic agents useful in treating infections in the oliguric patient. The physician must guard against candidiasis.[688]

Urinary tract

Measures taken to prevent urinary tract infection are important. For example, reverse isolation techniques are used to prevent hospital-borne infections from being carried to the patient, especially if the patient is in a multibed intensive treatment unit. Reverse isolation techniques are used when the patient undergoes peritoneal dialysis. On the other hand, the patient's infections must not be disseminated to the hospital environment. Other methods to prevent infections are positive-pressure ventilation, proper housecleaning methods, especially in floor and laundry care, and the use of a Stryker frame to prevent tissue breakdown in patients suffering from injury caused by extensive trauma.

Instrumentation of the urinary tract by cystoscopy, ureteral catheterization,

Table 3-2. Data on antibiotics in patients with renal failure*

Antibiotic	Renal clearance	Probable renal mechanism‡	Half-life in serum of patient with anuria
Amphotericin B	?	?	?
Bacitracin	159 ml/min	G?T	?
Cephaloridine	0.9 × Cl creat (Dog)	G	1 day
Cephalothin	1.8 × Cl creat (Dog)	G+T	2.9-18 days
Chloramphenicol	24 ml/min	G	3.2-4.3 days
conjugate	340 ml/min	G+T	3-6 days
Chlortetracycline	0.3 × Cl creat	G	6.8-11.0 days
Colistin	32-78 ml/min†	G	2-3 days†
Cycloserine	?	?	?
DMC Tetracycline	0 3 × Cl creat	G	?
Erythromycin	0.76 × Cl creat (Dog)	G	4.8-5.8 days
Gentamycin	0.9 × Cl creat (Dog)	G	Prolonged
Isoniazid	41 ml/min	G	?
Kanamycin	0.8-1.6 × Cl creat	G?T	3-4 days
Lincomycin	43 ml/min	G	10-13 days
Methacycline	0.3 × Cl creat	G	?
Methicillin	4-6 × Cl creat	G+T	4 days†
Nitrofurantoin	3.2 × Cl inulin	G+T	?
Novobiocin	?	?	?
Oxacillin	Cl creat (Dog)	G+T	2 days†
Oxytetracycline	0.85 × Cl creat	G	?
PAS	140 ml/min	G+T	?
Penicillin G	560-1,050 ml/min	G+T	7.2-10.5 days
Polymyxin B	?	G	2-3 days†
Ristocetin	0.67 × Cl creat (Dog)	G	?
Streptomycin	30-70 ml/min	G	4-5 days
Tetracycline	0.62 × Cl creat	G	2-4 days
Vancomycin	0.69 × Cl creat (Dog)	G	9 days†

*Modified from Kunin. [650-655]
†Calculated from data presented in literature.
‡G = Glomerular filtration, T = Tubular secretion.
§Rare complication probably caused by allergic reaction.
#Does not appear to be related to renal function.
¶Glucuronic acid conjugate of chloramphenicol is not known to be toxic.
‖With anesthesia.

retrograde pyelography, and the urinary bladder catheter predispose the genito-urinary tract to infection.[611] These infections may occur anywhere along the urinary tract. They include acute pyelonephritis, renal abscesses, necrotizing papillitis, cystitis, and ureteritis. Pyelonephritis and renal abscesses are more likely to occur in patients with complete anuria caused by bilateral renal corti-cal necrosis or by obstructive uropathy. Necrotizing papillitis occurs more fre-quently in patients with obstructive uropathy, especially if they have diabetes mellitus. Infants receiving exchange whole blood transfusions and patients with acute and chronic alcoholism are also prone to have papillary necrosis.

Potential toxicity in uremia	Modified dose
Nephrotoxicity	Major
Nephrotoxicity	Major
Not significant	Minor
Not significant	Minor
Gray syndrome in newborn, erythropoietic failure when liver disease also present¶	None except newborn and liver disease
Liver damage, prerenal azotemia due to negative nitrogen balance, riboflavinuria	Avoid
Nephroxtoxic, apnea#	Major
Cerebral irritation	Probably major
	Major
Hepatic damage associated with propionate ester‖	Minor
Labyrinthine damage	Major
Peripheral neuritis	Probably minor
Nephrotoxic, cochlear deafness, neuromuscular blockade#	Major
	Minor
	Major
Hematuria and proteinuria§	Minor
Peripheral neuritis	Avoid
	Minor
	Minor
	Major
Oral agent, not necessary for uremics	Unknown
Convulsion with very high levels	Minor
Nephrotoxic, apnea#	Major
Thrombocytopenia	Major
Labyrinthine damage, occasional deafness	Major
	Major
Deafness	Major

Although instrumentation of the urinary tract must be performed to differentiate obstructive uropathy from other causes of acute renal failure, the urinary catheter should be avoided whenever possible. The physician is usually tempted to use the catheter to drain the urinary bladder and to measure the urine flow, especially when the uncatheterized patient with absolute anuria develops symptoms of cystitis and urethritis. I have frequently observed this. If the bladder is catheterized, closed urinary bladder drainage and rinsing of the bladder with a weak solution of neomycin may help to prevent urinary tract infection.

Septicemia

Septicemia proved by positive blood cultures develops subsequent to infection elsewhere in the body such as in burns, renal abscesses, and septic abortions.[250] Septicemia occurs with increasing frequency and is directly related to an increased duration of oliguria and to the severity of uremia. In patients with burns, the portal of entry for bacterial infection is the damaged, exposed skin.[527] Following surgery, the portal of entry for septicemia is a surgical wound or traumatized tissue. The peritoneal cavity is a portal of entry for secondary gram-negative bacterial infections such as *Pseudomonas aeruginosa*. When reverse isolation measures are omitted in patients undergoing peritoneal dialysis, hospital-borne gram-positive organisms commonly produce peritonitis.

The bacteria associated with septicemia are usually *Staphylococcus aureus* (coagulase-positive), *Proteus vulgaris*, *Enterobacter aerogenes*, *Escherichia coli*, Pseudomonas organisms, *Clostridium perfringens*, and *Chromobacterium janthium*.

Peritonitis

Peritonitis usually occurs as a complication of peritoneal dialysis or as a result of a ruptured viscus. Gram-negative bacteria usually produce peritonitis secondary to peritoneal dialysis, especially if the peritoneal cannula remains in the peritoneal cavity for periods exceeding 72 hours. Peritonitis is more likely to occur when 7% glucose dialysis fluid is used. It is quite possible that the hypertonic glucose solution "pulls" gram-negative organisms through the gut wall into the peritoneal cavity.[989] This should be investigated with labeled bacteria given by mouth and, subsequently, the organisms recovered in the peritoneal cavity should be studied. The use of oral antibiotics such as neomycin may reduce the bacterial flora of the gut and subsequently either reduce the incidence of peritonitis or prevent it.

The peritonitis that occurs secondary to peritoneal dialysis is entirely different from the peritonitis caused by perforation of a viscus. The peritonitis secondary to peritoneal dialysis responds more readily to appropriate antibiotic treatment. On the other hand, perforation with spillage of fecal material into the abdominal cavity carries a grave prognosis. Folowing peritoneal dialysis, loculated infection within the peritoneum has resulted in formation of subdiaphragmatic abscesses or other intra-abdominal abscesses.

Respiratory system

The patient with acute renal failure has an increased accumulation of bronchial secretions in the upper respiratory airway as well as inadequate respiratory excursions. The mucus secretion becomes dry and crusts the mucous membranes. This interferes with cilia action and drainage of bronchial sections. This condition serves as a portal of entry and predisposes the patient to infection.

Pulmonary complication occurs in a large number (50 to 85%) of patients with neurologic complications.

A purulent bronchitis occurs in 50 to 60% of patients with acute oliguric renal failure. Although approximately one-third of the patients have a tracheostomy, pneumonia and bronchitis usually progress in severity and may be fatal. An airway may improve oxygenation of the patient and reduce cerebral anoxia. Early and frequent prophylactic dialysis is very important in resolving resistant infections.

Pneumonia frequently occurs and may complicate pulmonary edema. It may develop secondary to prolonged bedrest and in association with the inability of the patient to properly fill his lungs. In such a situation, bronchopneumonia occurs and is usually extremely difficult to cure. The early and frequent mobilization of patients with acute renal failure is the best prophylactic measure to prevent pulmonary infection.

Infected wounds

Infection and delayed wound healing are common in patients with acute renal failure. In uremia the body defenses are unable to control infections and wound healing is delayed. Infected wounds produce a high catabolic process as a result of tissue necrosis and infection. The uremia is intensified and the following cycle impairs wound healing: uremia ⟶ delayed wound healing ⟶ infection ⟶ increased catabolism ⟶ uremia.

The inability of wounds to heal makes heparinization as well as therapeutic measures for infection control difficult. In patients with acute renal failure the bacterial, fungal, or yeast organisms are difficult to treat and they are usually antibiotic-resistant. If high doses of prednisone are used, the physician should make certain that tuberculosis, yeast, fungi, and nocardia infections are absent. Finally, proper debridement of infected wounds is most important in eliminating local wound infections.

Primary illness

If a chronic hemodialysis unit is available as an effective replacement for kidney function, death of patients with acute renal failure would then result from the primary illness. At present, approximately one-third of the patients with acute oliguric renal failure die from the primary illness. There are several kinds of primary illness—trauma, infections, disorders of other organs, and protoplasmic poisons.

Trauma

According to battle statistics obtained during World War II, the Korean War, and the war in Vietnam, traumatic injury was the prime cause of death in patients with acute renal failure. In general, the mortality rate of battle casualties was directly related to the deaths resulting from acute renal failure. Deaths from acute renal failure have decreased percentage-wise from World War II to the war in Vietnam. This decrease is the result of rapid and more effective evacuation of the injured soldiers to areas of definitive medical treatment. Helicopter ambulances transport battle casualties from the front lines to a station hospital within 1 hour after the wound is inflicted. In addition to battle wounds, traumatic conditions include crushing muscle injuries, automobile injuries, surgical trauma, burns, electric shock, head trauma, traumatic hemorrhage with shock, traumatic perforations of a viscus leading to peritonitis, and mediastinitis with emphysema.

Infections

Infections are usually classified with trauma as the principle cause of death. When one considers all categories of infections, gram-negative septicemia with endotoxemic shock is the foremost; it occurs secondary either to biliary tract surgery or to gastrointestinal surgery. In general, sepsis is usually caused by antibiotic-resistant organisms. In some patients who have had a criminal abortion, uterine infections caused by *Clostridium perfringens* produce an endotoxin that leads to a fatal massive hemolysis. These infections may follow prolonged labor or instrumental delivery. Intravascular hemolysis may occur without bloodstream invasion by *Clostridium* organisms. On the other hand, patients with demonstrable bacteremia may not have acute renal failure. *Clostridium perfringens* can occasionally produce localized intrauterine infections of a purulent nature with little if any gas. Such infection may resemble infection by *Staphylococcus aureus*. True gas gangrene produces an acute and sudden anaerobic myositis. The muscle is painful and the patient develops tachycardia and shock with oliguria.

In the presence of acute oliguric renal failure, the patient with severe acute pyelonephritis is difficult to treat. If papillary necrosis and septicemia accompany the kidney infection, the chances for recovery are very slight. The patient usually dies of multiple renal abscesses and embolic abscesses throughout the body, especially those of the brain, lungs, and liver.

Disorders of other organs

Primary illness of other organs can produce acute renal failure and death. Acute myocardial infarctions with sufficient muscle injury may produce a rupture of the heart wall, and cardiac tamponade ensues. Severe acute myocardial infarction produces fatal congestive heart failure with cardiac dysrhythmia, including cardiac standstill. I observed a middle-aged laborer who had "alcoholic myocardiopathy" and a single kidney.[784] He was treated for congestive heart failure with digitalis and meralluride and was confined to bed. He improved greatly until an associated mural thrombus of the left atrium became embolic to the renal artery (Fig. 2-39, A). Death resulted not from the biochemical complications of acute renal failure but from an uncontrollable cardiac dysrhythmia with a second episode of congestive heart failure.

Hemorrhagic pancreatitis producing acute renal failure is usually a fatal condition. This condition can occur spontaneously or it can be the result of trauma, both accidental and iatrogenic. Death has occurred from either a severe fulminating peritonitis or multiple pancreatic abscesses with secondary septicemia.

In some patients acute yellow atrophy or advanced liver disease associated with a hepatorenal syndrome has been fatal. Involvement of the brain by head injury, neoplasm, leukemia, or infection has produced a fatal acute renal failure. The patient dies not from the complications of acute renal failure but usually from some severe and irreversible primary disorder involving the brain.

Spontaneous rupture of an abdominal viscus due to a variety of causes such as trauma, peptic ulcer, drug-induced ulcer, diverticulitis, or neoplasm has resulted in spillage of fecal material into the peritoneal cavity. Peritonitis develops and is subsequently followed by acute renal failure. Death results not from acute renal failure but from the fulminating primary illness—an irreversible fatal peritonitis.

Acute massive pulmonary emboli induced by oral contraceptives have resulted in acute tubular necrosis.[762] Although acute renal failure was treated satisfactorily, death resulted from the massive pulmonary infarction.

Regardless of how successfully acute renal failure is treated, the primary illness may be severe and difficult to resolve and the patient usually dies. This is discussed in the following case presentation.

CASE PRESENTATION

A 72-year-old lady entered the hospital with progressive jaundice, fever, and right upper quadrant abdominal pain. She related episodes of abdominal bloating to eating "heavy meals." Chronic cholecystitis was diagnosed. On the eleventh hospital day a surgical exploration of the gallbladder and biliary ducts was done. A carinoma of the common duct was found. A T tube was inserted into the common duct.

The postoperative course was uncomplicated until the T tube was removed by the patient. She became jaundiced and a second exploration was done. On the thirty-second hospital day, a cholecystojejunostomy was performed. The patient developed acute oliguric renal failure, fever, shock, and a leukocyte count of 21,500/cu mm. Metaraminol bitartrate (Aramine) and hydrocortisone sodium (Solu-cortef) were given and the acute renal failure was treated effectively by using conservative measures (Fig. 3-7). In spite of an excellent diuresis the patient died. At autopsy, peritonitis was found to have been caused by an anastomosis separation of the cholecystojejunostomy. Findings of kidney studies were normal.

Protoplasmic poisons

Patients with severe and fulminating systemic protoplasmic intoxication sometimes develop an associated acute oliguric renal failure. This can be observed in patients who become deeply comatose as a result of overwhelming barbiturate intoxication. They quickly lapse into shock and develop anuria. Pulmonary edema follows, and death ensues.

Acute carbon tetrachloride intoxication sometimes produces acute tubular necrosis. In some patients it also leads to extensive hepatic damage and in others

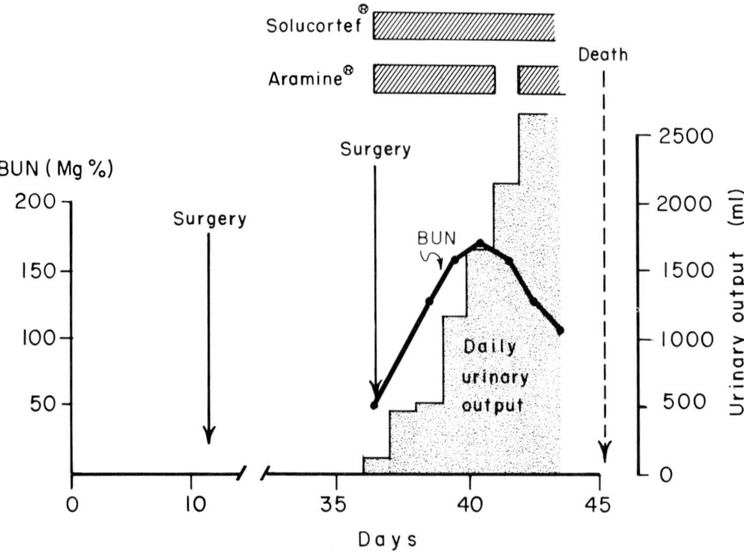

Fig. 3-7. Hospital course of patient with acute renal failure following cholecystojejunostomy. A 72-year-old woman entered the hospital with jaundice caused by carcinoma of the common bile duct. On the eleventh day exploration of the abdomen was done and a T tube was inserted into the common bile duct. Twenty-five days later the patient pulled out the T tube. A cholecystojejunostomy was done. She developed a severe gram-negative endotoxemia and subsequent acute oliguria. Large dosages of Solu-Cortef and Aramine were given. The daily urinary output increased step-wise; however, the BUN reached 164 mg per 100 ml before it dropped to 96 mg per 100 ml. In spite of a diuresis the patient died on the forty-fifth day. At autopsy peritonitis was found to be caused by a leak in the cholecystojejunostomy anastomosis.

to acute yellow atrophy. Although acute renal failure is successfully treated, the patient usually dies in coma caused by hepatic failure. Other lethal protoplasmic poisons are arsine vapors, aniline, bichloride of mercury, and methanol. The finding of amino aciduria indicates tubular damage.[346]

Biochemical abnormalities

Numerous biochemical abnormalities[506,518] result from acute oliguric renal failure.[291,330,981] These include hyperkalemia,[293] hypermagnemia, metabolic acidosis, hypernatremia,[309] uremia, and water intoxication.* If these abnormalities go uncorrected the patient dies.[508,509,886]

Hyperkalemia

In acute renal failure the serum potassium level rises because of infection, formation of pockets of blood, hemolysis, protein catabolism, dead and dying tissue, and tissue destruction.[282,560] Each of these processes constantly releases potassium into the extracellular fluid, and this potassium is not excreted from the body by the kidneys.[293,341] The catabolic processes are augmented by fever,

---

*See references 73, 278, 333, and 501.

infections, trauma, toxins, and adrenocortical steroids.[497] In the diuretic stage potassium deficiency is the prime hazard.

Neuromuscular effects. Significant hyperkalemia may be present without any clinical symptoms. When symptoms occur they are related to the neuromuscular system. Clinical symptoms of hyperkalemia are paresthesia, mouth numbness, muscle weakness, and, in some instances, paralysis, generalized weakness, and decreased tendon reflexes. The muscle weakness can progress into paralysis if the patient actively exercises.

The neuromuscular symptoms include a large spectrum—from vague weakness to gross flaccid paralysis of all extremities. In some patients paralysis involves muscles of phonation and respiration.

Myocardiotoxicity. In recent years most authors have reported a decrease in potassium intoxication as a complication of acute renal failure. However, it still remains a serious biochemical hazard. The complex disturbance produced by potassium intoxication affects the myocardial conducting system. Its myocardial toxicity is aggravated by other factors such as hyponatremia, hypocalcemia, and acidosis. The constant monitoring of the patient by means of electronic equipment is the preferred method to detect cardiac conduction disorders caused by hyperkalemia.[249] The electrocardiogram of all patients with acute renal failure is constantly monitored. I have been completely surprised by unsuspected transitory dysrhythmias. Hyperkalemia may be associated with depressed atrial activity or increased intraventricular conduction time that results in a slow idioventricular rhythm, which may terminate in cardiac arrest during diastole (Fig. 3-2).

Potassium intoxication causes the T waves on the electrocardiogram to be peaked and tall.[541] However, they may not be tall if they are superimposed on previous inverted T waves. At this point, it is worthwhile to mention the Sharpey-Shaeffer effect. T waves in this phenomenon are the change of inverted T waves to normal T waves in the presence of hyperkalemia. For example, patients with left ventricular hypertrophy or patients on digitalis therapy have inverted T waves. These abnormal T waves may become upright in the presence of potassium intoxication. In fact, the T waves may appear normal. When the serum potassium levels are reduced by removing potassium from the body, the T waves revert back to the previous inverted state.[216]

The electrocardiogram changes of hyperkalemia can be accentuated by other biochemical abnormalities such as hypocalcemia, hyponatremia, and acidosis; therefore, one must carefully evaluate the ECG tracing of patients with acute renal failure. For example, the biochemical abnormalities of uremia can produce ECG changes compatible with those resulting from subendocardial ischemia. If the physician is not aware of this fact he may incorrectly treat the patient for an acute myocardial infarction.

Teschan and his colleagues studied soldiers with acute renal failure resulting from war wounds sustained in Korea.[1073] They found hyperkalemia frequent and of special clinical importance in treating battle casualties. Their patients' serum potassium levels were usually unaffected by treatment with cation exchange resins.

Metabolic acidosis

Progressive metabolic acidosis is a characteristic biochemical change in patients with acute renal failure.[342] It results through several metabolic mechanisms —the retention of metabolically generated hydrogen ions of endogenous acids derived from the oxidation of sulphur-containing amino acids,[526] incompletely metabolized organic acids, loss of bicarbonate, and the metabolism of isoelectric phosphoprotein substances. It is associated with a lowered bicarbonate concentration, low blood pH, and a CO_2 combining power well below normal probably as the result of hyperventilation. Attempts should be made to keep the CO_2 combining power from falling below 12 to 15 mM/L. In extreme acidosis it is necessary for the body to "blow off" carbon dioxide, which results in Kussmaul-Kien respirations.

Acidosis is seen less frequently in patients who vomit frequently or in patients who are undergoing gastric suction. The loss of hydrogen ions from the body through gastric suction helps correct uremic metabolic acidosis. The prognosis is grave if severe metabolic acidosis goes uncorrected.

Uremia

The rate of the daily rise in the BUN or creatinine[281] is a good measure of tissue breakdown and of the mildness or severity of the disorder.[208] Elevated BUN levels have no damaging effect to body tissue and are insignificant in producing the toxic uremic clinical features.[1096]

Uremia can produce death by massive hemorrhage from the gut or by a massive fatal hemorrhage into the pericardial sac; in the latter, death results from cardiac tamponade. When the BUN was not permitted to exceed 200 mg per 100 ml by early and frequent dialysis, Scribner and associates found better therapeutic results and less complications from uremia.[986] This is supported by Barsolv's report.[71] He found a difference in mortality rate between the patients with a blood urea of 500 mg per 100 ml and those patients in whom the blood urea was not allowed to reach 300 mg per 100 ml. The mortality rate was significantly reduced when the blood urea level was controlled.

Water intoxication

Water overload is the chief danger in the early stage of acute renal failure.[1141] It occurs when patients with undiagnosed acute renal failure are loaded with water or when excessive electrolyte-free fluids are given to patients with acute renal failure. Water intoxication produces muscle twitching, disorientation, stupor, convulsions, and acute pulmonary edema.[452] In some patients the latter condition is fatal.[502] In patients with water intoxication, it is necessary to restrict fluids and to give hypertonic solutions of sodium chloride to correct this serious and sometimes fatal intoxication.[113,985] In the diuretic stage water depletion becomes a chief danger.[503]

COMPLICATIONS

The vast knowledge of the pathophysiology of acute renal failure has led to sound therapeutic principles. The application of this knowledge in the management of patients with acute renal failure has greatly reduced complications and morbidity caused by uremia, especially the complications caused by abnormalities in fluid and electrolytes.[124] However, extrarenal complications occur and constitute the largest percentage of the morbidity and mortality of patients with acute renal failure. In addition to hemorrhage and anemia, there are neurologic, gastrointestinal, cardiovascular, and nutritional complications.

Neurologic complications

To date, attempts at isolation of a single neurotoxic substance in uremic patients have met with failure. Numerous biochemical abnormalities contribute to the neurologic complications of uremia. These are acidemia, alkalemia, potassium intoxication, water intoxication, calcium deficit, and magnesium excess. No single biochemical alteration in uremic patients could account for the neurologic changes.

In 1839, Thomas Addison, a colleague of Richard Bright at Guy's Hospital, described the classic neurologic symptoms observed in patients with chronic renal failure.[9] These identical neurologic abnormalities are noted in patients with acute renal failure. In Addison's classic paper, he described "sluggishness of manner, inability to concentrate, dullness of the intellect, visual impairment and drowsiness going into quiet stupor and ending in coma." Transient disturbances such as monoplegia, hemiplegia, asphasia, deafness, and amaurosis occur.

In 1941, Wilson described "ethnic uremia" and included catalepsy, psychic derangement, and disorders of speech, hearing, and vision.[1132] It may be impossible for the physician to differentiate between the neurologic effect of acute renal failure caused by uremia, water abnormalities, or electrolyte abnormalities and that of a primary underlying illness. For example, water intoxication produces strange behavior, loss of attention, confusion, delirium, aphasia, convulsions, disorientation, and coma. For a comprehensive review of the neurologic complications of acute renal failure, I suggest the work of H. Richard Tyler.[1091]

Aberrations of mental status

The more rapid the onset of catabolic mechanisms leading to uremia the earlier the mental aberrations occur. Mental aberrations and emotional responsiveness are the earliest and most sensitive criteria useful in detecting cerebral impairment. The patient's personality becomes flat and sometimes appears paranoid. If patients older than 41 years have catatonia one should rule out uremia.

Their emotions may swing between euphoria and depression.[47] The patient's intellectual awareness varies from periods of complete orientation as to self, time, and place to episodes of marked dullness in intellect. Osler described mania as being characterized by noisiness, talkativeness, restlessness, and sleeplessness.[854] He wrote on the ideas of persecution and suicides.[853] The patient's lethargy may persist, reverse, or progress into marked disorientation and death.

The patient with acute renal failure may develop an acute psychosis with or without catatonia. This is similar to other acute toxic psychoses and is probably caused by uremia, water intoxication, cerebral anoxia, and/or electrolyte imbalance. The psychotic behavior can be made worse by certain therapeutic agents such as prochlorperazine (Compazine), meperidine (Demerol), and barbiturates.

Following recovery or after dialysis the mental aberrations subside in a reverse order. Schreiner and Maher emphasized the delay in clinical improvement following a chemical improvement: chemical azotemia $\longrightarrow$ lag phase $\longrightarrow$ clinical uremia $\longrightarrow$ dialysis $\longrightarrow$ chemical reversal $\longrightarrow$ clinical reversal.[978]

I have observed in some patients a deterioration of their clinical status following a return to normal of serum electrolytes and BUN. Patients who recover from the mental abnormalities caused by prolonged oliguria or anuria develop either complete or partial amnesia of events that occurred during the oliguric and diuretic stages.

Convulsions

Spasmodically occurring coarse twitching is common in uremia caused by acute renal failure. Prior to convulsions a flapping tremor or asterixis can be noted in most patients. This is similar to that seen in prehepatic coma. It can be detected when the patient extends his arm and then extends his hand at the wrist. A fine tremor of the fingers occurs, followed by a quick falling or jerking of the hand.[1091]

Muscle twitchings progress to convulsions. Seizures are multiple and are usually Jacksonian, tetanic, and grand mal in character. Most common are generalized convulsions. They are more prone to occur in association with hypertension, usually during the early diuretic stage. The electroencephalograms range from "coma" type, with loss of background alpha activity, to a predominant rhythm in the delta range.[623]

Early and frequent dialysis is the best way to prevent convulsions. Either 0.1 to 0.2 gm amobarbital sodium (Amytal) or 10 mg diazepam (Valium) given intravenously is effective. Convulsions in the postpartum woman can result from infarcts in the hypothalamic-pituitary area. If hypocalcemia is present, 20 to 30 ml of 10% calcium gluconate should be injected intravenously.

Tetanic neuromyopathy

Muscle weakness is present in the patient with acute renal failure. When the BUN is greatly elevated, fasciculations occur and are usually gross and widespread. They may be repetitive in some muscle groups. In other patients with acute renal failure, jerking muscle movements occur and are referred to as "myoclonus." This tetanic neuromyopathy usually occurs in patients with chronic renal failure; however, it has been observed in patients with acute renal failure.

The condition is characterized by severe myospasm that produces a rigid extension of the legs and a talipes equinovarus position of the feet. The myospasm may be so severe that it ruptures large muscle bundles such as the abdominal rectus muscle. In some patients, convulsions occur; in others, myospasm produces unrelenting pain and precedes death by a few hours.

Merklen and Gounelle described "uremia myotonique" in a uremic patient who had myospasm of the abdominal muscles. Because of the severe pain and rigidity, an acute surgical abdomen was simulated. Uremic myospasm must be differentiated from infections by *Clostridium tetani* as well as from the pyramidal tract clonus caused by the adverse effects of prochlorperazine.

Dialysis disequilibrium syndrome

The vast majority of patients with acute oliguric renal failure undergo dialysis without developing symptoms of cerebral dysfunction. However, a few patients develop headache, confusion, disorientation, muscle twitchings, and convulsions. This condition is known as the "dialysis disequilibrium syndrome" and has occasionally been fatal.[618,941] It usually occurs after hemodialysis, but has followed peritoneal dialysis, at a time when there is improvement in the patient's biochemical status.

This syndrome can be explained by the biochemical barrier between the blood-cerebrospinal fluid and the brain. After dialysis, the cerebrospinal fluid urea remains high while the plasma urea nitrogen falls. Electroencephalographic studies of patients with the dialysis disequilibrium syndrome reveal characteristic bursts of high-voltage rhythmic delta waves. These changes are nonspecific and are similar to those seen in patients with cerebral edema.

The disequilibrium syndrome may result from one of several causes. The first is the reverse urea shift theory: during dialysis, urea is removed rapidly from the blood; however, the cerebrospinal fluid urea has a barrier that retains it.[867a] Therefore, there is a delayed clearance of urea from the cerebrospinal fluid and brain cells. Water is drawn by the osmotic gradient of urea into the cerebrospinal fluid, and subsequently the brain becomes edematous. The cerebrospinal fluid to plasma urea gradient persists for at least 24 hours.[399] Thus, cerebral edema occurs any time during the first 24 hours postdialysis. This edema was evident in a patient with a "skull flap" studied by Scribner. After dialysis the patient had swelling of the brain through the skull flap. Postmortem studies of two fatalities revealed the presence of marked cerebral edema.[941]

There is also a gradient between the cerebrospinal fluid and the plasma for uric acid, inorganic phosphorus, creatinine, and bicarbonate.[212] The disequilibrium syndrome can usually be prevented by diminishing the speed of dialysis during the first few hours or by adding extra glucose (2%) to the dialysis bath. However, the syndrome has occurred when extra glucose was added to the bath.

Another hypothesis is that an increase of carbon dioxide produces the cerebral dysfunction.[618] The blood pH, which is low before dialysis, is alkaline after dialysis. This may result from persistent overactivity of the respiratory center under the effects of a delayed correction of the low intracellular pH. The carbon dioxide fails to reach normal levels and the bicarbonate increases by a considerable amount to normality.

Autonomic nervous system

Clinical symptoms of uremia have been attributed to disturbance in the autonomic nervous system. Miosis results from parasympathetic irritation to the occulomotor nerve or the occulomotor center. Sialorrhea results from irritation of the chorda tympani and can be blocked with atropine.

Vagal stimulation may produce a rhythmic bradycardia, which may be associated with the Cheyne-Stokes respirations. Vagus irritability can produce nausea, vomiting, and gastrointestinal hyperactivity. Diarrhea may result from loss of sphincter tone at, for example, the pylorus, the ileocecal valve, and the rectum.

Cranial nerve abnormalities

Cranial nerve involvement is striking and varies in intensity in acute renal failure. The olfactory, optic, auditory, and vestibular nerves are usually involved. The physician may have difficulty in differentiating the adverse effects of drugs from the effects of renal failure. For example, antibiotics such as streptomycin, neomycin, and colistimethate sodium (Coly-Mycin) produce nystagmus because of ototoxicity to the vestibular nerve. Nystagmus is common in acute renal failure. Certain nephrotoxic drugs or chemicals may produce acute optic neuritis.

The sudden loss of vision or uremic amaurosis is more likely to occur in patients with chronic renal failure. However, it can occur in patients with prolonged acute renal failure. The pathogenesis of "uremic blindness" can be traced to three specific mechanisms, the first of which is a direct retinal damage such as papilledema or retinal hemorrhage caused by malignant hypertension. The second is involvement of the visual cortex in patients with prolonged seizures resulting from uremia; this may subsequently result in cortical thrombophlebitis. Retinal lesions caused by hypertension, as well as biochemical changes, produce blindness. Amaurosis with severe potassium deficiency has produced edema of the optic nerve. The third mechanism is caused by an optic neuritis. I observed this mechanism in one patient with severe and prolonged arsine-induced anuria. Although the patient survived acute renal failure, he developed chronic renal insufficiency; the optic neuritis gradually cleared over several months.

Facial weakness with mild transitory facial asymmetries are common. In addition, hemianopia, hemeralopea, and diplopia occur; ptosis is rare.

Patients in uremia caused by acute oliguric renal failure may have transitory episodes of vision loss or aberrations of vision. No retinal changes are seen on funduscopic examination. It is very possible that these findings are caused by severe biochemical abnormalities and their effects on nerve tissue. Dysarthria and dysphagia have been observed after treatment with dialysis.

Gastrointestinal complications

Clinical symptoms of gastrointestinal complications are among the most severe and most aggravating symptoms occurring in patients with acute oliguric renal failure. The entire gastrointestinal tract is involved, from lips to anus—for example, monilia stomatitis and proctitis. The characteristic features of gastrointestinal involvement in acute renal failure are stomatitis, anorexia, nausea, vomiting, diarrhea, abdominal pain, pancreatitis, and gastrointestinal hemorrhage.

Uremic stomatitis

The increased salivary secretion of urea and other nitrogen breakdown products such as ammonia may result in uremic or aphthous stomatitis. [55] Hempstead and Hench found that the uremic patient has an increase in salivary urea.[536] They studied the morphologic lesions and found destruction of the superficial layers of mucosa. In some patients papillary body tops were destroyed and only the tips of rete pegs were seen.[91] Black studied uremic stomatitis and found increased levels of ammonia. This could be explained on a basis that urease within the mouth may convert urea to ammonia. This end product fosters the stomatitis. Acute parotitis can be prevented by proper oral hygiene.

Uremic stomatitis is treated by removing the tooth tartrate by scraping. A mouthwash containing lemon juice or a 0.5 to 1% hydrochloric acid, a 3% hydrogen peroxide mouthwash, and potassium chlorate tablets dissolved in the mouth are all used. The ingestion of hard candy stimulates salivary flow, prevents dryness of the oral mucosa, and may aid in preventing stomatitis.

Monilia stomatitis has occurred in some patients with acute renal failure caused by lupus nephritis when so-called immunosuppressive agents were used. Benzalkonium (Zephiran) chloride solution rubbed over the growth has been useful in eradicating the infection.

Gastroenteritis

Anorexia, hiccups, nausea, vomiting, and diarrhea are nonspecific symptoms that reflect gastrointestinal involvement.[582,746] Esophagitis can produce heartburn, substernal pain, and epigastric pains, especially when the patient lies flat. In some patients, esophagitis was mistaken for pericardial or myocardial pain. Symptoms are released by antacids and antispasmodics such as atropine or belladonna.

A progressive diffuse erosive gastritis can produce symptoms similar to those of esophagitis. However, the symptoms may be more pronounced and the pain is located periumbilically. Uremic gastritis has progressed to ulceration and massive gastrointestinal hemorrhages. In some patients a fatal hemorrhage has resulted from numerous gastric erosions. Treatment consists of antacids and antispasmodic agents. In some patients nausea and vomiting occur in the morning and diarrhea occurs at night. Diarrhea may result from excessive urea secretion into the gut lumen. Furthermore, ulceration of the colon by urea has resulted in massive hemorrhage. Paregoric or atropine sulfate (Lomotil) has been very helpful in giving relief to the patient with almost intractable uremic colitis.

Uremic pancreatitis

The physician will have difficulty in deciding whether pancreatitis or acute renal failure is the primary disorder.[44,318] I have observed acute uremic pancreatitis as a frequent complication of acute renal failure.[682] The diagnosis may be missed unless a serum amylase is elevated.[84,385] Meroney and associates found elevated serum amylase levels in patients with acute renal failure without pathologic evidence of pancreatitis.[770] Moreover, extensive pancreatic damage may result in diabetes mellitus. This occurred in three patients who had neither a family history of diabetes mellitus nor prior clinical evidence of diabetes.

At autopsy, healed uremic pancreatitis was found in four patients with acute tubular necrosis. The necrosis was caused by prolonged hypotension in two, by gram-negative endotoxemia in one, and by accidental trauma in one.

Cardiovascular complications

The cardiovascular complications of acute renal failure are the greatest factors that influence the prognosis and outcome of the patient with acute renal failure.[505] Complications of the cardiovascular system result from a variety of causes and greatly modify the treatment. These complications include the following:

Primary illness producing cardiovascular complications

1. Systemic lupus erythematosus (perivasculitis, pericardial effusion, myocarditis)
2. Scleroderma (congestive heart failure, hypertension)
3. Acute glomerulonephritis (congestive heart failure, hypertension)
4. Polyarteritis nodosa (hypertensive congestive heart failure)
5. Alcoholism (myocardopathy with mural thrombi)
6. Hypersensitivity angiitis (myocarditis, hypertension)
7. Malignant hypertension (pulmonary edema)
8. Generalized Shwartzman phenomena (myocarditis, hypertension)
9. Endotoxemia (congestive heart failure, shock)
10. Hemorrhage (shock, pulmonary edema)

Abnormalities of renal failure producing cardiovascular complications
1. Potassium intoxication (dysrhythmia)
2. Uremia (pericarditis)
3. Hypertension (pulmonary edema)
4. Water overload (pulmonary edema)
5. Salt overload (pulmonary edema)
6. Mannitol overload (pulmonary edema)
7. Anemia (congestive heart failure)
8. Hypoproteinuria (pulmonary edema)
9. Digitalis intoxication (cardiac dysrhythmia)

In addition, a primary disorder involving the cardiovascular system can complicate acute renal failure.

Cardiac dysrhythmia

Potassium intoxication is the main cause of abnormalities of cardiac conduction. The intoxication can be aggravated by an associated acidosis, hyponatremia, or hypocalcemia. Because potassium intoxication is not related to a specific elevated level of potassium, the electrocardiogram is the outstanding instrument for determining potassium intoxication. Because of the rapid sequence of biochemical changes, continuing electronic monitoring is more accurate in determining changes in the QRS-T wave. Serum potassium levels produce changes not only in the QRS-T segment of the electrocardiogram, but also in the cardiac rhythm.

If cardiac conduction abnormalities result from potassium intoxication, the patient should be monitored by electronic devices. This method may detect more accurately the dynamic fluctuations and intensity of potassium intoxication. The conduction abnormalities vary from ventricular extrasystole to ventricular fibrillation, which is often the precursor of cardiac arrest in diastole.

The initial electrocardiographic change for hyperkalemia is the development of tall, peaked T waves. With greater increments of serum potassium levels, the T waves increase in height and acquire a narrow base. Changes in Q-T interval may reflect hypocalcemia. In severe hyperkalemia the QRS complexes broaden, indicating intraventricular conduction defects. Cardiac dysrhythmias follow.

Cardiac failure

In some patients with acute renal failure, congestive heart failure is of the "high output" variety. It is not caused by vitamin deficiences such as beriberi or heart disease. It is characterized by a rapid pulse, high venous pressure, wide pulse pressure, and, in some patients, a poor therapeutic response to digitalis. Some patients have an increased venous pressure and a rapid circulatory time; these patients have the usual congestive heart failure findings of dyspnea, cyanosis, tachycardia, gallop rhythms, and pulmonary congestion.[408]

The two leading factors that precipitate congestive heart failure are water overloading and hypertension. Next in frequency are anemia, overloading with sodium chloride, and overloading with an osmotic diuretic agent such as mannitol.

Hypertension occurs in patients with acute renal failure when the blood volume is expanded with plasma and blood. Moreover, the juxtaglomerular apparatus undergoes hypertrophy, and increased levels of renin are found.[1089] If the patient with acute renal failure is effectively treated by conservative measures, hypertension is less likely to occur.

Pericarditis

Wacher and Merrill found pericarditis in 18% of seventy-seven patients with acute oliguric renal failure.[1106] The pericarditis was mild and usually did not produce circulatory failure. Although cardiac tamponade caused by uremic pericarditis has been repeatedly noted in patients with chronic renal failure, it is rare in those with acute renal failure. Guild, Bray, and Merrill reported two patients with uremic pericarditis in whom the diagnosis of pericardial effusion was made during life and in whom removal of pericardial fluid resulted in both objective and subjective improvement.[483] Hutt and Holmes reported a fatal pericardial effusion that resulted in cardiac tamponade.[572]

The recognition and removal of cardiac tamponade can be life-saving. A diagnosis of fibrinous pericarditis can be made on the basis of a pericardial friction rub, pulsus paradoxus, increased venous pressure with inspiration, and decreased cardiac pulsation on fluoroscopy. Once a diagnosis is made of cardiac tamponade caused by pericardial effusion, the patient's life can be saved by pericardiocentesis.

Uremic pneumonitis

The pathogenesis and morphologic findings of uremic pneumonitis have not been well defined.[23,112] However, patients with uremia caused by acute renal failure have characteristic roentgenologic lung changes consisting of symmetric bilateral increased pulmonary densities extending bilaterally from the hilar areas.[72] They result in butterfly rings and have been referred to as the "sunburst" pattern. The x-ray finding has been attributed by some physicians to pulmonary edema and by others to uremia in the absence of congestive heart failure.* On dialysis there is roentgenologically remarkable clearing of the lung[11a] (Fig. 3-8).

Henkein and associates studied a patient with five episodes of uremic penumonia; his prompt response to dialysis, lung clearing, suggested that uremic pneumonitis was a distinct clinical entity.[537] In 1911, Lange described the original morphology of uremic pneumonitis. He related the change as obliterative bronchitis and attributed it to acute or subacute inflammation of the bronchiolar walls. The lung is increased in weight, appears indurated, and has central pneumonic infiltrations.[157,306] Approximately 30% of cases are further complicated

---

*See references 54, 71, 306, and 529.

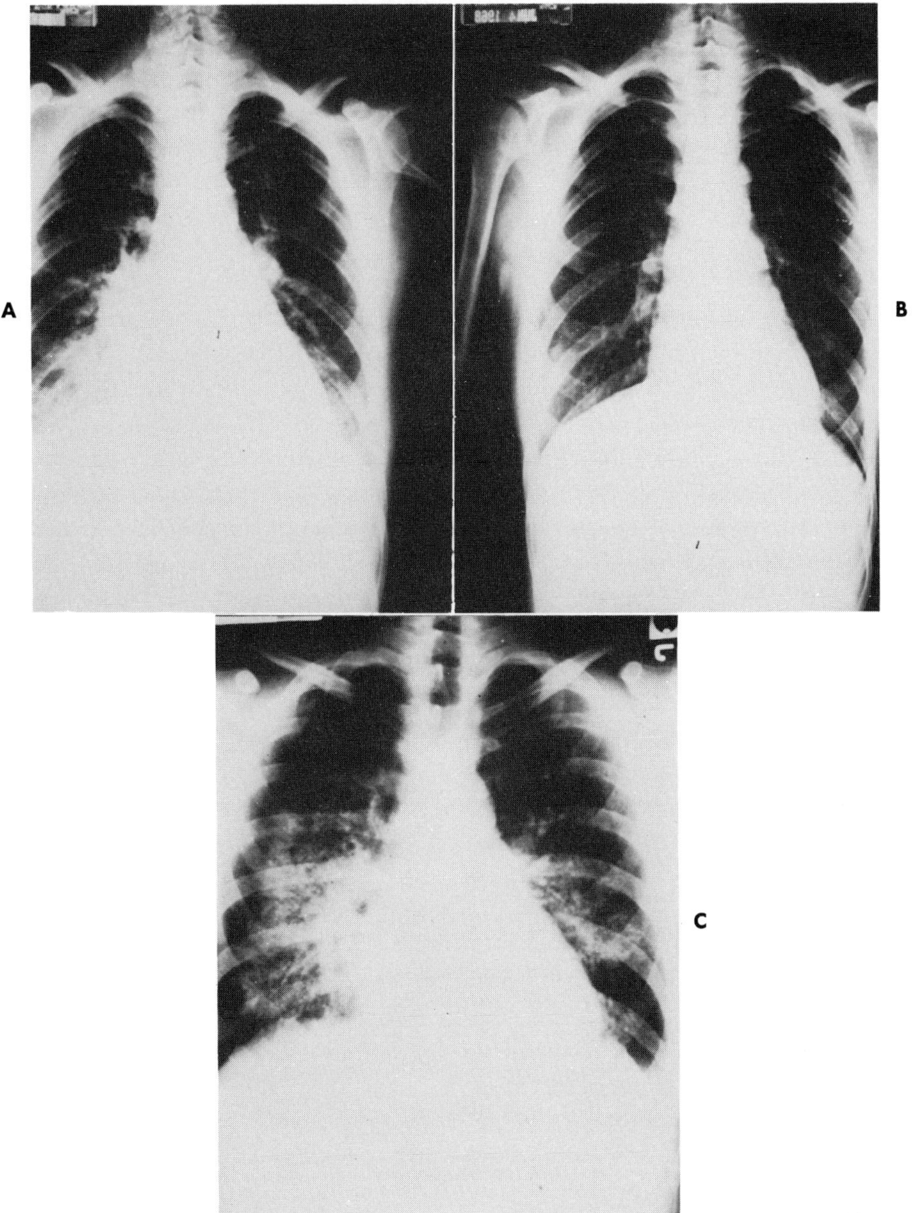

Fig. 3-8. A, Cardiomegaly and pulmonary edema caused by acute renal failure. A 40-year-old woman had acute renal failure caused by acute proliferative glomerulonephritis. She developed hypertension and congestive heart failure with pulmonary edema. On this chest x-ray, the heart is enlarged and the lung is edematous. **B,** Clearing of pulmonary edema and cardiomegaly following peritoneal dialysis. After 48 hours of peritoneal dialysis, the lungs cleared of pulmonary edema and the heart returned to normal size. Eleven liters of excess fluid were removed, using hypertonic (7.0%) glucose solution in peritoneal dialysis. **C,** Uremic pneumonitis. Uremic pneumonitis occurred in a 26-year-old male with acute renal failure caused by tubular necrosis. Following hemodialysis the pneumonitis, as noted in this chest x-ray, cleared.

by bacterial pneumonia, pulmonary infarction, passive congestion, or miliary atelectasis.[561]

Another factor regarding uremic pneumonitis is the central nervous system. In some patients pulmonary edema was noted to coincide with the generalized seizures. It is known that central nervous system activity can produce acute pulmonary edema; therefore, it is quite possible that some "unknown factor" present in patients with acute uremia produces central nervous system irritability.

Hypertensive encephalopathy

A slight rise in blood pressure usually occurs during oliguria.[441] Teschan found a considerable rise in blood pressure in 85% of both casualties. Hypertension during oliguria is common and is frequently found in overhydrated patients with acute oliguric renal failure. It is more likely to occur, however, when acute oliguria is caused by severe nephrosclerosis. Renin activity is increased in acute tubular necrosis.[1089] It has been associated with drug-induced glomerulonephritis, acute poststreptococcal glomerulonephritis, lupus nephritis, polyarteritis nodosa, and eclampsia and pre-eclampsia. Renin levels have been elevated during oliguria; this elevation has been associated with proliferation of the juxtaglomerular apparatus.

Parenteral hypotensive agents have been helpful in reducing the hypertension.[442] These include 2.5 mg of reserpine intramuscularly, 20 mg of hydralzine, and 500 mg of trimethaphan camphorsulfonate (Arfonad) diluted in 500 ml of 5% dextrose and infused at a rate of ten drops (0.5 mg) or more per minute. The latter method cannot be used when fluid is restricted. During oliguria parenteral injections of magnesium sulfate are very hazardous and should be avoided.

Nutritional complications

Before oliguria occurs, patients with acute renal failure are frequently but not always in a good nutritional state. If the patient survives the prolonged nutritional stress and metabolic demands on his body during oliguria, he enters the recovery stage in a state of severe nutritional and caloric bankruptcy. He is markedly depleted of proteins, amino acids, and energy stores. Severe anemia and vitamin deficiencies, usually of the water-soluble vitamins, are present. This is more pronounced if peritoneal dialysis is continued for a prolonged period and if body protein is removed in the dialysate. Deficiency of fat-soluble vitamins such as vitamin K and water-soluble vitamins such as folic acid[513] and vitamin B_{12} has occurred following prolonged peritoneal dialysis. Folic acid deficiency has occurred in patients with chronic renal failure undergoing chronic hemodialysis. Serum folate levels were below normal (7 to 15.9 μg/ml) in eleven of twenty-seven patients.[513] I observed folic acid deficiency in a postpartum patient with partial renal cortical necrosis. She had continuous peritoneal dialysis for 6 weeks. Her serum folate level was 9.5 μg/ml.

Hemorrhage

The uremic syndrome is complicated by hemorrhages in the skin (purpura), gastrointestinal tract (hematemesis and melena), or pericardial sac (cardiac tamponade), and from surgical wounds. Bleeding from the gastrointestinal tract is a common complication.

Hemorrhagic tendencies occur more frequently in patients with acute renal failure than in those with chronic renal failure.[844a,908] This is probably due to a variety of coagulation defects. The exact mechanism is not known. For example, thrombocytopenia was found in all patients with acute renal failure where bleeding caused death,[966] yet other patients had defects in the first stage of coagulation. Afribrinogenemia is common in patients with retroplacental hemorrhage.

Anemia

During the course of acute renal failure a moderate normochronic and normocytic anemia frequently develops early in the disorder and may approach a hematocrit of 28 to 30% in 10 to 14 days. Anemia is one of the cardinal findings in patients with acute renal failure, and it is well tolerated by the patients. The anemia reaches a low plateau near a hematocrit of 25% and remains constant. In general, the anemia results in part from suppression of hematopoiesis and in part from a hemolytic process.

In patients with acute renal failure anemia can result from hemolysis caused by the primary illness or by the initiating factor that produces acute renal failure.[1045] In addition, hemorrhage produces anemia caused by either the primary illness or by a defect that accompanies disruption in the coagulation mechanism.

Production and destruction

In patients with the uremic syndrome the metabolic abnormalities impair the production and secretions of an erythropoietic substance and thus inhibit the erythoid response of the bone marrow to exogenous erythropoietic-rich serum.

There is much confusion in the literature concerning the degree and importance of red blood cell destruction. Because many variables exist, it is difficult to ascertain the exact relationship of any one factor to erythrocyte destruction.

Primary illness

The primary illness or the primary precipitating factor of acute renal failure can produce severe anemias. This production occurs through many mechanisms, the outstanding of which is intravascular hemolysis. Second in importance is that which results from hemorrhage. The intravascular hemolysis of erythrocytes results from a variety of causes; these include primary diseases of the erythrocytes such as sickle cell disease, burns, drugs (sulfonamides, quinine sulfate), nephrotoxins (arsine), falciparum malaria, distilled water, radiation, and systemic diseases such as systemic lupus erythematosus. Hemolysis can also result from microangiopathic processes associated with the defibrination syndrome and consumption coagulopathy. These include the generalized Shwartzman reaction, sepsis, eclampsia with capillary thrombosis and fibrin deposition, arteriolar thrombosis as seen in the hemolytic-uremic syndrome dissecting aneurysm, and neoplasms, and in association with TTP.

Hemorrhage resulting from a surgical procedure or trauma, or spontaneous or undetected hemorrhage such as retroperitoneal bleeding can produce anemia with an associated renal ischemia and subsequent acute renal failure. Furthermore, hemorrhage can result from coagulation defects such as those associated with afibrinoginemia or from conditions in which factors of coagulation are utilized in formation of multiple thrombosis (eclampsia, sickle cell disease, arteriolar thrombosis). The consumption coagulopathy results in decreased fibrinogen, platelets, factor II, factor V, and factor VIII.

I have found marked prolongation of the prothrombin time in patients undergoing continuous peritoneal dialysis for periods of up to 4 weeks. Prior to dialysis these patients had normal prothrombin times. It is believed that excessive amounts of vitamin K were removed with the peritoneal fluid. Intramuscularly administered vitamin K restored the patients' prothrombin times to normal.

Another patient with renal cortical necrosis had continuous peritoneal dialysis for 6 weeks. She developed an anemia believed to be caused by vitamin B_{12} or folic acid deficiency. A hematologic study revealed a macrocytic anemia. On a bone marrow study, megaloblastic proliferation was noted. After vitamin B_{12} was administered, there was an increase in the red cell mass and reticulocyte count.

The physician may sometimes have difficulty in distinguishing what component of the anemia was caused by blood loss and what component was caused by acute renal failure. The anemia of acute renal failure is probably an adaptive mechanism of the patient. Unless the anemia reaches critical levels (hematocrit below 22%), produces symptoms, or contributes to heart failure, packed erythrocytes are not indicated and may be hazardous to the patient. Iron supplements and liver are of no benefit to correct the anemia. Following recovery from acute renal failure anemia may persist for months.

Chapter 4

The etiology and pathogenesis of "acute tubular necrosis"

Acute oliguric renal failure results from many etiologic conditions, the frequency of which varies from one country to another and from one age group to another.[808,1110] Precipitating factors are numerous and include shock, endotoxins, ischemia, infection, hemolytic crisis, nephrotoxins, acute hypersensitivity reactions, intrinsic renal disease, and renal vascular damage (Fig. 4-1). This variation of factors is exemplified in the words of Oliver: "There is no single 'cause' of oliguria but a great collection of them."[847]

Insults to the body at sites far remote from the kidney may reduce the renal blood flow to such low levels that little or no urine is formed. These etiologic factors disturb renal function, damage the kidney, and result in acute renal failure. In view of the etiologic uncertainties about acute renal failure, a number of terms are offered to describe this condition. They include traumatic uremia,[262,-188] lower nephron syndrome,[178] traumatic anuria,[43,191] posttraumatic anuria,[181,238] hemoglobinuric nephrosis, anoxic nephrosis, ischemic nephrosis, crush syndrome,[194] compression syndrome, lower nephron nephrosis,[265] shock kidney,[261] toxic nephrosis,[816] and acute tubular necrosis.[126]

In approximately 30% of all patients the etiology of acute oliguria is unknown. In other patients the etiology is quite specific, and in some the etiology is multiple. Therefore not only single mechanisms but combinations of mechanisms may explain the pathophysiology of acute oliguric renal failure.[394,395]

INTRODUCTION

When acute oliguric renal failure is caused by acute glomerulonephritis, necrotizing arteritis, or renal cortical necrosis, the extensive renal damage makes it easy to understand the pathophysiology of oliguria. Excluding primary parenchymal diseases of the glomeruli, interstitium, arteries, and arterioles, therefore, the pathogenesis of acute renal failure is difficult to explain. In general the patho-

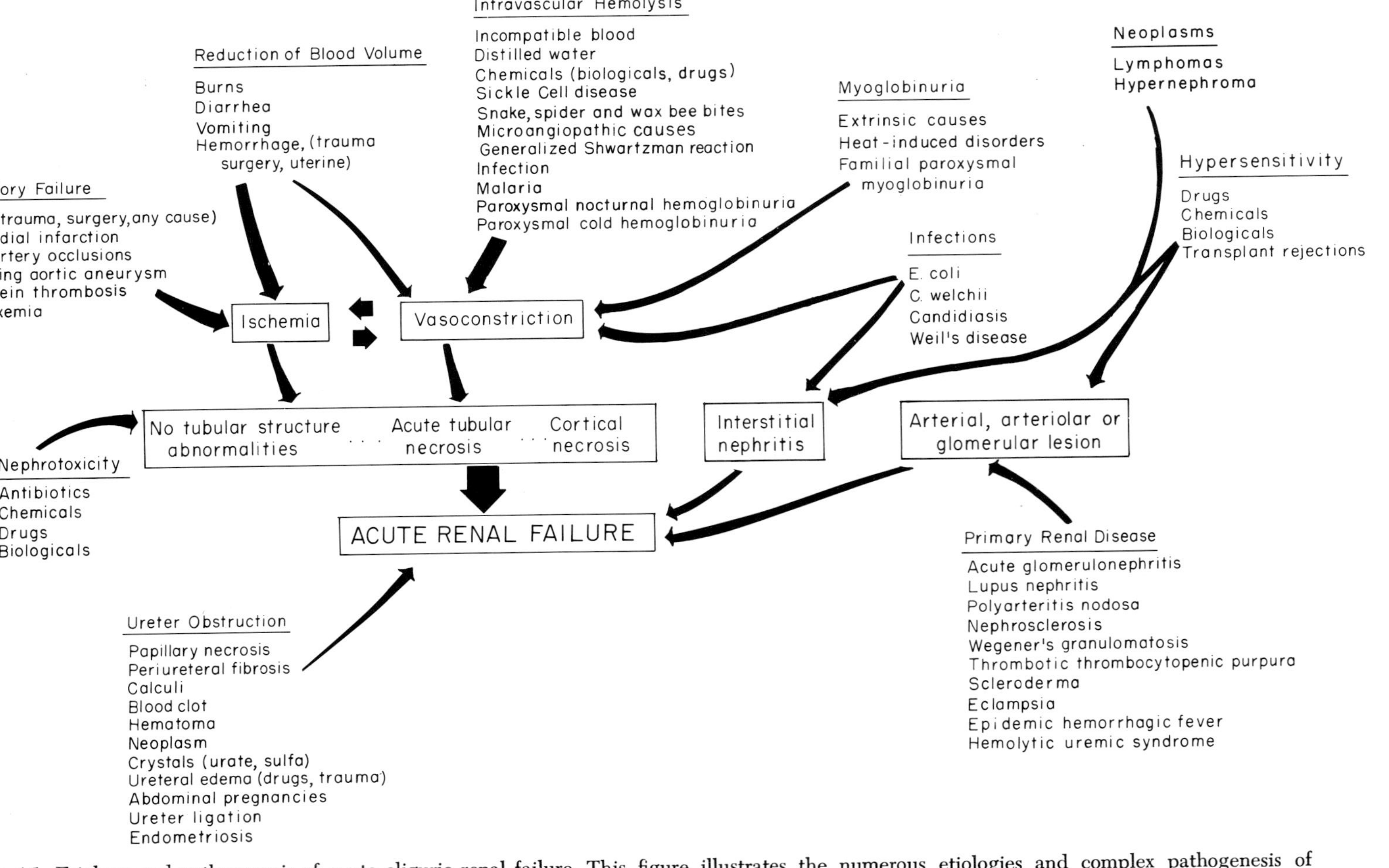

Fig. 4-1. Etiology and pathogenesis of acute oliguric renal failure. This figure illustrates the numerous etiologies and complex pathogenesis of acute oliguric renal failure. The reader is referred to the text for a detailed explanation.

genesis can be discussed from two major aspects—ischemia and nephrotoxicity. These were emphasized in a clearly defined manner by Oliver.[849] Classifying the pathogenesis of acute oliguric renal failure into two groups is an oversimplification of a complex disorder. Oliver studied the morphologic lesions produced by these two salient groups and found that in "severely damaged kidneys" not all nephrons were affected and that in some kidneys "only occasional ones" were affected.[849] He interpreted this finding as the effect of patchy renal vasoconstriction and ischemia. In addition, he found that ischemia (tubulorrhexis) produced complete disruption of the tubular epithelium with basement membrane fragmentation. When nephrotoxins produced acute oliguria, he found tubular necrosis without basement membrane changes (nephrotoxic). He believed that this structural finding was a major factor in the explanation of the pathogenesis of acute renal failure.

Theories for the pathogenesis of acute renal failure

Numerous hypotheses have been put forward regarding the pathogenesis of acute renal failure since Bywaters' first reports on the "crush syndrome" in 1941.[188] These hypotheses include renal ischemia, vasoconstriction, reduced renal blood flow, tubular obstruction, interstitial edema, and nephrotoxicity.[149]

Renal ischemia

Renal ischemia caused by reduction of the renal blood flow is the most common factor responsible for acute renal failure.[555] It is present when acute tubular necrosis occurs in association with severe circulatory failure. The concept of renal ischemia has been accepted without critical review and was first made known by Foy in 1943.[47,390] The exact pathogenesis of renal ischemia is a complex mechanism and is confused by experimental data. If ischemia were the sole factor in producing acute tubular necrosis, one would expect to find distal tubular necrosis as frequently as proximal necrosis; however, this is not the case. Furthermore, the role of ischemia in perpetuating oliguria once acute tubular necrosis has been initiated has been a point of great controversy.

Many individuals speak of ischemia in the same sense as they speak of decreased renal blood flow.[993] There are few observations available on renal circulation during acute renal failure. The renal blood flow determined by radioactive krypton has been reported as being normal in dogs with oliguria.[161,1082] Other investigators, who used a flowmeter in the renal vein and who took direct measurements, found a decrease in renal blood flow in acute renal failure. To measure renal blood flow, Bull and his colleagues used the direct Fick principle and PAH for determination.[173] They found that renal blood flow during oliguria was reduced in two patients to 3 to 5% of normal. They did not take into consideration that low A-V differences of PAH make this particular technique inaccurate. Moreover, not only did their observations lack controls, but no comparison was made with healthy individuals. In general, data on renal blood flow in various stages of acute renal failure are scanty; if more controlled data were available it might be possible to obtain a more exact solution.

Prolonged reduction in effective circulating blood volume with prolonged vasoconstriction is sufficient to result in renal ischemia.[512] When ischemia is intense and prolonged, renal damage usually occurs. This damage can vary from mild tubular abnormalities to diffuse complete renal cortical necrosis. Brun and Munk studied patients who had acute renal failure during oliguria caused by acute tubular necrosis. They found that renal blood flow frequently exceeded the levels considered necessary to produce irreversible tubular lesions.[161] Although ischemia is necessary in initiating the sequence of events leading to oliguria, it is not the only factor that causes acute tubular necrosis.

Current experimental data do not support the theory that hemorrhagic shock produces damaging renal hypoxia despite the marked reduction in renal blood flow.[562] Therefore, the belief that hypoxia initiates acute oliguric renal failure following shock must be challenged. Other factors associated with renal ischemia include catecholamines, epinephrine,[564] endotoxins, and pigments. A "shock-producing factor" capable of inducing anuria has been demonstrated in vessels from normal subjects. Such substances released from cells damaged as a result of trauma or prolonged hypotension might increase the sensitivity of blood vessels to substances such as catecholamines.

Waugh and associates believe that the earliest lesion in acute renal failure caused by ischemia is the infraglomerular epithelial reflex;[1115,1116] it is a detachment and upward displacement of uppermost epithelium of the proximal tubules. The detached pyknotic epithelial cells occupy a portion of the urinary space of Bowman's capsule. This lesion was first described by Councilman in 1857 and has been referred to as desquamative glomerulonephritis,[241] epithelial protrusions,[750] and penetration of convoluted tubular epithelium into the glomerulus.

The infraglomerular epithelial reflex was observed in kidneys of rats with serotonin experimental—induced acute renal failure. It lasts not more than 6 hours and is believed to be the result of the flushing of the upper nephron with the reestablishment of glomerular filtration. The reflex was found in six of seven adequately documented cases that showed evidence of terminal renal ischemia or acute oliguria.

Renal blood flow

When man is in a normal state of health, his abdominal organs receive about half the cardiac output; of this amount, his kidneys receive approximately 50 to 60%. If the cardiac output diminishes or if the blood volume decreases,[51] circulatory economy results from vasoconstriction and a subsequent reduction in the renal blood flow occurs, followed by reduction of urine flow. In patients with chronic renal failure the renal blood flow may be reduced to 20% of normal; however, they usually have a large urinary output. On the other hand, the patients with acute oliguric renal failure with a similar renal blood flow must have associated acute intrarenal changes of vasoconstriction to account for the reduced urine output. It is quite possible that shunting of renal blood occurs, bypassing the superficial cortical glomeruli. Pappenheimer postulated the "plasma skimming" mechanism to explain the redistribution of erythrocytes.[860] The patchy cortical ischemia observed by Oliver could be the result of focal renal ischemia caused by focal renal vasoconstriction or by plasma skimming.[849]

At rest, the normal renal blood flow is approximately one-fifth of the cardiac output, or about 1,100 ml per minute. The renal blood flow is reduced when the individual is upright, when he is exercising, when he is exposed to heat, if he is malnourished, after he receives epinephrine, and when he reaches old age. If the circulating blood volume is reduced or if the heart fails, the renal blood flow falls.[814] To economize, there is an associated compensating renal vasoconstriction.[121] This occurs even though the peripheral blood pressure remains unchanged. The compensating redistribution of blood flow after hemorrhage ensures almost normal blood flow to protect the integrity of the heart and brain.

Blackburn measured renal blood flow in patients with acute renal failure caused by infusions of distilled water.[116] He concluded that renal ischemia was present. Vasoconstriction with reduced blood flow to the kidney and liver results in maintenance of normal central blood pressure at the expense of the renal circulation. The reduced renal blood flow is associated with a reduced glomerular filtration rate and thus with a decrease in excretion of solutes such as sodium.

Tubular obstruction theory

Obstruction of the nephron by casts or cellular debris is another explanation of the pathogenesis of acute renal failure. Tubular obstruction has reportedly caused intratubular pressure and hence reduction of glomerular filtration, but this theory has been questioned. The nephron can be obstructed from within its lumen by necrotic cellular debris, by decomposed body pigments such as degradation products of hemoglobin and myoglobin, or by protein casts of multiple myeloma;[556] it can be obstructed externally by interstitial edema[821] (Fig. 4-2).

Yorke and Nauss in 1911 first recognized an association between hemolytic disease, acute renal failure, and hemoglobin casts in renal tubules.[1143] Fourteen years later, Baker and Dodds related acute renal failure to tubular obstructions in rabbits caused by the precipitation of acid hematin in acid urine of high sodium concentration.[49,108] They suggested alkalization of the urine to afford protection against cast formation and subsequent renal injury. In other rabbit experiments, Bywaters and Stead found that the deposition of myoglobin within renal tubules and the production of oliguria were also enhanced in acidotic states.[195] It was believed that intrarenal tubular obstruction produced tubular lumen dilatation above the obstruction with partial collapse of the glomerular structure. The most significant argument against this mechanism is that both

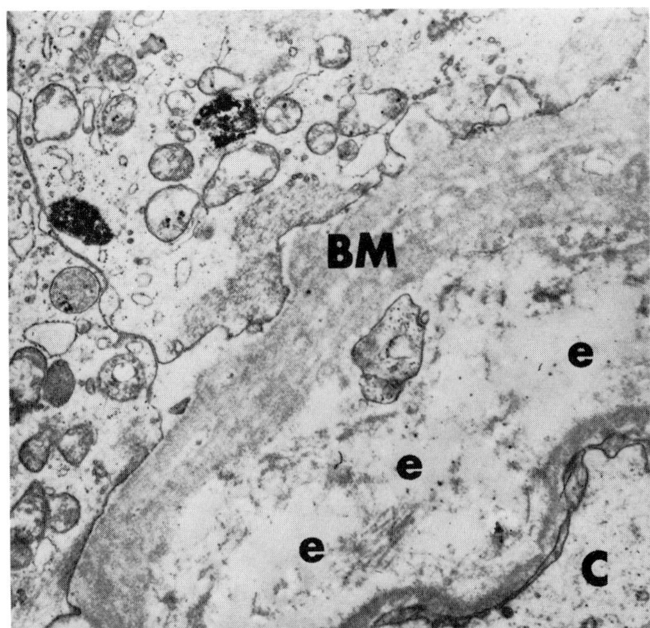

Fig. 4-2. Interstitial edema in acute tubular necrosis. A renal biopsy was obtained from a patient with acute tubular necrosis during acute anuria. The tubular basement membrane (BM) was thickened. A peritubular capillary (C) was noted (right bottom). Between the tubular basement membrane and the peritubular capillary was a striking interstitial edema (e) with a few collagen fibers. (×13,000.)

biopsy and necropsy findings indicate an insufficient overall number of affected nephrons to account for massive nephron failure and to produce oliguria.

Meroney and Rubini explained the pathogenesis of acute renal failure as the precipitation of protein and cellular debris within the lumen of collecting tubules, distal tubules, and the ascending loops of Henle.[771]

The theory of renal tubular blockage by pigmented debris forms the basis for some physicians to give large quantities of fluids to dissolve, dilute, and "flush out" the pigmented casts. The severely dehydrated patient or the patient with prerenal failure may be helped. However, many patients given excessive fluids for oliguria have drowned "in their own fluid" because of iatrogenically induced acute congestive heart failure with pulmonary edema.

Interstitial edema and interstitial pressure

In 1945, Peters and associates attributed oliguria to an increased interstitial pressure produced by interstitial edema.[879] Although interstitial edema is a frequent finding in renal biopsy sections from patients with acute tubular necrosis (Fig. 2-20), it is not usually present in the kidneys of patients with oliguria caused by glomerular or vascular renal disease. The importance of interstitial edema is that it may be a morphologic reflection of increased interstitial pressure. Therefore, an increase in the renal interstitial pressure may explain alterations such as suppression of glomerular filtration, decrease in urinary flow, and subsequent oliguria.[1057,1113]

The renal interstitial pressure may be defined as the hydrostatic pressure exerted at the tip of the needle containing fluid that is inserted into the renal interstitium. Winton refers to this pressure as the "needle pressure."[1134] Reubi measured the needle pressure in eight patients with a variety of renal diseases.[918] Five patients had elevation of the blood nonprotein nitrogen. The intrarenal pressure ranged between 23.5 and 41.5 mm Hg, with a mean pressure of 34.0 mm Hg. There was no significant difference in renal pressure between the patients with azotemia and those without it. Intrarenal interstitial needle pressure more correctly reflects the result of the damage to local capillaries, tubules, and renal interstitium.

Brun and associates used an indirect method to measure the intrarenal pressure.[162] They wedged a cardiac catheter into an interlobar vein. The external catheter end was attached to a condenser manometer. Because the renal interlobar veins had no direct anastomoses between the arcuate veins and the calyceal veins, the pressure at the catheter tip occluding an intralobar vein could not be less than or greater than that in the arcuate veins. Brun and associates referred to this pressure as the "wedge renal vein pressure" (WRVP). They believed that this pressure approximated the pressure within the interlobular veins and the peritubular capillaries. Thus, the resulting pressure should be similar to the renal interstitial pressure. The WRVP found by Brun and associates was significantly lower than the intrarenal pressure noted by Reubi.

Munck believed that pressure in a catheter wedged into a renal vein was the true intrarenal pressure.[813] However, wedged renal pressure of healthy individuals was similar to that of patients with acute oliguric renal failure. Flanigan and Oken found no difference between the hydrostatic pressure of the tubule and of the peritubular capillaries in normal rat kidneys.[380] These data suggested that no significant hydrostatic pressure gradient existed between cortical tubules and renal interstitium. The tubules were both collapsible and distensible. The interstitial fluid was a ready source of fluid coming from renal lymphatics and veins. These two facts should result in an equilibrium of pressure differences between renal interstitium and tubules.

Oliver observed that interstitial edema disappeared as the tubular lesion healed.[849] Merrill emphasized the reabsorption of the interstitial edema to decompress the nephron before renal function was restored.[773a] Although Brun observed interstitial edema in 25% of his patients with acute renal failure,[164] in our laboratory most renal biopsy specimens obtained during the oliguric phase from patients with so-called acute tubular necrosis revealed the striking presence of interstitial edema. This edema occurred secondary to tubular injury and was the forerunner of a more serious pathologic process—diffuse interstitial fibrosis. When tubular repair and healing were slow and oliguria was prolonged, the interstitium was more prone to undergo interstitial fibrosis that in time resulted in irreversible impaired renal function.

Several hypotheses are present regarding the development of interstitial edema. Some believe that it is the result of fluid leaking through damaged tubules into the interstitium, but I do not share this view. A uniformly diffuse and severe interstitial edema has been observed in kidneys during prolonged oliguria when normal tubules were found by electron microscopy (Fig. 2-11).

Interstitial edema probably occurs secondary to the primary renal insult and appears to increase quantitatively with the duration of oliguria. The massive interstitial edema accounts for the increase in renal size and mass (Fig. 2-5). The correct hypothesis for interstitial edema is probably that it results from and accompanies an inflammatory renal response to some insult or injury to the renal parenchyma. The insult may be ischemia or a nephrotoxic agent.

If interstitial edema is diffuse and is associated with tubular obstruction, one may postulate an overall decrease in glomerular filtration rate. This increased interstitial pressure effect on the peritubular capillaries may cause a decrease in renal blood flow. Hinshaw observed that the effective blood flow driving force is the difference between the renal arterial pressure and the interstitial pressure.[549] This may account for the marked reduction in renal blood flow and the congestion of the renal medullae.

Vascular shunts

During World War II, Trueta and associates investigated the renal vascular response of rabbits to trauma.[1088] In addition, they stimulated the sciatic and splanchnic nerve endings and observed a shunting of renal blood flow from the cortical glomeruli to the juxtamedullary glomeruli. They postulated that renal blood was diverted from cortical glomeruli to juxtamedullary glomeruli and that this mechanism explained a decreased urinary output. They did not offer the shunting of renal blood as an explanation for the mechanism of acute renal failure caused by acute tubular necrosis. They were probably observing the effects of severe renal vasoconstriction.[1088]

From other animal experiments, in which tourniquets were applied to the hind limbs and the animals bled massively, conclusions were derived that the renal cortex became ischemic because the blood was shunted to the renal medullae.[235] This mechanism accounted for a pale cortex and a dark, blood-rich medulla. Other investigations indicated that the total renal blood flow must be greatly reduced to obtain a pale cortex and dark medulla. Still other studies indicated that a dark medulla may be a congested medulla with little blood flow.[447] This is similar to the trapping of the blood in veins when vasoconstriction occurs. If renal medullary blood flow is reduced to such a degree that hypoxia occurs, structural damage may result.

In a series of rabbit experiments, Trueta demonstrated that intense anoxia and hypercapnea produce diversion of blood flow away from the renal cortex with subsequent blanching of the renal cortex and concomitant oliguria.[1088] This reflex originates centrally, probably through chemosensitive spinal cord centers below the fourth thoracic vertebra, and mediates through the sympathetic nerves that accompany the renal arteries.[448]

Flanigan and Oken induced anuria in rats with mercuric chloride and, using micropuncture techniques, studied the nephron.[380] They believed that decreased glomerular filtration rate was caused by any one of or a combination of the following: preglomerular vascular constriction, postglomerular dilatation, and preglomerular shunting.

Nephrotoxins

The kidney, because of its rich blood supply and its ability to concentrate substances, is especially vulnerable to toxic agents. Nephrotoxins are chemicals, drugs, and biologic products in any physical form that, when inhaled, ingested, injected, or absorbed into the body, result in toxic degradation products that circulate in the bloodstream to disrupt the kidney function.[1001] They act directly on the renal cells to interfere with their functional and structural integrity.[704]

Nephrotoxins can inflict damage on any one of the four major renal components—the glomeruli, the tubules,[820] the vessels, and the interstitium.[719] This damage occurs through one or more of several specific mechanisms: through immunologic mechanisms, through hypersensitivity mechanisms, directly as a protoplasmic poison, or indirectly through hemolysis, electrolyte imbalance, or dehydration. Moreover, nephrotoxins may aggravate preexisting disease. Nephrotoxins will be discussed in greater detail on pp. 203.

Experimentally induced acute renal failure

Numerous animal experiments have been done in an attempt to produce the syndrome of acute oliguric renal failure.* Nephrotoxins and ischemic hemolytic mechanisms have been used, and shock has been induced. Under such experimental conditions the kidney has been studied by light and electron microscopy, by micropuncture, by microdissection, by immunopathology, by histochemical methods, and by ultramicrochemical techniques.[1105]

Shock

Investigators have used dogs, rabbits, and rats without success.[589] One exception is a dog experiment by Conn and associates.[232] They produced shock in dogs by serial infusions of human blood; they made simultaneous measurements in renal blood flow by using a bubble flow meter and by determining kidney uptake of inert nitrous oxide gas. One dog developed acute renal failure that lasted for several days. In general, most of the animals had anuria during shock; as a result

---

*See references 239, 254, 366, and 589.

of recovering from shock, they made a complete recovery and their renal function returned to normal.

Nephrotoxicity

Since Pavy's first report in 1860 on animal experimentation with mercury salts, there has been considerable controversy about the level of the nephron affected by this nephrotoxin.[869] In 1929, Richards studied the effects of mercury on the nephrons of frogs.[924] He found apparently normal glomerular circulation and function. He concluded that anuria resulted from the reabsorption of the glomerular filtrate by the tubules. He did not mention his method in recording the glomerular filtration rate. Oliver perfused 10 ml of 1:10,000 corrosive sublimate in Locke's solution into the renal arteries of frogs.[845] He noted a prompt decrease in urinary output to about a third of central values. When he perfused mercury through the peritubular circulation by way of the renal portal vein, the urinary volume increased fourfold. Oliver's results were directly opposite to Richards' observation of decreased urinary output.

Edwards[334] and others* have localized the renal lesion in rats to the proximal convoluted tubules, particularly the terminal segment.[836] Edwards found a similar location in guinea pigs, rabbits, and frogs. Simonds and Hepler localized these lesions in dogs to a similar segment.[1015] On the other hand, Oliver placed the mercury-induced lesion of rats in all cortical tubules.[846,849] Others used dogs and described damage to the ascending Henle's loops as well as to the proximal convoluted tubules.[570] Burmeister and McNally implicated the subcapsular tubules in dogs given bichloride of mercury.[179]

Harmon[517] and Oliver and associates[849] described in patients with mercury poisoning degenerative changes in Henle's loops and in convoluted tubules. The previously mentioned conflicting observations may result from a variation in experimental factors such as dose of mercury or method of determining the level of damage.

Ischemia

Renal artery occlusion also fails to produce acute oliguric renal failure. The animals usually develop multiple large renal infarcts. The extensive literature dealing with induced renal failure in animals and the ability of the renal tubules to withstand ischemia emphasizes species differences and the variation in animal reaction to the ischemic insult.[882,1071] Dogs appear to be more resistant to prolonged ischemia than are man and rats. Infusion of epinephrine into dogs produces extensive renal ischemia and subsequent anuria, while in rabbits epinephrine produces acute bilateral renal cortical necrosis. For some unknown reason rabbits tend to develop renal cortical necrosis rather than tubular necrosis.[571] This may be explained by the fact that rabbits have juxtamedullary shunts.

---

*See references 538, 766, 937, and 938.

In man, if the renal veins are clamped before the renal artery is occluded, anuria of several days' duration occurs. However, if the renal artery is occluded and draining of the renal blood is permitted prior to occlusion of the renal vein, a diuresis occurs that lasts for 45 to 65 minutes.

Teschan has produced acute renal failure in rats without subjecting them to prior ischemia.[818,1070-1072] He injected them with methemoglobin and sodium ferrocyanide. It is important to stress his exact techniques and sequence of methods that produced acute renal failure. Details of the Teschan model can be found elsewhere.[1070] In general, he induced acute renal failure in rats by means of an "induction injection" of a "methemoglobin (0.5 mg/kg) and sodium ferrocyanide (14.3 mg/kg) mixture." The rats were pretreated with an acid-ash diet for 4 days, were dehydrated for 24 hours, and were given unrestricted access to the same diet and water approximately 1 to 4 hours following injection. Forty-eight hours later, Teschan used the plasma urea nitrogen level as an index of acute renal failure.

The Teschan model of acute renal failure in rats has a clinical course comparable to that seen in man and also has renal morphologic abnormalities similar to those in man. This was pointed out by Schaefer,[959] who repeated Teschan's work and made a comparison of the pathologic findings of the rat kidneys with the lesions in man described by Mallory and by Lucke.[712] Schaefer found a great similarity between changes.

ISCHEMIC ETIOLOGY OF ACUTE RENAL FAILURE

Renal ischemia is a prominent feature of acute oliguric renal failure and is the result of circulatory failure. Reduction in the effective circulating blood volume reduces circulation restriction and vasoconstriction caused by body pigments.[1098] Circulatory failure can result from massive myocardial infarction, from a dissecting aortic aneurysm, from traumatic shock after an automobile accident, from intra-abdominal catastrophes, from electric shock therapy,[223] from crushing muscle injuries, from gram-negative endotoxemia, from massive pulmonary embolism, and from surgical shock. Reduction in the effective circulatory blood volume results from plasma loss such as that caused by burns, from electrolyte and water loss associated with severe and prolonged vomiting or diarrhea as seen in Asian cholera, from loss of whole blood during surgery,[128] and from massive hemorrhage caused by trauma or by internal hemorrhage.

The common pathophysiologic pathway to all of these conditions is initiated by ischemia and is aggravated by unknown factors. It is followed by a series of compensatory homeostatic reactions (Fig. 3-10): decrease in blood volume $\longrightarrow$ decrease in cardiac output $\longrightarrow$ renal vasoconstriction $\longrightarrow$ renal ischemia $\longrightarrow$ disruption of renal tubular integrity $\longrightarrow$ acute tubular damage $\longrightarrow$ acute tubular necrosis $\longrightarrow$ acute oliguric renal failure. If ischemia is severe, sudden, and prolonged, renal damage may extend to a diffuse bilateral renal cortical necrosis.

Acute circulatory failure

The common pathogenesis in the development of acute oliguric renal failure is circulatory failure, which could be associated with either a reduced central venous pressure or an elevated central venous pressure. The causative factors of circulatory failure can be divided into three categories—hypovolemic factors, cardiogenic factors, and low circulatory resistance. Initially they produce acute renal circulatory failure. If not effectively treated, acute renal circulatory failure can progress to renal parenchymal lesions of acute tubular necrosis and bilateral renal cortical necrosis.

Hypovolemia

Hypovolemia results from a reduction in circulating blood volume, which is caused by either fluid loss or blood loss. It can be determined more exactly by measuring the circulatory blood volume and by monitoring the central venous pressure.

Hypovolemia caused by fluid loss. Fluid loss can occur either acutely or gradually. An example of the latter is the chronic use of oral diuretic agents that produce hypovolemia and sudden oliguria.[104] Hypovolemia can follow acute fluid loss[504] that occurs into the abdominal cavity from acute inflammatory disorders such as peritonitis, pancreatitis, and perforation of the gut. In addition, acute fluid loss commonly results from gastrointestinal disorders such as severe gastroenteritis—for example, Asiatic cholera.[90] Severe fluid loss can occur through the skin as a result of extensive body surface burns.[118]

Asiatic cholera. Vibrio cholerae produces a profuse watery diarrhea, thirst, vomiting, dehydration, and shock. Despite proper rehydration, a late and often fatal complication of Asiatic cholera is acute renal failure. In 1921, Rogers suggested that hypotension and impaired circulation produced acute anuria in patients with cholera.[939a] In 1941, Tomb related the renal pathology of cholera-induced acute renal failure to that of renal anoxia.[1084]

Acute tubular necrosis is commonly seen in patients with anuria caused by cholera.[90,730] In addition, acute tubular changes of superimposed hypokalemic changes may be seen (Fig. 4-6). De, Sengupta, and associates clarified the pathogenesis by differentiating between the initial anuria of hemoconcentration and that of circulatory collapse.[272] Patients with acute cholera may lose excessive water in the stool and may develop very severe shock and/or hemoconcentration. Acute oliguria usually occurs within the first few hours of the severe diarrhea. In addition to fluid loss, as much as 131 mEq of potassium can be lost daily. This loss is increased if large quantities of sodium are given.[472]

Fluids and electrolytes must be replaced hourly. Accurate measurements of body weight serve as a guide in fluid replacement. In addition to replacing fluids and electrolytes, one must supplement an adequate carbohydrate and fat diet.

Burns. Body burns can result from flash fires, steam, electricity, lightning, and scalding liquids. Severe body burns are complicated by infection, septicemia, coma,[527] pneumonia, cardiac arrest, acute renal failure, pulmonary edema, hepatitis, pulmonary embolism, and/or Curling's ulcer.[746] The prime cause of death of burn patients is usually septicemia.[444]

Oliguria is common in burn patients; it usually results from a combination of factors.[856] (A rare cause is fibrin thrombi within glomerular capillaries.[745]) These factors, which include dehydration, ischemia, burn toxin, a reduced blood volume, and hypovolemia,[233] play a large role in the pathogenesis of acute renal failure. Both acute oliguric and nonoliguric renal failure are directly related to the body surface burned.[458] One must differentiate between oliguria caused by prerenal causes and that caused by intrinsic renal disease. Moreover, one must consider the possibility of a rapidly rising BUN as the result of overwhelming urea production from the breakdown of injured tissues and from infected areas. A rapidly rising BUN can also result from dehydration caused by the large loss of extracellular fluid through the exposed body surface.[516]

Septicemia is common and is usually caused by *Escherichia coli* or by *Pseudomonas aeruginosa*. Microscopic hematuria is an almost constant finding in burn patients. Hemoglobinuria occurs as a result of a burn toxin or disseminated infection.

Shortly after the burn the urinary specific gravity is high (1.035 or more). This level reflects dehydration, sodium chloride depletion, or prerenal circulatory failure. Once renal damage occurs the urinary specific gravity is fixed near 1.010.

Hypovolemia caused by acute hemorrhage. Hypovolemia caused by blood loss usually results from spontaneous hemorrhage into the gastrointestinal tract, abdominal cavity, and pleural cavity. The hemorrhage results from a ruptured abdominal aortic aneurysm, from accidental trauma, from postpartum uterine hemorrhage, and from surgical hemorrhage.

Cardiogenic factor

Insufficient cardiac output can result from cardiac tamponade, congestive heart failure, cardiac dysrythmia, acute myocardial infarction, dissecting thoracic aortic aneurysm, and pulmonary embolism. Central venous pressure measurements are usually elevated. In addition to the treatment of acute oliguria, treatment is directed toward the correction of the primary precipitating disorder. Acute oliguric renal failure from cardiogenic factors carries a very grave prognosis; the mortality rate varies between 65 and 90%. Death occurs as a result of the precipitating illness.

Reduced circulatory resistance

Reduced circulatory resistance results from gram-negative endotoxins, hypersensitivity reactions, acidosis, hyponatremia, and adrenal insufficiency. Other factors that reduce circulatory resistance include drugs such as barbiturates and anesthetic agents. There are vasodilation, hypotension, and a reduced central venous pressure. Oliguria caused by reduced effective circulatory resistance can be rapidly reversed. Therefore, effective treatment must be started soon after the onset of oliguria. If precipitating factors are not corrected, parenchymal damage usually results. Monitoring of central venous pressure is very important in early detection so that effective treatment can be initiated.

Surgery

Acute oliguria is a relatively rare complication of major surgery, and for this reason is often overlooked.[128,801,834] Although the primary condition may carry a high mortality risk, delay in diagnosis of renal failure and inadequate treatment of oliguria make the total condition much worse.[540] Numerous mechanisms, occurring either singly or in combination, can explain oliguria following operative surgery.[496] These include fluid restriction, use of drugs and anesthetic agents,[128] infection, surgical trauma, and blood loss.[977]

Severe vasoconstriction occurs during surgery, especially during abdominal laparotomy. For example, manipulation of the intra-abdominal viscera with resultant reduction of the effective circulating blood volume sometimes produces oliguria. Blood loss and sequestration of blood in flaccid muscles and liver with impaired venous return can singly or in combination reduce the effective circulating blood volume.

An additional and important factor in vasoconstriction is the handling of trigger areas that excite the abdominal sympathetic nervous system. It is prone to occur during extensive surgery of the pancreas or of the abdominal aorta. Prolonged hypertension as a result of injury can be responsible for vasoconstriction. Several anesthetic agents such as ether will increase antidiuretic hormone secretion and will result in subsequent transient oliguria. The postoperative oliguria associated with sodium retention must be emphasized.[690]

Vasoconstriction of the intrarenal venous system can increase vascular resistance to a relatively greater degree than the afferent arteriolar resistance. Thus the peritubular capillary blood is dammed back; this damming produces an increase in the total volume of renal medullary blood. The renal mass is therefore increased and the medulla takes on a dark congested appearance. The renal interstitium becomes edematous and cellular infiltrates and fibrosis occur.

The prognosis of patients with acute renal failure of surgical origin is significantly worse than that of other patients, and the management is much more complicated and demanding.[997] This difference is explained by the high rate of protein breakdown, age of the patient,[948] infections, and demands of wound healing. The treatment of the surgical patient with acute renal failure is made more difficult by gastric aspiration, wound drainage, wound dehiscence, and hemorrhage,[643] but gastric aspiration aids in removal of excessive fluids, hydrogen ions, and large quantities of potassium.

Aortic surgery

Surgical operations involving the temporary occlusion of one or both renal arteries occur with repair of abdominal aortic aneurysms and disease of the celiac, superior mesenteric, and renal arteries.[310,311,1083] The brief temporary occlusion of the renal arteries during a surgical procedure predisposes the kidney to the potential dangers of renal ischemia. Hypothermia has increased the period during which surgeons can safely occlude the renal artery.

Cross clamping of the abdominal aorta distal to the renal arteries and manipulation of the aorta have led to acute oliguric renal failure in approximately 30% of cases.[388] This incidence of acute oliguria can be reduced by intravenous infusion of mannitol and by lowering the blood pressure with trimethaphan camphorsulfonate (Arfonad).[64] In addition, central venous pressure monitoring has detected hypovolemia and has led to early and adequate correction of the defect and prompt diuresis.

Open heart surgery

A significant number of patients who undergo open heart surgery develop acute renal failure.[301] Some patients may have a transitory oliguria and a slight elevation of BUN, while others have a progressively fatal anuria. The incidence of fatal renal failure varies between 3 to 8% and 20%. This high incidence can be explained on several bases, such as extensive surgery, multiple transfusions, chance of dislodging emboli to the kidneys, and nephrotoxic effects of anesthetic agents.

The intravenous administration of mannitol has been helpful in preventing oliguria and in reducing the number of fatalities from acute oliguric renal failure.

Accidental trauma

Accidental trauma can result from road accidents involving vehicles such as automobiles, trains, tractors, or wagons, from crushing injuries caused by earth cave-ins or heavy and massive objects, from gunshot wounds, from falls, and from fractures.

Injuries to the intra-abdominal organs are usually multiple visceral injuries. These include fractures of ribs, pelvis, and long bones, and rupture of liver, spleen, or kidneys. Massive fat emboli from fractured flat bones can produce oliguria.

Acute renal failure results from ischemia, from shock, or from a combination of these two,[251] in addition, muscle trauma may result in release of myoglobin into the blood and subsequently into the urine. This myoglobinuria in the presence of reduced blood volume leads to subsequent renal damage.

The following case presentation discusses the clinical events of a patient with acute renal failure caused by massive blunt abdominal trauma.

CASE PRESENTATION

On May 6, 1960, C. K., a 36-year-old laborer, fell two stories from a scaffold and struck his right side in a jackknife fashion across a board. He was unconscious and in shock. His fellow-worker immediately rushed him to Presbyterian–St. Luke's Hospital. At 9:30 AM he was admitted to the emergency room and was found to be in shock, agitated, and inco-

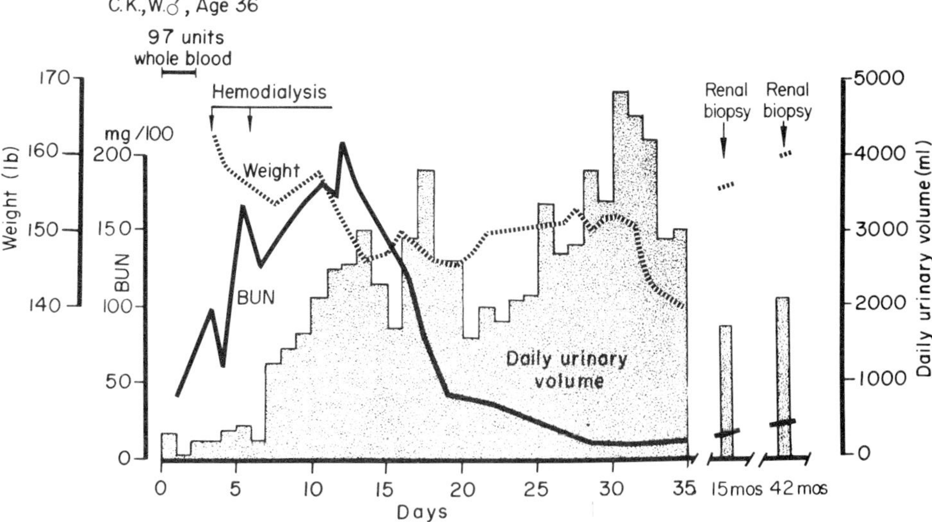

Fig. 4-3. Hospital course of patient with acute renal failure following trauma. A 36-year-old laborer fell from a scaffold and ruptured his liver. He arrived at the hospital in shock. Multiple whole blood transfusions were given and the ruptured liver was repaired at operation. Hemodialysis was done on the third and fifth postsurgical days. On the seventh day a step-wise diuresis occurred. On the twenty-eighth day the BUN was normal. Renal biopsy was done 15 and 42 months after acute oliguria occurred.

herent. Blood was coming from his mouth and was in his urine. A whole blood transfusion was started and he was sent to the intensive care unit in preparation for surgery. A total of thirty-six units of whole blood was transfused. (His hospital course is plotted in Fig. 4-3.)

At 11:50 AM he underwent surgery. Lacerations of the hepatic and portal veins were sutured, and a severely lacerated liver was repaired. The chest was opened and a drain was inserted. An additional seventeen units of cold whole blood were transfused. The body temperature dropped to 89° F. Following surgery he was found to have hypofibrinogenemia; he received an additional eight units of blood. Adrenocortical steroids, vitamin K, and chloramphenicol were given. His blood pressure stabilized; he was confused but responsive. On May 7 a tracheotomy was done to aid respiration. The BUN increased from 42 mg% on May 7 to 100 mg% on May 8, and the serum potassium increased from 6.6 mEq/L to 7.5 mEq/L. On May 8 he underwent hemodialysis for 6 hours with the twin coil unit. On May 10 the 24-hour urinary output was 450 ml and the patient was confused. On May 11 he underwent a repeat hemodialysis; after 4 hours of dialysis he went into shock, his abdomen was distended, and blood came from the intra-abdominal drains. A diagnosis was made of a delayed rupture of the spleen. He underwent surgical exploration and the ruptured spleen was removed. He received an additional nineteen units of whole blood. On May 13 he entered the diuretic stage of acute oliguric renal failure with a stepwise increase in urinary output. Four days later he had hypertension. The adrenocortical steroids were stopped and mecamylamine hydrochloride (Inversine) was given. A daily dose of 50 mg of norethandrolone (Nilevar) was started.

On May 19 he had uremic frost and muscle twitching. The 24-hour urinary output was 1,650 ml. The serum calcium was 6.6 mg% and the BUN 108 mg%. Two days later his blood pressure was 230/108 mm Hg. Parenteral reserpine, 0.5 mg, and magnesium sulfate were given.

On May 22, 750 ml of serosanguineous fluid was removed through the chest tubes. The BUN was 114 mg%. Salt-poor human serum albumin was given. In addition, whole blood transfusions were given to make a total of ninety-nine units. A subdiaphragmatic abscess was treated by drainage and antibiotics.

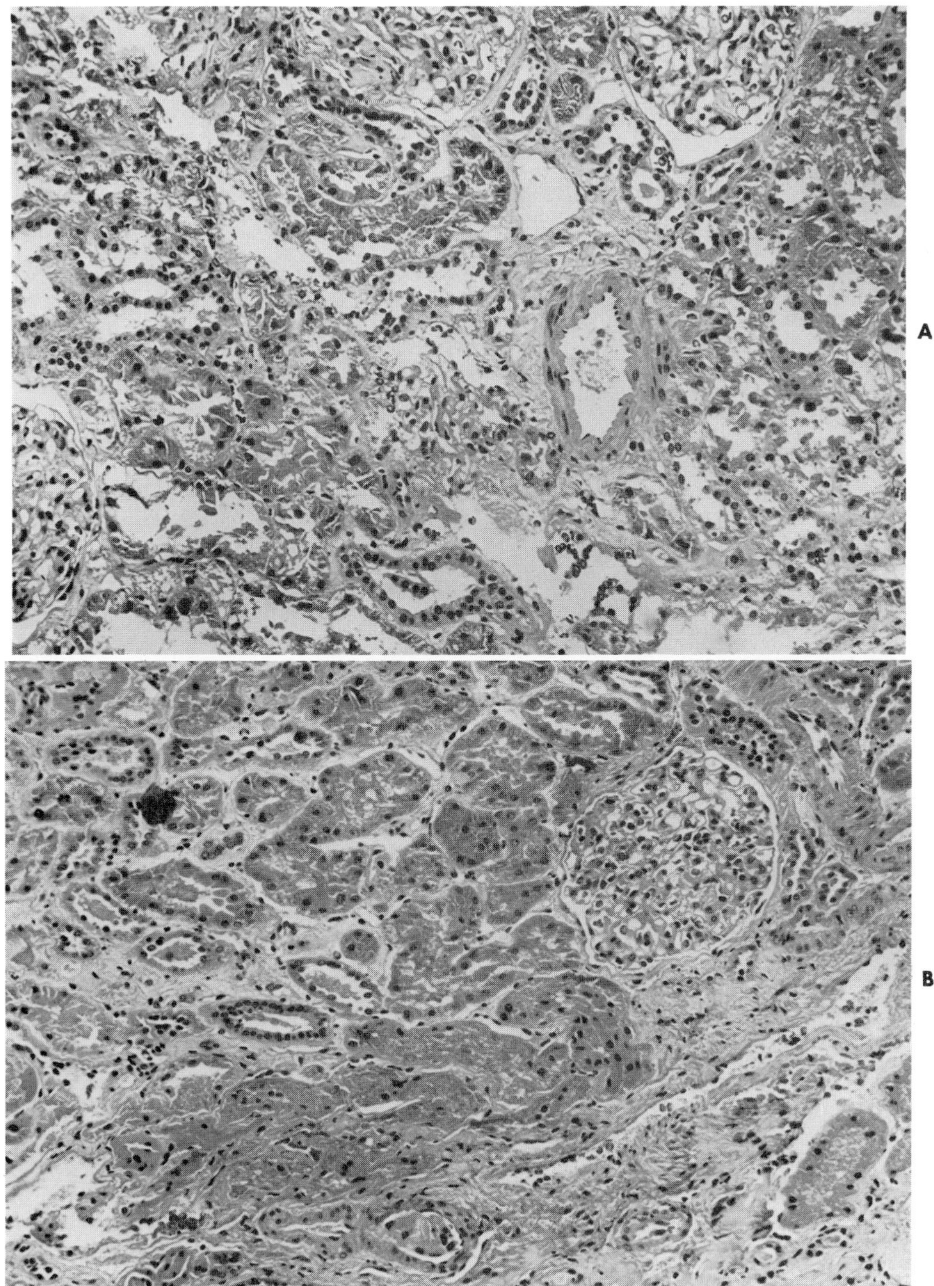

Fig. 4-4. A, Focal interstitial fibrosis following trauma-induced acute renal failure. This microphotograph illustrates focal interstitial scarring following recovery from acute renal failure. The glomeruli were normal. Electron microscopic study revealed a mild diffuse interstitial fibrosis. (H&E ×440.) **B,** Progression of interstitial fibrosis following trauma. As illustrated in this microphotograph, interstitial fibrosis is denser around the glomerulus in the second renal biopsy of patient described in Fig. 4-3. The fibrosis appears increased. There was reduction in the 24-hour creatinine clearance from 84 ml/min, when the first biopsy was obtained, to 54 ml/min at the time of the second renal biopsy. (H&E ×440.)

The patient required intensive nutritional rehabilitation. A gastric tube was inserted and 3,000 calories were given daily. Later his diet consisted of 4,500 calories with 275 gm of proteins. On August 4, 1960, he was discharged.

On September 17, 1960, he was readmitted to the hospital for evaluation of his renal injury. His blood pressure was 110/58 mm Hg. Funduscopic examination findings were normal. There was no peripheral edema. Urinalysis revealed 10 to 15 WBC in the urinary sediment and a trace of proteinuria. The hematocrit was 38%. The 4-hour oral glucose tolerance test was of the diabetic type. A percutaneous renal biopsy was done on September 23, 1960, and diffuse interstitial fibrosis was found (Fig. 4-4,A). On October 27, 1961, he had a trace of proteinuria and the creatinine clearance was 78 ml/minute. A renal biopsy study revealed interstitial fibrosis and complete healing of the renal tubules (Fig. 4-4,B).

THE ROLE OF BODY PIGMENTS

The massive liberation into the circulation of either hemoglobin or myoglobin, which ultimately reaches the kidney, produces a disturbance in kidney function,[364] damages the nephron, and subsequently results in acute oliguric renal failure.[237] The exact role of pigment in the pathogenesis of renal failure is not clearly understood.[224]

For a long time the morphologic finding of intratubular hemoglobin and myoglobin casts was considered the most important factor in producing oliguria. It led to the "tubular obstruction" theory as first described by Bywaters.[195] The finding of obstructing pigment casts in dissected nephrons from patients with acute renal failure gave additional support to this belief. One can easily visualize how one large pigmented cast in a large collecting duct could dam the urine flow from many nephrons. As Oliver said: "In the last analysis, water cannot flow through stopped pipes." Currently, the tubular obstruction theory does not explain the role of body pigments in producing acute renal failure. Moreover, blood pigments may not be nephrotoxic per se.

Many conflicting opinions have been expressed about the effects of hemoglobinuria and myoglobinuria on the kidney. For example, intravenous injections of purified crystalline hemoglobin preparations do not induce acute renal failure.[146] On the other hand, untreated hemolyzed whole blood induces marked vasoconstriction and acute renal failure. It appears that some by-product of the hemolytic process may cause renal ischemia and subsequently acute renal failure. This substance could be the erythrocyte wall or a cytoplasmic constituent with vasoconstrictive properties. Conn and colleagues believe that this renal ischemia is secondary to an overall increase in peripheral vasoconstriction.[231,232] Schmidt and Holland showed that the antibody complex with the blood group antigen on the erythrocyte membrane can induce acute oliguric renal failure.[965] Delayed anuria after transfusion of blood containing Kell-positive stroma is a good example of this phenomenon.[872] In 1900, Bell first reported four patients who had acute renal failure after receiving Kell-incompatible whole blood transfusions.

Dog experiments of DeMarin and Harris[275] support these concepts and also give support to Schmidt and Holland's[965] earlier observations. When vasodilatation was produced by the use of magnesium sulfate, the infusion of hemolyzed erythrocytes did not produce oliguria. It is very likely that a vasoconstrictor substance is released by the hemolyzed erythrocytes. This consequently results in a discontinuation of renal blood flow and oliguria. Large and excessive amounts of pigment in the glomerular filtrate may damage the tubular cells in the resorption process. Finally, in the presence of water deprivation, dehydration, ether, anesthesia, or anoxia, only a relatively small amount of injected hemoglobin is necessary to produce acute oliguria.[382] Therefore, clinical acute renal failure associated with hemoglobinuria may result in patients in shock in the absence of urine discoloration. Moreover, hemoglobinuria through release of erythrocyte membrane antibodies may be a more common cause of acute oliguric renal failure than is now diagnosed.

In the presence of dehydration or lack of fluid intake either hemoglobinuria or myoglobinuria forms a proteinic gel within the tubular lumen and subsequently produces tubular obstruction. It is quite possible that the obstructed pigment cast may exert a nephrotoxic effect on the nephron.[116]

Hemoglobinuria

Free hemoglobin in the urine is abnormal and indicates abnormal hemolysis of erythrocytes in the blood, the kidney, or the urine.[224,277,1149] This finding is not a specific disease but is the reflection of a variety of pathologic conditions.[203] Hemolysis with subsequent hemoglobinuria and acute oliguric renal failure occurred in 121 (11%) of 1,345 patients with acute renal failure due to a variety of causes. Hemoglobin has a molecular weight of 68,000 and accounts for 97% of the solid content of the erythrocyte. More is known about hemoglobin than about any other body protein. It is made up of four ferroprotoporphyrin complexes bound to globin.[31] Therefore, plasma hemoglobin combines with haptoglobin and makes a relatively stable compound that does not pass through the glomerular filter. In a healthy person the haptoglobin can bind only 100 to 135 mg of hemoglobin per 100 ml of plasma; therefore, hemoglobinuria does not occur until the plasma hemoglobin concentration exceeds a threshold level of approximately 135 mg per 100 ml. Once hemoglobinuria occurs it may continue until the plasma hemoglobin concentration has fallen to 30 to 50 mg per 100 ml. The hemoglobin/creatinine clearance ratio is 0.023, as compared to the greatest myoglobin/creatinine clearance ratio of 0.58.

The circulating concentration of hemoglobin abnormally increases from a variety of adverse conditions that lead to intravascular hemolysis.[185] These include transfusion of mismatched blood,[116] microangiopathic hemolytic anemias, paroxysmal nocturnal hemoglobinuria, paroxysmal cold hemoglobinuria, march hemoglobinemia, black-water fever, and favism.

Intravascular hemolysis

The most common cause of intravascular hemolysis is the infusion of mismatched blood.[26,27,56] In addition, intravascular hemolysis can result from one of the following distinct mechanisms.[175,285]

1. A direct toxic effect of a drug or chemical on the erythrocyte (erythrocyto-toxin), such as the effect of arsine vapors, biologic poisons, distilled water, burn toxin,[1053] or bacterial toxins
2. A hypersensitivity mechanism (immunohemolysis) such as incompatible blood transfusions, quinine sulfate, phenylbutazone, penicillin, and sulfonamides[910]
3. The mechanical fracture of erythrocytes such as the microangiopathic hemolytic anemias, falciparum malaria, and distilled water

Genetically susceptible individuals with a glucose-6-phosphate dehydrogenase deficiency can develop hemolysis, especially if they are given specific antimalarial agents.

Incompatible blood transfusions. Approximately 6 million units of whole blood are given annually in the United States. In spite of rigid precautions, at least 120,000 recognizable reactions may occur. Transfusion reactions include incompatible blood transfusion reactions,[440] contaminated blood, bacterial pyrogens, unexplained fever, circulatory overload, air embolism, allergy, sensitivity to donor leukocytes, sensitivity to donor platelets, and sensitivity to donor plasma.[19,88]

Intravascular hemolysis following blood transfusions usually results from three factors:[410] (1) destruction of the donor's erythrocytes by the recipient's antibodies, (2) destruction of the recipient's erythrocytes by acquired immune antibodies in the donor, and (3) destruction of transfused erythrocytes that became fragile when stored.[406] Human errors have been the cause of incompatible transfusions; these include errors in grouping the recipient, transcribing the main results, and labeling and choosing bottles.

An incompatible blood transfusion has the most serious prognosis of all transfusion reactions.[77,210,259] It occurs in significant frequency, produces shock and acute renal failure,[457,809] and carries a high mortality risk if not treated properly. Early symptoms of an incompatible blood transfusion reaction are chills, fever, headache, and backache.[456] Later the patient has gross hematuria, jaundice, and oliguria.[135] In a patient under general anesthesia, intravascular hemolysis caused by incompatible blood transfusions may be difficult to diagnose. The earliest finding will be oozing of blood from the operative site. The hemorrhagic tendency is usually associated with hypofibrinogenemia,[403] which results from intravascular clotting in response to two factors:[248,515] a thromboplastic substance liberated from the hemolyzing erythrocytes, and complications of increased fibrinolysis.[404]

Castle first demonstrated that in vivo incompatible erythrocytes first agglutinate and produce capillary stasis, ischemia, and anoxia.[210] The occurrence of this mechanism in the renal capillaries when acute oliguric renal failure results was emphasized by Merrill and his colleagues.[773] Incompatibilities in minor blood groups as well as major ABO groups and Rh system can lead to acute renal failure. In addition, Kell, Duffy, Kidd, and X and S incompatibilities have led to renal failure. I have successfully used mannitol infusions to promote an osmotic diuresis and to sustain an excellent urinary output when incompatible blood transfusion reactions occur.

Distilled water–induced hemoglobinuria. In the past, sterile water (tap or distilled) has been used for irrigation of the open prostatic field during trans-urethral prostatectomy.[3,445] Water has gained access into the blood through the venous channels of the raw prostatic surface.[245,246] Water produces a hypotonic environment for the red blood cell (the heat factor has also been implicated[362]). Subsequently, it produces an osmotic intravascular rupture of erythrocytes. The patient will experience chills, loin pain, and, later, nausea and vomiting, followed in a few hours by oliguria or anuria.[489] The oliguria or anuria probably results from a fall in cardiac output and a decrease in renal blood flow. Currently, distilled water–induced acute renal failure is rarely seen. Urologists are well aware of this precipitating factor and use nonelectrolyte irrigating fluid that is iso-osmotic to the blood.

Hemolysis caused by drugs and chemicals. Chemicals and drugs that produce severe hemoglobinuria and acute renal failure are arsine, tribromoethanol (Avertin), quinine sulfate, quinidine sulfate, hydroquinine-pyrogallic acid, benzene, hydralazine, fava beans, djenkol beans, sodium chlorate, methyl chloride, and coal tar products.

Arsine-induced acute renal failure. Arsine (hydrogen arsenide) is evolved when hydrogen generated by the wetting of metallic dross reacts with arsenic con-taminants.[796,804,1036] Arsine (AsH_3) is one of the most toxic gases known. It is colorless, inflammable, heavier than air, unstable, and a strong reducing agent. The toxic properties of arsine were first described by Gehlen in 1815.[422a] Arsine enters the bloodstream through the lungs. Because of its strong reducing prop-erties it rapidly combines with hemoglobin within the erythrocytes.[566] Hemolysis occurs within 2 to 24 hours.[422]

The clinical symptoms of arsine poisoning result from erythrocyte hemolysis.[590] The sequence of symptoms is as follows: first there is a vague sick feeling and nausea; then the patient suffers from cramping abdominal pains, from vomiting, from weakness, from tingling of the face, hands, and feet, and from headache;[828] pain over the kidneys is followed by passage of dark urine; finally, the patient complains of extreme weakness and fatigue and becomes feverish, dyspneic, and lethargic. He may develop an intense coppery-bronze skin color. Pulmonary edema and cyanosis appear and are followed by lethargy, coma, and death.[287,619,1130]

In general, the treatment of patients with arsine-induced anuria has not been successful because the arsine-hemoglobin complex does not cross either the peritoneal membrane or the cellophane membrane of the extracorporeal hemodialysis unit; therefore, it cannot be removed by either peritoneal dialysis or hemo-dialysis. A whole blood exchange transfusion given early in the treatment reduces the circulating arsenic-hemoglobin complex, may restore the patient's erythrocyte mass to normal, and prevents the additional hypoxic insult of anemia to the nephron. The patient's life should be sustained by peritoneal dialysis or by hemodialysis until the nephron function is restored.[885]

The mortality rate of patients with arsine poisoning is reported by Locket as being 20%.[702] Once anuria develops, the mortality rate approaches 100%,* and death occurs between the fourth and twelfth days. Arsine produces acute tubular necrosis, with the greatest damage to the proximal and distal tubules. This damage can result from any of the following conditions, either singly or in combination: hemoglobinuria, anemia with renal ischemia, or the toxic effects of arsine on the respiratory enzymes of the nephron. Severe interstitial edema and fibrosis occur.[806a] Tubular healing is extremely slow, and the patient may be left with impaired renal function.[833,1092]

Quinine sulfate. Acute intravascular hemolysis with subsequent acute renal failure has followed treatment with quinine sulfate in patients with falciparum malaria and in patients in whom quinine sulfate was used as an abortifacient during early pregnancy, usually in the first trimester. Quinine can also induce purpura.[534] In a review of the literature, Terplan and Janert found eight patients with acute renal failure caused by quinine-induced hemolytic anemia.[1068] They reported a ninth patient who had received quinine sulfate as an abortifacient. All died from acute oliguric renal failure. Schreiner, Vartan, and Discombe reported other patients with fatal quinine-induced renal failure. Lang and Jones reported a 28-year-old woman who, in her eighth week of pregnancy, ingested 1.2 gm of quinine sulfate.[664] She developed acute oliguric renal failure. A renal biopsy study done at the peak of her diuresis revealed acute tubular abnormalities. Although tubular necrosis was not present, tubular regeneration and areas of tubular basement membrane disruption were seen. They concluded that acute tubular necrosis was the cause of oliguria. On review of their microphotograph, a marked diffuse interstitial edema and fibrosis were also noted.

Other hemolysis. Sodium chlorate may be ingested or inhaled; it produces hemoglobinuria and methemoglobinuria with subsequent acute renal failure caused by acute tubular necrosis.

The djenkol bean has produced acute intravascular hemolysis with acute anuria.[914] The broad bean (*Vicia fava*) has also produced acute hemolytic anemia with subsequent hemoglobinuria and acute renal failure.[940] Apiol poisoning has produced intravascular hemolysis, thrombocytopenia, and fatal acute renal failure associated with tubular necrosis.

Sickle cell disease. In 1910, Herrick reported a young Negro patient with anemia characterized by "queer elongated sickle-shaped and oat-shaped erythrocytes."[541a] He attributed this abnormality in shape to some unrecognized change in the corpuscle itself. The unusual form of hemoglobin (hemoglobin-S) found within the erythrocyte has led to the concept that disease can result from a

---

*See references 303, 436, 446, 563, and 1130.

familial-determined defect in protein synthesis. A basic hemoglobin abnormality of the sickle erythrocyte is its increased mechanical fragility. The cell is really phagocytosed and easily destroyed. A fall in oxygen tension that occurs at high altitudes (10,000 to 15,000 feet) has precipitated sickling of erythrocytes and has led to intravascular thrombosis and hemolysis.[801,1021] Sickle cell disease is occasionally serious and is variable in nature.[895,1067]

Approximately 8 to 10% of Negroes in the United States have this familial heterozygous condition characterized by the presence of hemoglobin-A plus hemoglobin-S.[868,1078] The latter is present in a concentration of less than 40%. Sickle cell disease can involve the kidney by proteinuria, hematuria, cylinduria, repeated urinary tract infection, fixed specific gravity of urine, renal thrombosis, renal infarction, and acute oliguria.[103,741] Acute renal failure is a rare complication of sickle cell disease.[971] It is more likely to occur associated with anoxia and hemolysis of the sickled erythrocyte. The associated renal lesion is tubular necrosis. In addition, intravascular thrombosis of renal arterioles has also resulted in acute renal failure. I observed resolution of renal vein thrombosis and the nephrotic syndrome in a patient with sickle cell anemia and other evidence of

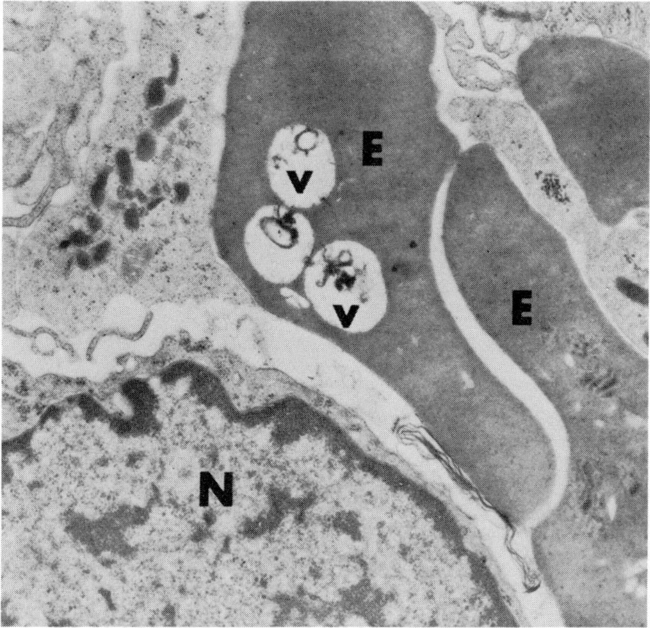

Fig. 4-5. Vacuoles within erythrocytes of patient with sickle cell anemia. This electron microphotograph illustrates a renal biopsy from a 13-year-old schoolgirl with sickle cell anemia. A renal biopsy was done during anuria. Within the glomerular capillary lumen are portions of three erythrocytes (E). Within the center erythrocyte are three vacuoles (V). Myelin bodies were seen within the vacuoles. An endothelial cell nucleus (N) was seen at the bottom. Between the epithelial cell and the large erythrocyte are strains of myelinoid material. (×17,000.)

thrombosis. Further damage results from hemolysis caused by intravascular sickling with a subsequent mechanical fracture of erythrocytes (microangiopathic anemia).[840] Acute renal failure due to sickle cell crisis can be complicated by central venous system injury. This is caused by arterial thrombosis.

Salisbury reported a 32-year-old nurse who recovered from sickle cell–induced acute renal failure.[951a] She was given adrenocortical steroids and heparin. In view of excellent results following heparin treatment in patients with microangiopathic anemia with acute renal failure, this patient may have recovered in spite of adrenocortical steroid treatment. I studied a 13-year-old Negro schoolgirl who had sickle cell anemia and who developed poststreptococcal glomerulonephritis. She developed a fatal acute renal failure. Electron microscopic study of her kidney early in oliguria revealed severe and active lesions of poststreptococcal glomerulonephritis. Erythrocytes within the glomerular capillaries contained laminated myelin vacuoles and were sickled (Fig. 4-5).

Snake, spider, and wax bee bites. Acute renal failure induced by bites of snakes, spiders, and wax bees have been reported from Lima, Peru, by Piazza and associates[883] and from Sao Paulo, Brazil, by Silva and associates.[1031] Acute intravascular hemolysis was common in all afflicted patients and probably had an immunohemolytic basis. During the oliguric-anuric phase the urine was iso-osmolar with a high urinary sodium concentration (above 50 mEq/L) and urea urine/plasma ratio under 10.

Snakes. Of all the snake species in the United States, approximately 10% are venomous. Snakebites inflicted by the pit viper, *Crotalus terrificus* (rattlesnake),[387] and *Brothrups zararaca* species usually produce local pain and swelling. The greater the area of edema and erythema around the fang marks, the greater the venomation. Severe venomation may cause twelve or more inches of surrounding edema and erythema within the first 12 hours after the snakebite. The *Ancistrodon contortrix mokeson* (copperhead),[865] the *Ancistrodon piscivorus* (water moccasin), and the *Micruroides* (coral snake) are other important venomous snakes. Their venom usually contains a variety of enzymes, cytolysins, and neurotoxins that produce a variety of neurologic disturbances, circulatory collapse, shock, and acute renal failure. Other clinical features are dizziness, severe headaches, visual impairments, paralysis of neck muscles, respiratory depression, and urinary findings of myoglobin, proteinuria, and hematuria.

Snakebite-induced oliguria occurs in a small percentage of those patients suffering a greater degree of renal damage. When acute renal failure develops, acute tubular necrosis is the common renal lesion found. One patient with a fatal bite by a brothrups species developed bilateral renal cortical necrosis with an associated afibrinogenemia.

Treatment should start with immobilization of the patient and application of a constricting band (tourniquet) to the bitten extremity and several inches above the fang marks. The tourniquet should be tight enough to permit arterial blood to reach the extremity and to prevent the superficial venous and lymph flow to reach the systemic circulation. Incision and suction effectively remove venom for up to 2 hours after a bite. Suction should be continued for at least 1 hour. Antivenom, antitetanus prophylaxis, and antibiotics are the "three A's" to consider in the treatment of patients poisoned with snake venom. Adrenocortical steroids do not affect the survival rate of animals poisoned with venom. Hemodialysis has been used to treat patients with snakebite-induced oliguria.[396] Antihistaminics are contraindicated. Shock should be treated with infusion of blood, plasma, antibiotics, and vasopressor agents. Analgesic drugs are given for relief of pain. Exposure to cold and treatment with it should be avoided.

A bite of the *Echiscarinatus* (sand viper), which is found near Lake Rudolph in Kenya, produces bilateral renal cortical necrosis. The bite of the *Atracepaspis microlapidata* (small African snake) can result in severe tubular necrosis with complete anuria. Snakebites can produce other renal lesions leading to clinical syndromes other than acute oliguric renal failure. For example, bites of the *Enhydrina schisdossa* (sea snake) can result in hematuria and proteinuria. Still other snakebites can produce a nephrotic syndrome.

Spiders. The *Loxosceles reclusus* and *Loxosceles laeta* (tarantula) spiders live in homes, outdoor privies, and in gardens, and they seldom bite man. When such a spider does bite a human, the injected "poison" produces a local necrotic and angry cutaneous lesion, usually in buttocks and genitalia. Some bites have caused extensive tissue sloughing at the site of the bite. In others the lesion has healed locally in several weeks and has left a healed scar. The spider's poison, a "toxalbumin," usually affects the nerve endings. If it reaches the systemic circulation a marked hemolysis occurs. This is followed by anemia, jaundice, and acute oliguric renal failure. The *Loxosceles laeta* spider produces a prolonged anuria that is usually fatal.

In addition to present accepted methods of treating acute renal failure, use of antiloxoscele serum is most helpful in neutralizing the spider antigen. The bite of the *Amanrobius ferox* results in severe intravascular hemolysis with production of a dark urine, as seen in black-water fever. Methemoglobinuria and hemoglobinuria occur. Intravenous injections of calcium gluconate and antivenom have been helpful. The *Latrodectus mactans* (common black widow spider) predominately produces a neurotoxin. The patient experiences pain in the kidney area similar to that of renal colic, and in addition has severe dehydration and oliguria.

Wax bee. Immunohemolytic anemia and subsequent acute oliguric renal failure have followed the bite of a wax bee (*Appis mellificus*). Multiple bites can produce fatal anuria. The patient's skin becomes edematous, red, painful, and itchy. The clinical course and renal lesions of acute renal failure are not as severe as those produced by snakebites or by spider bites. Immediately after exposure, the use of antihistaminics, epinephrine, adrenocortical steroids (prednisone, 30 mg), and local skin treatment have been helpful.

Portuguese man-of-war stings. The sea nettle (Portuguese man-of-war) produces a sharp sting at the site of its tentacle strike. The toxin injected into the skin has resulted in local swelling, local secondary infection, and angioneurotic edema. Hypersensitivity reactions include anaphylactic shock, urticaria, and eosinophilia. Patients have had gastroenteritis with severe abdominal pain and generalized muscle cramps and spasms.

Acute oliguric renal failure and less severe renal disease have followed sea nettle stings. These usually occur in the unsuspecting tourist who swims or bathes in ocean waters. Adrenocortical steroids have produced a diuresis and have suppressed the hypersensitivity reaction of the sea nettle sting.

Microangiopathic hemolytic anemia. Dacie and associates coined the term "microangiopathic anemia"; they believed the condition to be produced by repeated contact of erythrocytes with pathologically altered small blood vessels.[147] The striking morphologic characteristics of the erythrocytes on a peripheral blood smear are red cell fragmentation, distortion, and crenation. These red cell abnormalities usually suggest an underlying serious systemic disorder that is similar to the "mechanical anemia" that follows the insertion of Teflon patches or prosthetic valves into the heart.

The predominant clinical features associated with microangiopathic anemia are jaundice, anemia, acute oliguric renal failure, and abnormal erythrocytes on a peripheral blood smear. The combination of a mechanical hemolytic anemia[147] and thrombocytopenia should lead the physician to suspect TTP.

The clinical features of microangiopathic hemolytic anemia must be differentiated from the hepatorenal syndrome, the generalized Shwartzman phenomenon, and hemolytic uremic syndrome and other causes of intravascular hemolysis.

The Shwartzman reaction. Acute oliguric renal failure caused by renal glomerular capillary thrombosis[758] and acute renal cortical necrosis[551a] are morphologic criteria suggestive of a generalized Shwartzman reaction. These abnormalities have developed in pregnant women either at delivery or postpartum as the result of a generalized Shwartzman reaction.[1011] Hypercoagulability of the blood caused by eclampsia occurs during the postpartum period. Fibrin thrombosis extends into the glomeruli and results in acute renal failure. A similar lesion of thrombosis of the afferent glomerular arterioles occurs in the hemolytic-uremic syndrome.[147]

In man, the generalized Shwartzman reaction commonly develops from one of two mechanisms. The first is from an underlying infection with an endotoxemia usually resulting from a gram-negative bacteria of the coli groups such as *Escherichia coli, Aerobacter aerogenes, Proteus* species and possibly *Pseudomonas aeruginosa.*[579,1035] The endotoxin is found within the O somatic antigen present in the cell wall of gram-negative bacteria. The mechanism by which the endotoxin triggers intravascular clotting to produce fibrin thrombi is not known.

Endotoxin shock is produced by a high molecular weight. Lipo-protein-carbohydrate complex is released by the cell wall of gram-negative bacteria. The toxicity of the pseudomonas bacteria is probably not caused by a true endotoxin but by a slimy "capsule-like" material. Patients with endotoxemia are usually acutely ill and are suffering from a fatal illness associated with severe shock.

The second mechanism leading to the generalized Shwartzman reaction occurs in pregnant women, particularly in the postpartum period. Either renal cortical necrosis or glomerular fibrin thrombi can result from an intravascular clot formation caused by hypercoagulability of the blood. Later a generalized bleeding tendency usually occurs. The hypercoagulability starts from an intrauterine hemorrhage or from retained fragments of placenta. The uterine condition is usually undiagnosed.

The pathogenesis is as follows: degeneration of the labyrinth and giant cell trophoblasts of the placenta occur. Focal deposits of fibrin form in the maternal spaces, followed by extension from the parauterine thrombosis. On separation of the placenta, a coagulative substance is released into the systemic circulation. This is followed by generalized thrombosis and hypofibrinogenemia. A clot-producing agent escapes into the circulation, and intravascular thromboses subsequently occur. This substance could be a thromboplastin material. Fibrin accumulates in the afferent renal arterioles with extension of the thrombosis into the glomerular capillaries and other renal vessels. Subsequently, acute oliguric renal failure develops.[218] With the use of electron microscopy, fibrin deposits are seen below the glomerular basement membrane; in TTP the fibrin is within the capillary lumen.

Microangiopathic anemia results from the mechanical fragmentation of erythrocytes passing through the narrowed capillary lumen. These fragmented red blood cells can be seen on a peripheral blood smear. The anemia is associated with an elevated reticulocyte count, elevation of serum lactic dehydrogenase (isoenzyme V), and elevation of the total serum bilirubin level.

McKay and Waile observed the generalized Shwartzman reaction in nine infants.[761] *Escherichia coli* caused diarrhea, which was followed by irreversible shock. Diffuse thromboses were found in the smaller renal vessels. The glomerular lesions were similar to those seen in children with the hemolytic-uremic syndrome and in patients with the generalized Shwartzman reaction. The evidence to support a generalized Shwartzman reaction is the fact that *E. coli* produces a potent endotoxin. This endotoxin is known to cross the gut wall into the systemic circulation. The infants developed a fatal shock very suggestive of endotoxic shock observed in adults. The final evidence is finding the morphologic lesion of fibrin thrombi not only in the kidneys but in other organs as well.

Diffuse deposits of fibrin in the glomerular capillaries have been observed in a patient with *Serratia marcescens* septicemia complicated by a fatal burn.[457a] Because fibrin thrombi consume factors and other constituents in coagulation, blood coagulation studies in those patients reveal a marked decrease in factors V and VII, reduction of platelets, and some prolongation in the prothrombin time. Deficiency in blood coagulation leads to widespread purpura and tissue hemorrhage.[107a]

The Shwartzman reaction must be recognized as being a result of complicating primary disorders. These disorders must be recognized and effectively treated. The patients are usually in shock from either massive hemorrhage or endotoxemia; in many patients both are present. The process of shock must be reversed by use of adrenocortical steroids. Above all, heparin should be used to treat the generalized Shwartzman reaction. If heparin cannot be used, then adrenocortical steroids should not be used. Some observation suggests that adrenocortical steroids intensify the generalized Shwartzman reaction. Heparin has been found to be effective in stopping the intravascular coagulation reaction; thus, the generalized Shwartzman reaction may be arrested.

Falciparum malaria. Parasitic infection with *Plasmodium falciparum* may result in such fatal complications as acute oliguric renal failure, black-water fever, cerebral malaria, and pulmonary involvement.

"Black-water fever" is the clinical term applied to renal involvement caused by *Plasmodium falciparum*.[271] It has a high mortality rate, about 20%, with acute renal failure as a mode of death. It is the hemoglobinuria and other breakdown products of hemoglobin that blacken the urine (the condition is a hemoglobinuric syndrome). Both oliguric and nonoliguric renal failure can occur as a complication in approximately 1% of those afflicted with falciparum malaria.

The pathogenesis of renal failure can result from any one of several mechanisms. For example, McGraith and Findlay suggested a shunting of blood flow from the renal cortex to the medullary and papillary vessels.[217] They based this theory on finding ischemic glomeruli at autopsy. The second mechanism is massive intravascular hemolysis and subsequent hemoglobinuria resulting from severe parasitemia (ranging from 20 to 90%). The third mechanism occurs following treatment of falciparum malaria with quinine. A drug-induced hemolytic reaction resulting in hemoglobinuria and acute oliguric renal failure subsequently occur. The fourth mechanism was made known by Sitprija and associates[1018a] They believe that acute oliguric renal failure can develop in patients with malaria as a result of the massive parasitemia without dehydration, intravascular hemolysis, or hemoglobinuria. Finally, the toxicity and dehydration with reduced blood volume associated with black-water fever may be an important precipitating or etiologic factor. Approximately one-fourth of the patients with acute renal failure have a "high output" (nonoliguric) renal failure. They usually recover by means of antimalaria treatment with quinine.

Nausea, vomiting, confusion, mental changes, hyperpnea, hyperreflexia, and twitching could be caused by either severe falciparum malaria or impending acute renal failure. A sudden weight gain in the febrile patient with falciparum malaria may be a signal of impending renal failure. Daily observation should be made of urinary output, urinary specific gravity, and BUN. The patient with acute oliguric renal failure caused by falciparum malaria should be adequately hydrated and given sodium bicarbonate to alkalinize the urine. A dose of 25 gm of mannitol in a 20% solution should be given early to promote a diuresis and possibly to prevent the progression of the disorder to tubular damage.[433] Treatment should consist of conservative management of acute oliguric renal failure and the early and repeated use of renal dialysis. The overall survival rate of patients with acute oliguric renal failure is approximately 60%. If oliguria or anuria persists, the most important facet of treatment is the administration of antimalarial drugs to eliminate the infections and to ensure recovery. This is the foremost goal in treating the patient.

In certain areas of the world, such as the Magdalena Valley of Colombia, Thailand, Laos, and Vietnam, the falciparum malaria parasite was found to be resistant to chloroquine. Despite strict malaria discipline and the mandatory use of weekly chemoprophylaxis (chloroquine, 300 mg, and primaquine, 45 mg), clinical malaria developed in 5 to 50% of the military personnel in the remote forested areas of Ia-Drang and Vinh-Thanh Valleys of central Vietnam. Ninety-eight percent of the infections were caused by *Plasmodium falciparum*. A combination of chloroquine and quinine successfully treated these clinical infections. Therefore, the drugs of choice are a combination of quinine and pyrimethamine. Their prompt and appropriate use has been most beneficial in the treatment of chloroquine-resistant falciparum malaria.[123,789] The dose level of quinine must be maintained by determination of blood quinine levels; otherwise, toxicity may occur. A dose of 25 mg of pyrimethamine is given three times daily for 3 days, and a dose of 650 mg of quinine sulfate is given three times daily for 14 days.

The cause of death of oliguric patients with falciparum malaria who were treated in a renal dialysis center is either uremia or bacterial sepsis. This has been borne out by the experience of the United States Army medical teams in Vietnam.[1005] The soldier afflicted with malaria is flown from the combat area to medical centers for treatment. If acute oliguric renal failure develops, he is promptly and effectively cared for at dialysis centers. Peritoneal dialysis and hemodialysis have been equally effective.

Grossly, the kidneys are enlarged. The glomeruli appear ischemic early in acute renal failure, but they have actually undergone no apparent morphologic change. This ischemic finding has led some authors to postulate that cortical blood is shunted to the medullary areas of the kidney. It is difficult for me to accept this reasoning, since bloodless glomeruli are seen in kidneys from patients with normal urinary output. Later there is interstitial edema, followed by focal to diffuse interstitial fibrosis with cellular infiltrates of fibroblasts. Numerous histiocytes containing iron-positive pigment are found in the interstitium.

The tubular findings vary from normal to the more severe changes of acute tubular necrosis. During healing tubular repair is usually rapid. As a result of intravascular hemolysis, hemoglobin casts and casts containing degenerated erythrocytes are noted in the tubular lumen, within the tubular cytoplasm, and in the edematous interstitium. In patients with prolonged oliguria interstitial fibrosis becomes severe and diffuse and may be associated with tubular atrophy.

Plasmodium malaria in the peripheral blood has been found to be associated with the nephrotic syndrome in children from the Gold Coast area of West Africa. They have a nonspecific glomerular patchy lesion of varying severity associated with tubular degeneration.[1112a] This nephropathy has no direct evidence of a malarial etiology.

Paroxysmal nocturnal hemoglobinuria. Paroxysmal nocturnal hemoglobinuria is a nonfamilial condition that afflicts individuals during their third or fourth decade of life. The disorders characterized by chronic intravascular hemolysis with increased hemolysis during sleep. Therefore, the early morning urine specimen contains large quantities of hemoglobin. Patients with paroxysmal nocturnal hemoglobinuria die as a result of anemia, intercurrent infections, thrombosis, or splenectomy. Erythrocytes from patients with paroxysmal nocturnal hemoglobinuria are especially sensitive to hemolysis by both isoantibodies and the abnormal antibodies of a general hemolytic anemia. Electron microscopic studies of erythrocytes reveal a pitting of the cell surface. There are few case reports of acute oliguric renal failure occurring in patients with paroxysmal nocturnal hemoglobinuria. Once acute renal failure occurs, the prognosis for recovery is excellent. The renal cortex is a dark color, and there is deposition of iron pigment within the proximal convoluted tubular epithelial cell.

Paroxysmal cold hemoglobinuria. Paroxysmal cold hemoglobinuria (PCH) rarely results in acute oliguric renal failure. Sussmand and Kayden reported a patient with PCH who died in uremia caused by acute oliguric renal failure.[1054] At autopsy, tubular necrosis was found with hemoglobin casts filling the tubular lumen. Diffuse interstitial fibrosis was prominent. Oliver and associates did a microdissection study and found tubulorrhexis surrounded by granular tissue adhesions.

Heptinstall studied the kidneys of an elderly Negro lady who had latent syphilis.[539] She had a combination of frostbite and a bleeding peptic ulcer. She developed acute renal failure and died. Her kidneys were enlarged and dark. Microscopic study revealed acute tubular necrosis, large numbers of pigmented casts, and considerable diffuse interstitial fibrosis.

March hemoglobinuria. A benign intravascular hemolysis occurs in young men after the strenuous exercise of running and is entirely different from heat stress, which is associated with myoglobinuria. March hemoglobinuria is transient and is akin to exercise proteinuria. Neither anemia nor acute renal failure has been reported as a result. This acquired disorder must be differentiated from myoglobinuria that is induced by heat stress. The method to differentiate the two conditions is described in the following paragraphs.

Myoglobinuria

Acute oliguric renal failure occurs in approximately 45% of patients with myoglobinuria. Of the cases published, eleven patients had acute oliguric renal failure and five patients died. The remainder appear to have recovered without residual damage. There are two main categories in classifying patients with myoglobinuria. The first is myoglobinuria produced by extrinsic causes such as trauma or toxic substances.[190,464] The second is familial paroxysmal myoglobinuria. (A third type occurs in draft horses and is known as "equine myoglobinuria.")

Myoglobinuria must be differentiated from other diseases characterized by the passage of dark urine. These include paroxysmal nocturnal hemoglobinuria, paroxysmal cold hemoglobinuria, march hemoglobinuria, and porphyria. The differentiation of myoglobinuria from hemoglobinuria is plotted in Table 4-1.

Myoglobinuria is characterized by a spontaneous onset of weak, tender, painful, and swollen muscles.[192] The muscles most frequently involved are those of the calf and the thigh. However, the abdominal, thoracic, cervical, and upper extremity groups are also involved. Associated clinical findings include fever, vomiting, diarrhea, abdominal pain, and pseudoparalysis.

Myoglobin is not appreciably bound to haptoglobin; therefore, haptoglobin is not depleted in myoglobinuria.[850] Moreover, the finding of a normal or increased haptoglobin identifies the urine pigment as myoglobin. On the other hand, a decrease or absent haptoglobin identifies the pigment as hemoglobin. A simple test to differentiate myoglobin from hemoglobin is to dilute the urine to an 80% solution of ammonium sulfate. Hemoglobin precipitates out, while myoglobin remains soluble (Table 4-1).

Table 4-1. Difference between myoglobinuria and hemoglobinuria*

	Myoglobinuria	*Hemoglobinuria*
Clinical signs and symptoms	Painful, tender, swollen muscles with limitation of motion	Muscles normal
Appearance of serum	Not hemolytic	Hemolytic
Serum bilirubin	Normal	Rises
Reticulocyte count	Normal	Rises
Spectral characteristics of urinary pigment:		
Nonoxygenated	Rapidly changes to met-form giving spectrum almost identical with that of methemoglobin	Does not usually change to met-form spontaneously
Oxygenated form	Maximum absorption peak at 582†	Maximum absorption peak at 577†
Carbon monoxide complex	Maximum absorption peak at 579	Maximum absorption peak at 570
Electrophoresis	Myohemoglobin (metmyohemoglobin) migrates at about half the speed of hemoglobin in barbital buffer pH 8.6	
Solubility in urine 80% saturated with ammonium sulfate	Myohemoglobin largely remains in solution	Hemoglobin completely precipitated

*Large differences in molecular weights and oxygen dissociation curves of myoglobin and hemoglobin might also be of value in their differentiation.

†Fluorescent lamp as source of light aids in differentiation based on this spectral difference.

Myoglobin is a respiratory pigment containing iron-compounded prosthetic groups—protoporphyrin, together with globulin. It has a molecular weight of 17,500, approximately one-fourth the molecular weight of hemoglobin (68,000). Moreover, it is 25 times more filterable by the kidney than is hemoglobin. Myoglobin released into the bloodstream filters through the glomeruli; myoglobinuria subsequently occurs. If the myoglobinuria is excessive, if the patient is dehydrated by diarrhea or other causes, or if the urine is acid, acute oliguric renal failure is likely to be precipitated. Death may occur within hours from hyperkalemia or within days from acute renal failure and its complications.

Extrinsic causes of myoglobinuria

Myoglobinuria can result from one of four specific extrinsic etiologies: (1) traumatic crushing muscle injuries such as in the crush syndrome, flogging, electric shock, and femoral arterial occlusion;[195] (2) heat injury, heat stress, and heat exhaustion; (3) myotoxins such as barbiturates, fish myotoxins (Haff disease), ethanol, and viruses; and (4) severe myositis.

Trauma. The crush syndrome, as described during World War II, is characterized by a severe crushing muscle injury resulting in release of myoglobin and subsequent myoglobinuria. Fischer and Rossier reported patients with severe electric shock who developed myoglobinuria and subsequent acute renal failure.[372] Early in oliguria, myoglobinuria was accompanied by hyperkalemia. In 1945, Bywaters and Snead reported a 63-year-old lady with femoral artery thrombosis.[195] She had a low serum potassium and myoglobinuria. At autopsy, muscle necrosis and other abnormalities similar to muscle findings in the crush syndrome were noted.

Heat-induced disorders. Acute renal failure can result from heat-induced disorders such as heat stress and physical exertion. The prompt recognition of this disorder leads to a more optimistic prognosis. Heat-induced disorders result from disturbed physiology of thermoregulation. Some heat disorders may result from an indirect physiologic factor in water and salt imbalance or from circulatory collapse.

Heat stroke. Heat stroke must be treated as a disease entity caused by collapse of the temperature regulatory mechanism. It occurs in individuals who lack acclimatization. It is characterized by sudden unconsciousness, hyperpyrexia, and absence of sweating. Cessation of sweating may be a prodromal symptom. After the patient regains consciousness he may complain of headache, numbness, dizziness, nausea, and visual disturbances. On examination his skin is found to be flushed, hot, and dry. His pulse is rapid, weak, and perhaps irregular. Rectal temperature may be as high as 106 to 110° F.

Patients with heat stroke must receive supportive management, and negative heat balance must be established. To avoid brain damage, immediate and effective treatment must be started. For rapid body cooling, a cold water bath or cold spray to the body is effective. The stagnation of blood by peripheral vasoconstriction must be corrected by massage of the extremities. Treatment should be maintained for at least 1 week, when sweating will return. If the high temperature is not reduced within 4 hours acute renal failure occurs. Serum potassium levels should be carefully followed since hypovolemia occurs initially.

Renal damage is more prone to occur in those patients who survive more than 24 hours. Approximately one-third of these patients probably had acute tubular necrosis. Knochel and associates noted acute renal failure in approximately 9% of their patients who survived heat stroke. They related acute hypokalemic tubular changes (hydropic vacuole degeneration) as an added factor in producing acute renal failure (Figs. 4-6 and 4-7).

Heat exhaustion. Heat exhaustion follows sustained exposure to heat, salt depletion, strenuous exercise, and dehydration; in some patients hydration may occur. Subsequently there is a collapse of the peripheral circulation. The patient complains early of fatigue, confusion, weakness, stupor, headache, and dizziness. Later the patient suffers from anorexia, visual disturbances, and vomiting, and he may or may not have muscle cramps. Physical examination may reveal peripheral vascular collapse, mental confusion, profuse sweating, and muscular incoordination. The skin is usually cool and pale, the blood pressure is reduced,

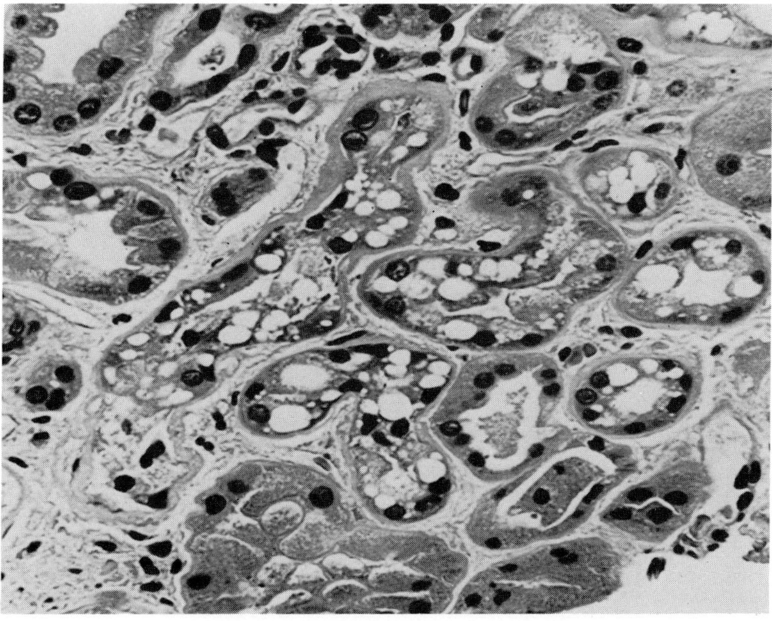

Fig. 4-6. Hypokalemic nephropathy. This photograph illustrates the renal biopsy of a patient aged 39 years with severe potassium deficiency. She took large quantities of phenolphthalein as a laxative. The renal biopsy was taken when the serum potassium was 1.9 mEq/L. Hydropic vacuoles were noted in the proximal tubular cells near the tubular basement membrane. The nucleus was pushed to one side. (H&E ×400.)

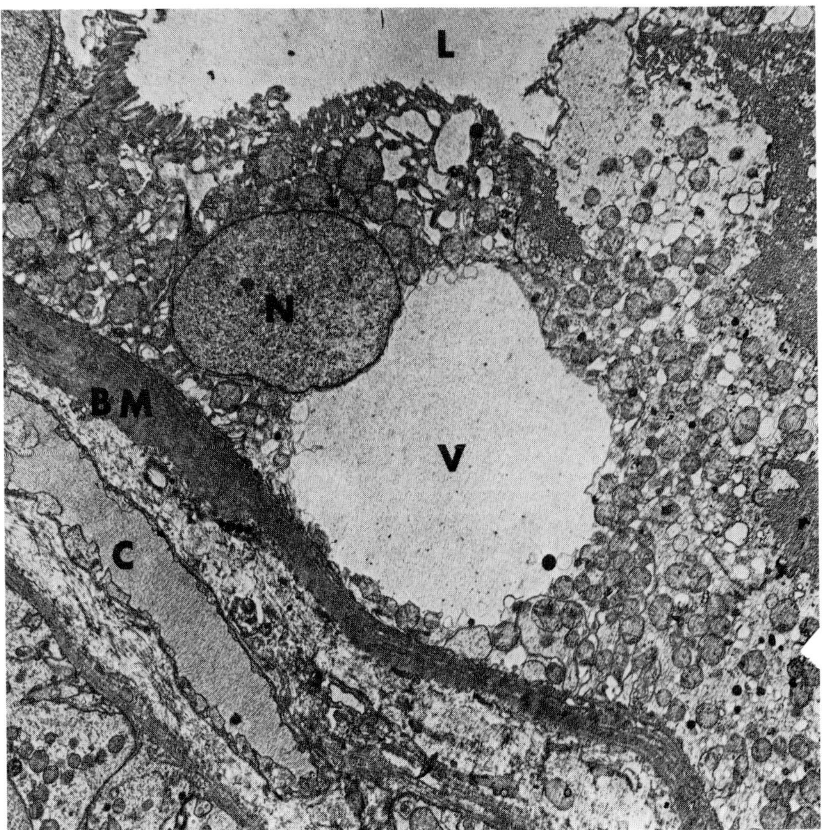

Fig. 4-7. Hypokalemic proximal tubular abnormalities. This electron microphotograph is taken from a patient with severe hypokalemia. A proximal tubule cell is seen with a hydropic vacuole (V). The tubular lumen (L) is above. The brush border appears crew-cut. The nucleus (N) is to the left of the vacuole. The tubular basement membrane (BM) is thickened. A portion of a distal tubule is seen at the left bottom. A peritubular capillary (C) is enveloped by fibrous tissue. (×4,144.)

and the body temperature is normal. Oliguria and tachycardia occur later in heat exhaustion.

In general, hyperkalemia is present in patients with heat exhaustion; however, hypokalemia can occur if patients sweat profusely and ingest large quantities of sodium chloride. Two distinct physiologic mechanisms can explain this potassium deficiency. The first mechanism is excessive potassium loss through sweat. As the amount of sweating increases the sweat potassium concentration is unchanged; however, the sweat potassium loss is increased. An acclimatized individual can lose as much potassium in sweat as some patients lose through diarrhea.

The second mechanism is the urinary loss of potassium, especially if excessive sodium chloride is ingested to replace the body salt lost through sweating.

Although the sodium chloride deficiency is rapidly corrected, there is an excessive sodium exchange for potassium at the distal tubule segment. This leads to urinary potassium wasting and still further potassium deficiency.[230] A potassium-depleted individual undergoing violent muscular activity is more prone to develop rhabdomyolysis—thus the release of myoglobin into the muscular spaces and the subsequent acute oliguric renal failure.

Heat stress and physical exertion. Prolonged periods of anuria are unique characteristics of heat stress and physical exertion. In hot weather, strenuous muscle exercises such as push-ups, squatting, and jumping as performed by army recruits or athletes have led to myoglobinuria and acute renal failure.[565] Hypercatabolism is implicated, especially in the presence of extensive rhabdomyolysis with muscle vacuolization and degeneration. The cellular vacuolization results from dilatation of the endoplasmic reticulum and is similar to that found in skeletal muscle of patients with periodic muscular paralysis. The rhabdomyolysis is present in approximately 60 to 70% of the patients and leads to myoglobinuria with subsequent acute renal failure.

Patients with McArdle's myopathy may have myoglobinuria after vigorous exercise; the exact mechanism is not well understood. The metabolic demands of exercise are not met by anaerobic glycogenolysis. These patients have an abnormal oxidative phosphorylation. Elevated serum enzyme levels are found. These include aldolase, serum glutamic oxaloacetic transaminase (SGOT), and lactic dehydrogenase (LDH) activity. Results of tests for liver function are usually normal; the specific isoenzyme elevated is LDH-5. The elevation of LDH-5 is characteristic for skeletal muscle and/or liver damage. Renal histologic findings reveal frequent pigmented casts with interstitial edema but little or no evidence of acute tubular necrosis. In some patients, numerous thromboses are found in the renal arterioles.[1007] This condition consumes various factors of the coagulation mechanisms and results in thrombocytopenia and bleeding tendencies.

Myotoxins. In 1957, Fahlgren and associates described four patients with massive muscle necrosis following ingestion of excessive amounts of ethanol.[354] Two patients had myoglobinuria. Pilz described a veteran who on his thirty-fifth birthday drank "excessive" quantities of ethanol.[349] Massive myoglobinuria occurred and was followed by acute renal failure. Pilz' observation confirms other reports of ethanol-induced myoglobinuria and subsequent acute renal failure. He observed myoglobinuria in association with an elevated SGOT (280 units); his patient had thigh muscle pain and on biopsy study muscle necrosis was found.

Toxic myoglobinuria usually occurs in children. The episodes of myoglobinuria are usually associated with infections. The disease is more severe and more often fatal than the exercise-induced forms. Myoglobinuria has followed coal gas poisoning.[707]

Viruses can produce myoglobinuria by a fulminating muscle involvement. For example, Coxsackie virus produced muscle necrosis in a 9-year-old boy reported by Favara and colleagues.[358] They attributed the disease to a mechanism triggered by the infection. In man, upper respiratory infections are the common infections that precipitate myoglobinuria.

Haff disease. "Haff krankheit" (Haff epidemic disease) is characterized by muscle pain, stiffness, weakness, and tenderness.[584] It was reported in the middle of the 1920's and early 1930's as an epidemic disease at Frisches Haff (Bay) on the Baltic Sea near Königsberg, Germany. Patients had respiratory difficulties, and their urine became dark, "like dark beer." Myoglobinuria was noted and urination was painful. Acute oliguric renal failure followed. The symptoms usually lasted for three days and the patient either completely recovered or died in uremia. The etiology of Haff disease is a myotoxin that is ingested by eating a specific fish or small eels from waters polluted by industrial wastes released by cellulose factories. The disease occurred in people living along seashore areas of Königsberg Haff, Germany, and along a small inland Swedish lake.[96] Another epidemic occurred in Northwestern Russia. Birds and foxes also develop this disease as a result of eating these polluted fish and eels.

Familial paroxysmal myoglobinuria. This familial condition is relatively rare and occurs predominantly in white males, although it has been reported in one Negro male. It was first described in 1910 by Meyer-Betz in a 13-year-old boy who had recurring attacks for six years.[775a] The disorder is characterized by a spontaneous onset of weak, painful, tender, and swollen muscles. There is a relatively high incidence of muscular dystrophy associated with familial paroxysmal myoglobinuria. Therefore, patients with familial paroxysmal myoglobinuria can be divided into two groups: those with and those without overt muscular dystrophy. The dystrophy is frequently pseudohypertrophic muscular dystrophy. On rare occasions its has been called "progressive muscular dystrophy." Patients may have skin erythema or skin wheals. Muscle power returns slowly and may be complete in 1 to 3 weeks.

One of the possible mechanisms for this hereditary disorder is a muscle cell membrane defect similar to that seen in congenital hemolytic anemias. The defective muscle cell membrane undergoes rupture. This is precipitated by sudden exercise, cold exposure, fever, or infection. The ruptured muscle cell spills its contents into the surrounding environment, and myoglobin, LDH, and SGOT enter the bloodstream.

Grossly, the kidney is a pronounced light-brown color. The pyramids are usually slightly darker than the cortex. Tubular changes from mild to severe tubular necrosis are noted and the interstitium is edematous. The pathogenesis of acute renal failure cannot be attributed singly to the precipitation of myoglobin within the renal tubular lumen. For example, Schaar pointed out that acute renal failure was not caused by myoglobin but by some other factor, as yet unknown.[957]

Equine myoglobinuria. In 1930, Carlstrom first described a unique condition that occurred in healthy draft horses that were stabled and given high caloric feed over a weekend.[203] On Monday morning when the horses were vigorously worked the disease "precipitated out." The horse suddenly fell to the ground with severe weakness and apparent muscle pain in the hind limbs. Therefore, the name of "Monday morning disease" was given to this disorder, which is characterized by swelling and muscle tenderness in the hind legs, muscle tremor, lumbar muscle paresis, and collapse. A scanty, dark urine is passed, azotemia develops, and 25% of the horses may die in uremia caused by acute renal failure. Some horses eventually recover within 2 to 4 days, sometimes completely and sometimes with persistent weakness. The affected muscle resembles fish flesh, with almost complete loss of all cell structures. Renal lesions are acute tubular necrosis with numerous myoglobin casts.

NEPHROTOXIC ETIOLOGY OF ACUTE RENAL FAILURE

The kidney, with its rich blood supply and superior excretory function, is especially vulnerable to the adverse effects of chemicals, biologic products, and drugs.[176,979] The kidneys comprise 0.4% of the total body weight and require a high oxygen consumption. To achieve the amount of oxygen required, the kidneys receive approximately 20 to 25% of the cardiac output. In relation to their relatively small weight, the kidneys have the greatest surface area of endothelial cells when compared to other organs. The kidneys are second only to the liver in complexity of metabolic function. Finally, the kidneys have extremely vascular renal medullae and rete mirabile that function in the final dilution and concentration of the urine. This complex mechanism results in hypertonicity of the renal interstitium with concentration of nephrotoxic chemicals and drugs. Of 283 cases of acute oliguric renal failure that I treated, approximately 25% were induced by chemicals, biologic products, or drugs.

Nephrotoxic chemicals have exerted these adverse effects on the kidney either singly or through a combination of pathopharmacologic mechanisms. One mechanism is the direct action of the nephrotoxic substance as a protoplasmic poison. The nephrotoxic agent passes into the glomerular filtration in an amount proportionate to the filtered plasma water. Since the nephrotoxic substance is a foreign compound and has no specific renal tubular transport process, it is progressively concentrated within the tubular lumen. The concentration of the nephrotoxic agent is so great that it damages the tubular epithelial cells. Moreover, other nephrotoxic substances[887,970,1145] may increase in their concentration to reach toxic levels within the medullary interstitium by the osmotic concentration of fluids.* When sufficient quantity is accumulated, the kidney interstitium is damaged. Chronic phenacetin nephritis is one example of such a condition.†

Some nephrotoxic substances penetrate the cell to interact with cellular constituents and subsequently poison the cell. One example of this mechanism is

---

*See references 337, 360, 386, 432, 471, and 669.
†See references 29, 30, 168, 220, 524, 660, 692, 825, 973, and 980.

the nephrotoxic effect of meralluride (Mercuhydrin), which reacts with enzyme systems of the sulfhydryl groups within the wall of mitochondria. Other nephrotoxins couple with enzymes to inactivate them. Some nephrotoxins affect enzymes within the mitochondria, while other toxins affect cytoplasmic enzymes. This functional interference may result in no apparent tubular morphologic abnormalities when the tissue is studied by light or electron microscopy. Other protoplasmic toxins, when concentrated, may coagulate protein and may result in either severe tubular necrosis or diffuse bilateral renal cortical necrosis.

Other nephrotoxic agents produce their adverse effects through a pathopharmacologic mechanism of hypersensitivity. The sulfonamides are the best example of such a model. The morphologic site involved is usually the large endothelial surface of the glomerular capillaries, arterioles, and arteries. One important additional site involved by hypersensitivity reactions is the renal interstitium. This hypersensitivity interstitial reaction was reported more than 75 years ago by Councilman.[242] It is known as "Councilman's interstitial nephritis" and is characterized by interstitial infiltrates of plasma cells, small lymphocytes, and eosinophils. A few of the drugs that cause this hypersensitivity reaction are phen-

Table 4-2. Common chemicals that induce acute oliguric renal failure

Chemical	*Mean lethal dosage (Approximately per 70 kg)*
Aniline	10 gm
Arsine gas (AsH_3)	MAC* 30 ppm
Camphor	2 gm
Carbon tetrachloride	4 ml (MAC 25 ppm)
Chlordane	8 gm
Chloroform	25 ml
Copper compounds	15 gm
Creosote	10 gm
Essential (volatile) oils	1 gm
Ethylene dichloride	MAC 100 ppm
Ethylene glycol	100 ml
Formaldehyde (formalin)	30 ml
Guaiacol	2 gm
Mercury compounds	MAC 0.1 mg/M³
	1 gm
Naphthalene (mothballs)	5 gm
Oxalates	5 gm
Paradichlorobenzene	15 gm
Pentachlorophenol	1 gm
Phenol	10 gm
Phosphorus, yellow	0.05 gm (MAC 1 gm/M³)
Resorcinol	2 gm
Tetrachloroethane	MAC 5 ppm
Thymol	2 gm

*MAC—Maximum allowable concentration.

indione,[48] diphenylhydantoin (Dilantin), methicillin, phenylbutazone, and meralluride (Mercuhydrin).

In general, substances toxic to the kidney include chemicals in any physical state (liquids, solids, and gases*), biologic products such as horse serum, fungi (mushrooms), and vaccines and drugs given orally or parenterally[913] (Table 4-2). Drugs produce other clinical syndromes of renal disease, including the nephrotic syndrome,[269,547,553] chronic renal failure, tubular disturbances, and acute hemorrhagic glomerulonephritis.

Chemicals

The more common nephrotoxins producing acute renal failure are heavy metals, organic solvents, glycols, analine, insecticides, arsine, cresol, and a miscellaneous group of chemicals. They usually act directly on the tubular cells to disrupt their metabolic and morphologic integrity.

Mercury compounds

The inorganic salt bichloride of mercury (mercuric chloride) is also known as corrosive sublimate. Mercuric chloride is usually ingested accidentally,[725] in suicidal attempts,[138] or following its use as an abortive agent. The dose required to induce renal failure is difficult to assess.[307] In most reports the patients with acute renal failure had ingested two or three tablets (0.5 gm each).[567] When more than four tablets were taken, acute oliguric renal failure was fatal. Renal lesions developed within 3 hours after ingestion.[179,1095] Emetic and gastric lavage solutions can be made from a glass of skimmed milk with three to four teaspoonfuls of table sugar, two tablespoons of baking soda, and three eggs.

Schreiner and Maher described eleven patients who had mercuric chloride–induced acute oliguric renal failure.[976,979] Five patients who survived were treated within 48 hours after ingesting mercuric chloride; hemodialysis and dimercaprol (BAL) infusion were the methods of treatment.[597,705,707] Six patients were treated after uremia occurred, and only three of those six survived.[706] BAL appears to enhance the removal of mercuric ions by 7 to 11% with the use of hemodialysis.[75]

The clinical symptoms of inorganic mercury poisoning begin with a lingering bitter and metallic taste in the mouth. The patient experiences a sensation of throat constriction, suffocation, substernal burning, gastritis, abdominal pain, and, finally, nausea and vomiting.[439] Persistent vomiting leads to retching of blood. Ulceration may be noted in the palate. The patient goes into circulatory failure; the pulse becomes weak and rapid. Syncope and shock are followed by a scanty urinary output. Finally, a fatal anuria develops. Jaundice occurs in approximately 35% of the patients.

The kidneys of patients with inorganic mercury poisoning are usually enlarged and weigh up to 250 gm each. The renal cortex is pale and thickened. The renal

---

*See references 227, 615, 751, 897.

medullae are a slightly darker brown than normal. The most striking morphologic abnormalities occur in the proximal convoluted tubules.[398] There is extensive cellular necrosis; the lumina are filled with granular eosinophilic material believed to be derived from the cytoplasm of necrotic cells.[253] Less striking abnormalities are found in the ascending limbs, distal convoluted tubules, and collecting tubules. In approximately 1 week, the luminal necrotic debris clears, probably because of digestion by plasmolytic enzymes. In addition, the debris is washed down the nephron lumen by the glomerular filtrate. The proximal tubule appears to be dilated and lined by flat epithelial cells.[791] Patchy calcification may occur in severely damaged tubules. Interstitial edema is noted early; if oliguria is prolonged, interstitial fibrosis ensues. Mercurials have produced the nephrotic syndrome in some patients.[80]

Carbon tetrachloride

Carbon tetrachloride (CCl_4) is widely used as an industrial solvent, as a household cleaning agent, as a constituent in certain types of fire extinguishers, in some hair lotions, as an antihelmintic agent, and as a vermifuge.[8] It is a volatile, heavier than air liquid that accounts for the high incidence of exposure in poorly ventilated areas. Carbon tetrachloride is toxic in concentrations greater than 100 ppm.[353] It is absorbed through the lungs, the skin, and the gut. It concentrates in fatty tissue such as the brain and bone marrow.

Carbon tetrachloride is soluble in ethanol. Therefore, the drinking of alcoholic beverages and the simultaneous exposure to carbon tetrachloride tend to increase or enhance carbon tetrachloride absorption and subsequent toxicity. In vitro, carbon tetrachloride is oxidized to phosgene and later can condense with ethyl alcohol to form ethyl chloroformate. The later is an extremely nephrotoxic substance. In the absence of ethyl alcohol, phosgene condenses with ammonia to form urea.

Carbon tetrachloride appears to be more dangerous in obese or in undernourished individuals. In France, carbon tetrachloride was the commonest chemical producing acute renal failure. The clinical features of acute poisoning are variable. Males are more often afflicted than females—by a ratio of 14 to 1. Inhalation is the most frequent route of exposure. Toxicity caused by ingestion carries a grave prognosis. Initially the patient has surface or superficial irritation to the exposed skin and mucous membranes. Later the patient has headache, nausea, vomiting, abdominal pain, and mental confusion leading to convulsions and coma. Although liver damage is a very striking feature of carbon tetrachloride toxicity, acute renal failure is the most frequent cause of death.

The onset of oliguria is prolonged and may occur 7 to 10 days after exposure. Some patients may have forgotten their exposure to this solvent. Absolute anuria may last from 1 day to several weeks. One patient had carbon tetrachloride–induced oliguria for 67 days. In my experience, patients with acute renal failure caused by carbon tetrachloride were usually "do-it-yourselfers." They usually worked indoors, generally in the basement during the winter months; this meant that the windows were closed and there was no source of ventilation. They usually drank several cans of beer while they refinished furniture or cleaned outboard motors or clothes—usually neckties.

Morphologic abnormalities occur in the cortical convolutions and Henle's loops. Tubular necrosis is most prominent in the outmost cortical portion. Acute tubular necrosis may be severe with tubular coagulation and degranulation.[1139] Ultrastructural study of the glomeruli reveals them to be normal. Initially interstitial edema is common and, later, interstitial fibrosis occurs.[1017a]

Features of the clinicopathologic correlations are discussed in the following case presentation.

CASE PRESENTATION

T. W., a 54-year-old laborer, used carbon tetrachloride to clean his outboard motor one night in February, 1963. His workshop was in an enclosed basement. He drank several cans of beer while working. Seven days later he noted oliguria and consulted his physician. He was admitted to the hospital (Fig. 4-8). The BUN was 37 mg% and the urinary output was 76 ml in 24 hours. On the twelfth day following carbon tetrachloride exposure he was markedly edematous, his weight was 187 pounds, and his BUN was 108 mg%. There was no sign of liver damage.

Peritoneal dialysis was started with 7% glucose in the dialysate. His weight was reduced to

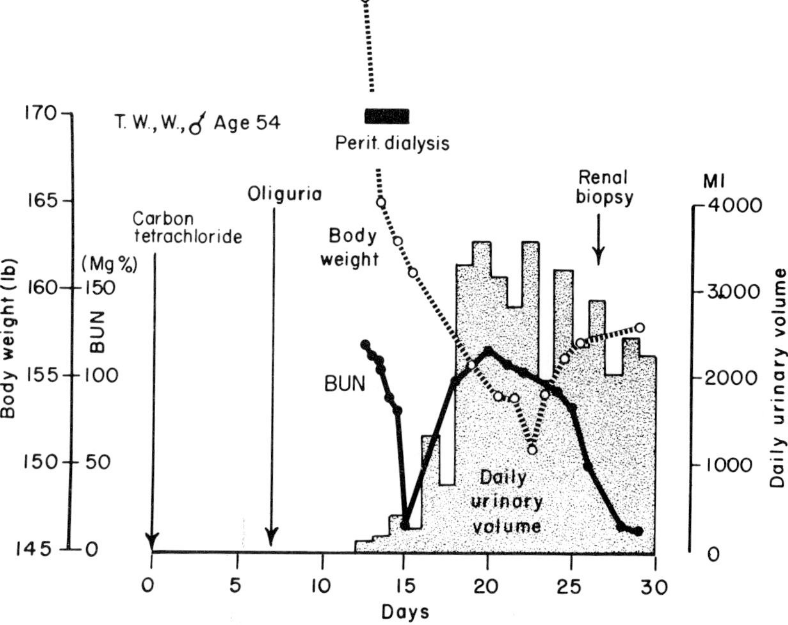

Fig. 4-8. Clinical features of patient with acute renal failure following carbon tetrachloride. A 54-year-old laborer was exposed to carbon tetrachloride while cleaning an outboard motor. Oliguria occurred on the sixth day. Peritoneal dialysis was done on the twelfth day. Spontaneous diuresis occurred on the seventeenth day. On the twenty-seventh day a percutaneous renal biopsy was taken. Tubular regeneration was found. The BUN was normal by the twenty-eighth day.

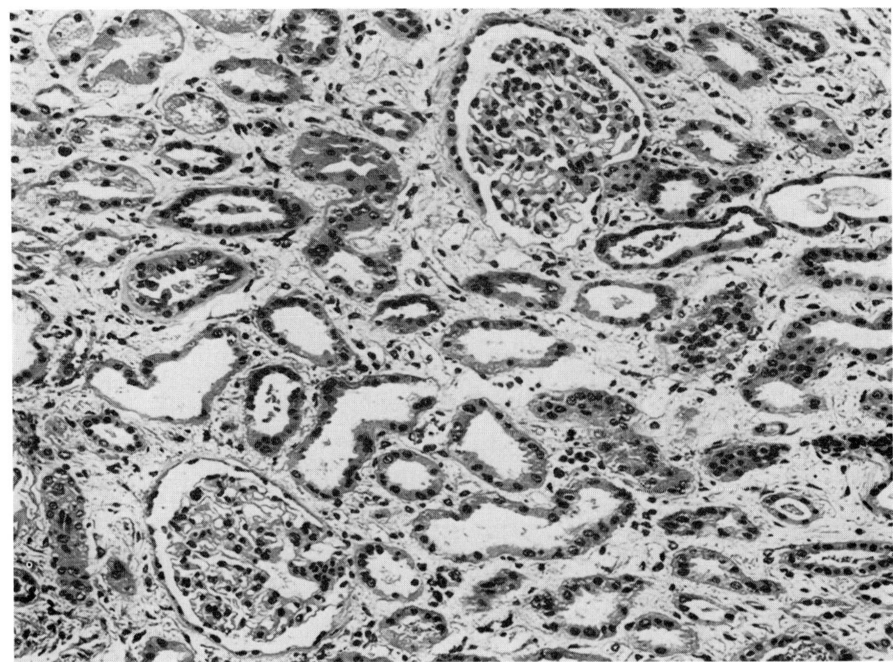

Fig. 4-9. Carbon tetrachloride–induced acute tubular necrosis. Renal biopsy was taken on the twenty-seventh day after carbon tetrachloride exposure from patient described in Fig. 4-8. There was tubular regeneration with diffuse interstitial fibrosis and edema. The juxtaglomerular apparatus was prominent. (H&E ×320.)

163 pounds and BUN to 18 mg%. He entered the diuretic phase on the seventeenth day. His body weight continued to fall. On the twentieth day, he reached a peak diuresis. The BUN was normal on the twenty-eighth day. A percutaneous renal biopsy was taken on the twenty-seventh day. The patient subsequently made a complete recovery.

Renal biopsy findings. Eleven glomeruli were noted in the sections; all appeared normal. Tubular regeneration was complete by ultrastructural studies. There was a diffuse interstitial edema with early but mild diffuse interstitial fibrosis. The morphologic diagnosis was interstitial edema (Figs. 4-9 and 4-10).

Comment. The patient was exposed to carbon tetrachloride in an enclosed, nonventilated basement. The absorption of carbon tetrachloride was probably increased by the alcohol content of the beer. Oliguria was late in onset and was not associated with liver damage.[280] His primary physician overhydrated him. Peritoneal dialysis and later conservative treatment were effective. Diuresis occurred with successful regeneration of renal tubules. Once again diffuse interstitial edema and fibrosis were the prominent morphologic findings.

Tetrachloroethylene

Tetrachloroethylene is a colorless liquid with an ethereal odor. It is soluble in organic solvents. Tetrachloroethylene has replaced carbon tetrachloride in the treatment of hookworm infestation. It is placed in soft gelatin capsules of either 0.2, 1.0, or 2.5 ml. Tetrachloroethylene produces inebriation, giddiness, and liver damage. It is less nephrotoxic than carbon tetrachloride but has produced acute oliguric renal failure from acute tubular necrosis.

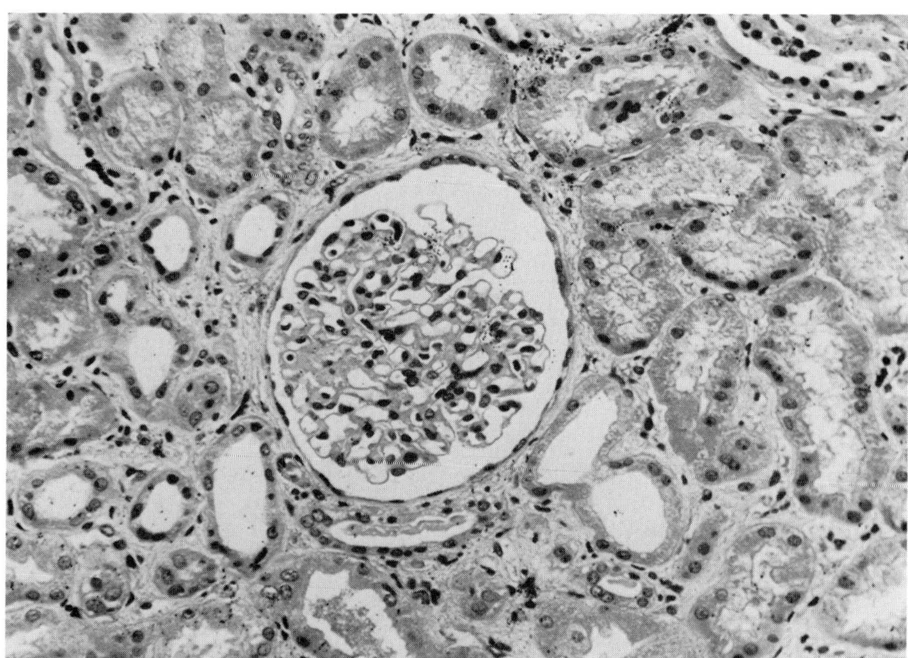

Fig. 4-10. Recovery from carbon tetrachloride–induced acute renal failure. Patient described in Fig. 4-8 had a second renal biopsy done on the sixty-first day after recovering from acute oliguric renal failure. The tubules have completely healed and are separated from each other by a diffuse interstitial fibrosis. (H&E ×375.)

Glycol toxicity

Glycols are found in automobile antifreeze, in solvents for plastics, in paints—especially lacquers, textiles, and cosmetics—and in flavoring extracts. Allen has classified the toxic glycols[14] (Table 4-3). The more important nephrotoxic glycols are ethylene glycol and diethylene glycol. Ethylene glycol dinitrite, a yellow liquid used in the explosives industry, produces symptoms resembling those of nitroglycerol toxicity. Methemoglobinuria and acute tubular necrosis are the prominent renal features. Propylene glycol produces hemoglobinuria and prolonged oliguria without crystals in the tubular lumen. Ethylene dichloride may produce shock, pulmonary edema, and tubular necrosis.

Ethylene glycol. Ethylene glycol is the main substance in antifreeze and was made popular during World War I. It is a colorless, odorless liquid and is ingested by mistake during "alcoholic bouts." Some describe its taste as unpleasant and waxy; others describe it as sweet.[694] When it is mixed with water and is drunk, it imparts a feeling of warmth to the mucous membranes and produces acute inebriation. Ethylene glycol is converted to the more nephrotoxic intermediaries—glycolaldehyde, glycolic acid, and oxalic acid.[598,891] Each of the intermediary compounds is a precursor of oxalate.

Table 4-3. The toxic glycols

Glycol	Formula
Ethylene glycol (antifreeze)	$HO \cdot CH_2CH_2 \cdot OH$
Ethylene glycol diacetate	$CH_3CO \cdot O \cdot CH_2 \cdot CH_2 \cdot O \cdot CO \cdot CH_3$
Propylene glycol	$HO \cdot CH_2 \cdot CH \cdot OH \cdot CH_3$
Diethylene glycol (diglycol)	$HO \cdot CH_2 \cdot CH_2 \cdot O \cdot CH_2 \cdot CH_2 \cdot OH$
Ethyl diethylene glycol (carbitol)	$C_2H_5 \cdot O \cdot CH_2 \cdot CH_2 \cdot O \cdot CH_2 \cdot CH_2 \cdot OH$
Methyl diethylene glycol (methyl carbitol)	$CH_3 \cdot O \cdot CH_2 \cdot CH_2 \cdot O \cdot CH_2 \cdot CH_2 \cdot OH$
Butyl diethylene glycol (butyl carbitol)	$C_4H_9 \cdot O \cdot CH_2 \cdot CH_2 \cdot O \cdot CH_2 \cdot CH_2 \cdot OH$
Diethylene dioxide (dioxane)	$\begin{array}{c} CH_2 \cdot CH_2 \\ O \qquad\qquad O \\ CH_2 \cdot CH_2 \end{array}$
Dipropylene glycol	$CH_3 \cdot OH \cdot CH \cdot CH_2 \cdot O \cdot CH_2 \cdot CH \cdot OH \cdot CH_3$

Although calcium oxalate crystals are found within the renal tubules and other organs, acute oliguric failure does not result from the simple obstructive effects of oxalate. It is the direct nephrotoxic effects of ethylene glycol or one of its intermediary products that induces acute oliguric renal failure. The most likely nephrotoxic product is oxalic acid. The lethal dose of ethylene glycol (100 ml) would be converted to 3 to 10 gm of oxalic acid. As small a dose of oxalic acid as 2 gm would be fatal.[402] Gastric lavage and sodium bicarbonate infusion are two important aspects of initial therapy.

When large quantities of ethylene glycol are ingested, the clinical features are dominated by three distinct stages.[694] The first extends from 30 minutes to 12 hours after ingestion and is characterized by central nervous system symptoms with initial hyperactivity progressing to coma. If the patient survives the initial complication he enters the second stage, which is characterized by cardiac and pulmonary features with tachypnea, cyanosis, and pulmonary edema. The third stage is caused by deposition of calcium oxalate crystals within the kidney; acute oliguric renal failure occurs. In the early stage of renal affliction the urine may contain oxalate crystals and protein.

Treatment includes the initial gastric lavage with a 5% solution of sodium bicarbonate. Intermediate dialysis is important to remove the glycol.[875] Intravenous ethanol is helpful in competing with liver enzymes (for example, dehydrogenase) that metabolize ethylene glycol. Morphologic abnormalities of epithelial cell destruction with intact basement membrane is common. Tubules are filled with masses of calcium oxalate crystals that are birefringent under polarized light. Intrarenal hydronephrosis is noted. Interstitial edema and focal cellular infiltrates of mononuclear cells are present. In addition, oxalate crystals are found within other organs such as the brain, the heart, and the lungs.

Diethylene glycol. Diethylene glycol is a colorless liquid that was used with catastrophic results as a medicinal vehicle in an elixir of sulfanilamide. During September and October of 1937, at least seventy-six patients died within a few days after taking the elixir which contained 72% diethylene glycol and a 10% solution of sulfanilamide. This drug-induced disaster occurred in an era before the United States Food and Drug Administration had its drug evaluation program in effect. The recommendation of Geiling and Cannon in a report on the toxicity of the sulfanilamide elixir can be used as an excellent guideline for the pharmaceutical evaluation of drugs.[423] Their report is recommended to individuals who have any doubts of the necessity for drug toxicity evaluation.

Grossly the kidney was pale, flabby, and swollen. Microscopically there was severe hydropic tubular degeneration similar to that seen in the proximal tubules of potassium-depleted patients. The epithelial cells were swollen and their lumina were patent. Spoke-like deeply basophilic crystals were seen in the distal convoluted tubules. Bilateral renal cortical necrosis was seen in a large group of individuals following sulfanilamide elixir ingestion.

Aniline

Aniline and its derivative, phenylhydroxylamine, have low molecular weights (93 and 109, respectively). They pass through the semipermeable membrane of the hemodialysis unit. Acute poisoning by pure aniline is rare.[511] However, poisoning does occur in industrial workers and in children exposed to inks, colored wax crayons, and shoe polishes. Diapers freshly stamped with aniline marking ink have resulted in fatal methemoglobinuria and acute renal failure in infants.

Aniline poisoning has been caused by the percutaneous absorption of aniline from freshly dyed shoes or blankets. Aniline and its derivative produce hemolysis, methemoglobinuria,[207] shock, cyanosis, anoxia, and acute renal failure. In patients who have sublethal poisoning the clinical manifestations are cyanosis, dyspnea, headache, dizziness, and blurring of mental functions. If the aniline poisoning is severe, the manifestations are shock, cyanosis, coma, anemia, and, finally, fatal anuria.[1144]

The diagnosis is made when methemoglobinuria is found. This is detected as a well-defined absorption band at 630 wavelengths and immediately disappears after the addition of a few drops of 5% potassium cyanide (KCN) solution. Diazo-reacting compounds can be found in the blood, urine, and hemodialysate. Comparisons of the diazo-reacting compounds in blood, urine, and dialysate are used to obtain an optimal clinical end point for dialysis.

Treatment is removal of aniline by gastric lavage, purges, and hemodialysis. This removal permits the reducing enzyme system of the erythrocyte to rapidly reconvert methemoglobin to hemoglobin. Intravenously injected methylene blue in doses of 1.0 to 2.0 mg/kg body weight should be given over a period of several minutes. This dose very rapidly reconverts methemoglobin to hemoglobin. It may be necessary to repeat methylene blue injections at hourly intervals. The blood pressure should be supported by whole blood transfusions, vasopressive agents, and hemodialysis. Dialysis should be maintained for longer periods than are usual for treating acute renal failure. Such treatment will remove toxic derivative mobilized as a lipid soluble material from body tissues. Acute tubular necrosis is the common morphologic change found in aniline poisoning.

Insecticides

The two main groups of nephrotoxic insecticides are the chlorinated hydrocarbons and the organophosphates. Acute tubular necrosis is the common morphologic finding in patients with acute oliguric renal failure.

Chlordane. The chlorinated hydrocarbon insecticides are stimulants of the central nervous system. They kill insects by overstimulation and may cause the death of man through the same mechanism. The chlorinated hydrocarbon insecticides penetrate the skin of man or are inhaled when the insecticide is in a fine aerosol spray.

Chlordane, one example of this group, has produced fatal anuria.[279] The initial clinical symptoms are dizziness, nausea, headache, and ataxia. Sudden unexpected convulsions similar to grand mal epilepsy occur and lead to stupor and coma. Pulmonary edema may occur between episodes of repeated convulsions. Shock may occur and may be followed by acute oliguria and death in uremia.

Parathion. Parathion is an organophosphate type of insecticide. Mann and associates observed that renal tubular malfunction occurred in individuals during occupational exposure to parathion. The chronic exposure to pesticides containing parathion produces a chronic irreversible renal tubular dysfunction that increases with duration of exposure.

Hexol

Hexol is a mixture of a steam-distilled pine oil derivative (70%) and neutral soap (30%). The pine oil derivative is a mixture of terpin alcohol, predominately terpineol, with 5 to 10% each of terpene, borneol, and terpene ethers. Hexol is used in the United States as a household disinfectant.

The common toxic effects of pine oil distillates are local irritation on the skin or burning pain in the mouth.[745] They produce central nervous system excitation and, later, depression. Hexol produces headaches, giddiness, ataxia, stupor, and death in respiratory failure caused by central nervous system depression.

The pine oil distillates have produced dysuria, hematuria, proteinuria, and glycosuria.[213,581] In general, renal damage is transient and completely reversible. Gornel and Goldman reported a 31-year-old woman who had Hexol-induced acute oliguric renal failure.[451] She used a syringe and catheter to instill into her uterus 3 to 6 ounces of 2:1 mixture of Hexol and water. The next day she had anuria, which lasted 4 days. A diuresis followed. Eleven months later her creatinine clearance was 47 ml per minute. Two renal biopsy studies were done, the first at 6 weeks and the second at 5 months after anuria. The prominent findings were a completely healed renal tubular lesion, atrophied tubules, and interstitial fibrosis.

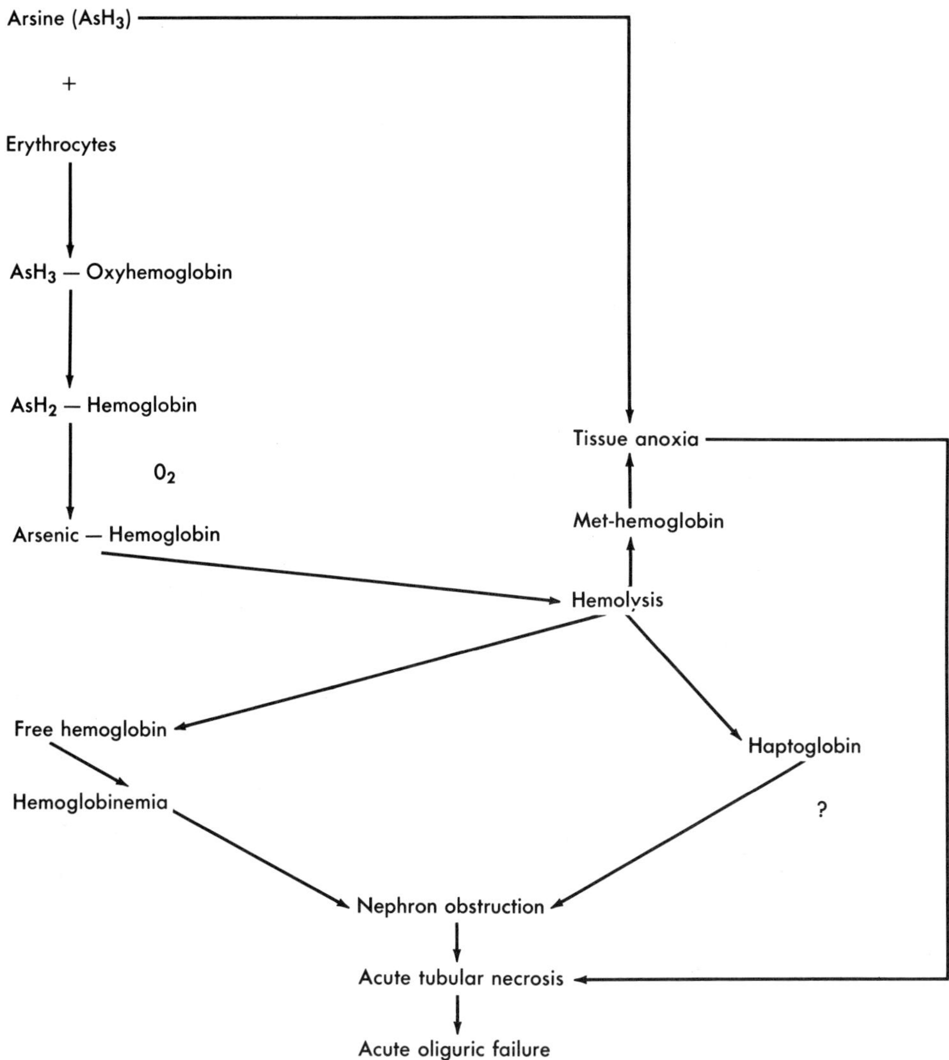

Fig. 4-11. Mechanism of arsine-induced anuria. Arsine is inhaled and rapidly enters the erythrocyte. Arsine (AsH₃) is reduced to AsH₂ when bound to hemoglobin. The arsine-hemoglobin complex causes rupture of the erythrocyte. Hemoglobinemia results with free hemoglobin converted to met-hemoglobin. If the serum hemoglobin exceeds 135 mg per 100 ml, hemoglobinuria occurs. The combined effects of tissue anoxia, erythrocyte, stroma, arsine effects on cellular respiration, and hemoglobin degradation products results in acute tubular necrosis with subsequent acute oliguric renal failure.

Arsine

Arsine (AsH_3)-induced renal failure was discussed previously. It usually occurs as an occupational hazard.[287,319] When anuria occurs the prognosis is grave.[134] The pathogenesis of arsine-induced renal failure is illustrated in Fig. 4-11. Arsine is inhaled and readily combines with the hemoglobin within the erythrocyte to form an arsine-oxyhemoglobin complex.[595] This is initially oxidized to AsH_2-hemoglobin. As the oxidation process continues an arsenic-hemoglobin–bound product occurs. Intravascular hemolysis occurs and results in methemoglobinuria and massive hemoglobinuria. Hemoglobin and erythrocyte casts fill the tubular lumen.[723] A number of simultaneous conditions occur. The ischemia caused by anemia, the presence of hemoglobin, methemoglobin, and erythrocyte casts, and the direct tissue anoxia of arsine on the respiratory enzymes of the nephron all, either singly or in combination, produce acute tubular necrosis.[763]

Cresol

Cresol shares the generalized nephrotoxicity of carbolic acid, naphtol, guaiacol, creosote, and other phenols. Lysol (cresol) has been taken for suicide purposes or in excessive concentrated solutions via vaginal douches to induce abortion.[371a] Cresol is lethal in a dose of 50 to 100 ml. It produces mucous membrane necrosis, but the patient is not aware of the toxic effect. The clinical features are nausea, vomiting, dizziness, ataxia, abdominal pain, and shock. Severe intravascular hemolysis occurs and is followed by hemoglobinuria, proteinuria, hematuria, acute cystitis, and acute oliguria caused by acute tubular necrosis. The penetrating smell of cresol makes the diagnosis easier. The mucous membrane of the mouth and tongue may be burned and may appear to be dull white with phenol and darker brown with cresol.

Treatment is lavage of the stomach with sodium bicarbonate, followed by a purge of magnesium sulfate (6 gm in 100 ml). Skin burns should be thoroughly washed with soap and copious amounts of water. This should be followed by a wash with a 10% solution of alcohol. The skin should be dressed with gauze soaked in a sterile solution of sodium bicarbonate (0.5%). Tracheobronchial secretions should be aspirated to prevent pulmonary infection. The patient may require dialysis.

Potassium bromate

Accidental poisoning with potassium bromate occurs in infants and children. Potassium bromate was the primary chemical constituent of the neutralizing solution used after Toni permanent wave or Coldwave. Dunsky reported a 17-month-old infant who had fatal acute oliguric renal failure following ingestion of the neutralizing solution.[326] At autopsy the patient had generalized edema and acute tubular necrosis. Warren and Gross reported a 2-year-old infant who was accidentally fed Toni neutralizer.[1114] After 38 days of anuria and oliguria, the child gradually recovered.

Chlorate compounds

Sodium chlorate and potassium chlorate are used in the manufacture of matches, explosives, toothpaste, and synthetic pigments, and they are used as weedkillers. Potassium chlorate is used as an oxidizing agent in lozenges and gargles.

If the patient develops acute renal failure, the onset stage varies from 3 to 15 hours. The clinical features are fever, hypotension, jaundice, abdominal pain, nausea, vomiting, diarrhea, extreme fatigue, nervousness, and headache. The skin and mucous membranes are deeply cyanosed with a brownish-gray color. The patient has massive hemolysis with hemoglobinuria. Acute tubular necrosis is the common morphologic lesion.[295]

A clinical test can make the diagnosis of chlorate poisoning. Ten grams of kidney obtained at autopsy is minced in 16 ml of warm distilled water and an equal volume of acetone is added. The mixture is centrifuged, the acetone is evaporated, and the mixture is filtered. The aqueous filtrate is decolorized by a few drops of a dilute solution of indigo sulfate followed by a few drops of sulfurous acid. Silver nitrate is added, then sulfurous acid. Silver chloride forms a white precipitate and is used for a quantitative estimate of the chlorates.

Miscellaneous chemicals

Acute oliguric renal failure has followed exposure to a wide variety of common chemicals.[89] Listed in Table 4-2 are these common chemicals, their maximum allowable concentration (MAC), and their mean lethal dosage (MLD). Some of the listed chemicals produce acute renal failure, but such a case is rare.[429] These include methyl chloride,[177,615] arsenic, phenols, copper sulfate,[953] paracetamol,[648] polyvinyl alcohol,[490] formalin, pyrogallol, dichromate,[45] tartaric acid, phosphorus,[468] and sodium tetrathionate.

Biologic products

Acute renal failure can result from biologic products of acute reactions such as anaphylactic allergic reactions, from delayed reactions to horse serum and vaccines, or from biologic toxins such as that found in mushrooms.[998]

Anaphylactic allergic reactions

Acute oliguric renal failure has resulted from anaphylactic shock caused by horse serum, penicillin, streptomycin, and other antibiotics. They produced sudden and prolonged hypotensive states resulting in acute tubular necrosis. Penicillin most often produces anaphylactic shock on a hypersensitivity basis. The management of patients with anaphylactic shock should be directed toward correction of the hypotensive state and interruptions of the hypersensitivity reaction. Patients with severe acute anaphylactic reactions should be given epinephrine subcutaneously (0.5 ml to 1 ml of a 0.001% solution). An adrenocortical steroid such as hydrocortisone (100 mg) should be administered intravenously and, if necessary, in multiple dosage.

A parenteral antihistaminic should be given. If the anaphylactic reaction is severe, vasopressive agents and adrenocortical steroids should be given by intravenous infusion. If a reduction of urinary output occurs, 25 gm of mannitol in a 20% solution must be given. If mannitol proves ineffective, ethacrynic acid (50 mg) should be given intravenously. If this is unsuccessful in producing diuresis, then the usual methods of treating acute oliguric renal failure must be employed.

Horse serum–induced fatal glomerulonephritis

In 1962, De LaPava and colleagues reported three patients who had malignant tumors and were treated with horse anti–human cancer serum.[274] All developed

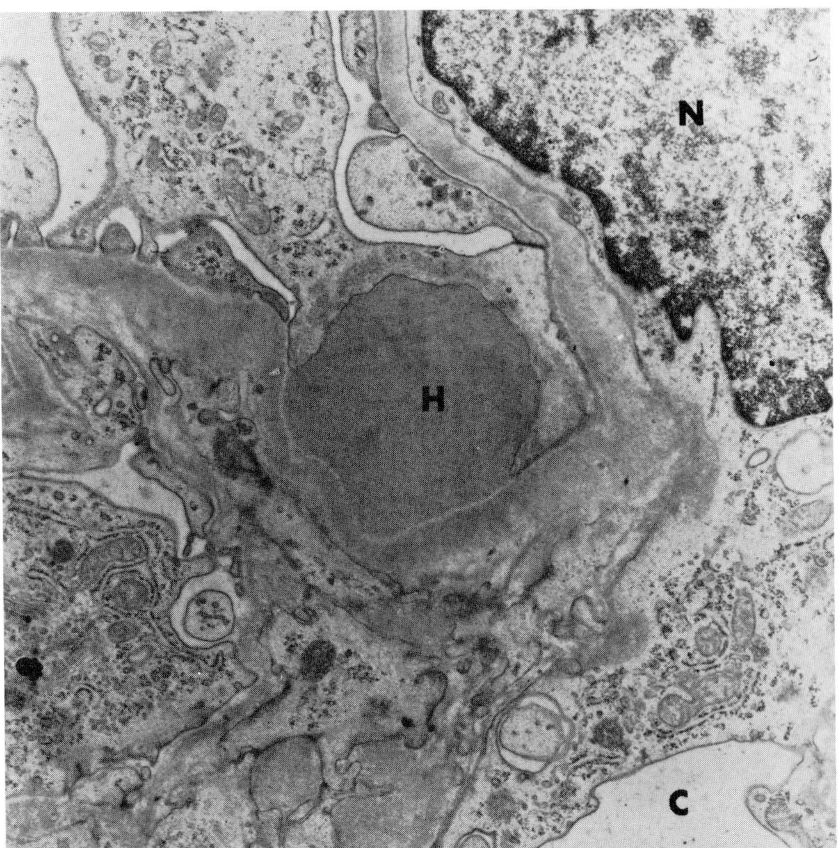

Fig. 4-12. Mechanism of soluble antigen-antibody complex–induced acute renal failure. Horse antihuman cancer serum has induced in patients a fatal proliferative glomerulonephritis with epithelial crescents. The mechanism for this renal lesion is a soluble antigen-antibody complex in antigen excess. This electron microphotograph illustrates a portion of a glomerular capillary loop. An epithelial hump (H) is noted on the epithelial side of the glomerular basement membrane. The glomerular capillary lumen (C) is seen below right. An endothelial cell nucleus (N) fills much of the cytoplasm of an endothelial cell. (×16,800.)

a fatal acute renal failure. At autopsy, a proliferative glomerulonephritis with epithelial crescents was present. The kidney was studied by electron microscopy. Epithelial humps on the glomerular lamina densa were found (Fig. 4-12). They were similar to humps of antigen-antibody complex seen in poststreptococcal glomerulonephritis, dextran-induced glomerulonephritis, and renal disease caused by syphilis. The use of large dosages of adrenocortical steroids has been most beneficial in resolving these lesions of drug-induced diseases.

A horse serum–induced disease was first observed by Rackemann, Longcope, and Peters.[901] They noted water retention, decreased urinary output, and retention of chloride. They were the first to point out that the mechanisms of horse serum–induced renal failure were immunologically based. Later, the specific immunologic reaction was bound to be caused by soluble antigen-antibody complexes in the presence of excessive antigen.

Pertussis vaccine

Acute oliguric renal failure caused by pertussis vaccine is rare.[110] Fatal renal failure has followed eight injections of pertussis vaccine over a 6-week period. One week after the eighth injection the patient developed fever, arthralgia, adenopathy, and progressive renal failure. On the eighth day he was comatose and had mild hypertension, and his BUN was 201 mg per 100 ml. A diffuse healing vasculitis was found to be involving the medium and small arteries, arterioles, and veins. The pathologic findings in the kidney were multiple infarction in the cortex and medulla. There were numerous antemortem thrombi and extensive papillary necrosis.

Typhoid vaccine

Four patients given typhoid vaccine intravenously for 2 to 3 days died in shock and acute oliguric renal failure. One patient died in acute renal failure 4 days after receiving the vaccine. Another patient developed the hepatorenal syndrome. The third patient died 6 hours following injection of the vaccine. Acute tubular necrosis and acute necrosis of the liver were noted.

The fourth patient, a 7-month-old boy who had hereditary agammaglobulinemia, developed complete anuria following one injection of typhoid vaccine. At autopsy acute renal cortical necrosis was found. In addition, there was diffuse thrombosis of the glomerular capillaries. This patient may have had an increased susceptibility to the typhoid vaccine in view of an inadequate or underdeveloped reticuloendothelial system.

Mushroom-induced acute oliguria

The terms "mushroom" and "toadstool" have no specific identifying meaning and are used interchangeably by some mycologists. There are approximately 2,000 species of mushrooms, of which about thirty are poisonous. Some mushrooms are toxic if eaten in excessive quantities, if eaten during certain seasons, if eaten at specific stages of growth, or if eaten by a susceptible individual.[169] In England and Wales there were thirty-eight fatal cases of mushroom poisoning between 1921 and 1949. In the United States the overall mortality rate is difficult to estimate. The common poison mushroom is the *Amanita phalloides.* It must be distinguished from the common field mushroom (*Agaricus campestris*). This distinction is made by noting the presence of the volva on the phalloides. I strongly recommend that "mushroom amateurs" purchase mushrooms from commercial sources and neither pick them nor accept them from a neighbor.

For more than a century, German and French biochemists have studied toxins from *Amanita phalloides.* Their investigations led to the finding of five crystalline toxins and the almost complete description of the structural formulas. These toxins are alpha, beta, and gamma amantin; phalloin; and phalloides.[5] When the toxins are fed to animals their effects vary widely. The pure toxins do not reproduce all the features of mushroom poisoning induced by the intact fungus. Phalloin and phalloides attach to susceptible cells, usually the liver and the kidney. The toxins' molecular weights are 1,072 and 898, respectively. They are poorly dialyzable in vitro, and they attach to albumin. During peritoneal dialysis, therefore, the addition of serum albumin (12.5 gm to 2 liters) to the peritoneal fluid may remove these mycetous toxins.

The toxins of *Amanita phalloides* produce a characteristic clinicopathologic course.[316] Initially gastrointestinal toxicity occurs and is followed by other conditions that are fatal to the patient. These dread complications are acute oliguric renal failure,[343] hepatitis, acute yellow atrophy,[267] myocardial injury, central nervous system disease, and hypoplastic anemia. The exact mode of action of mycetous toxins is not known. However, Wieland and Wieland suggested that mycetous toxins act as inhibitors of mitochondrial oxidative phosphoryl action with consequent interference with specific enzymes necessary for cellular metabolism.[1129]

Prolonged anuria may result from the mycetous toxins of *Amanita phalloides.*[824] Acute tubular necrosis is the common morphologic lesion and involves both proximal and distal convoluted tubules. The glomeruli are usually not affected. Following recovery from prolonged anuria, diffuse interstitial fibrosis develops and is associated with thickening of the cortical convoluted tubular basement membrane. The creatinine clearance remains reduced for several months until diffuse interstitial fibrosis becomes more focal in its renal distribution. Then the creatinine clearance may approach normal values.

Treatment is directed toward sustaining life by the use of conservative measures and dialysis. Peritoneal dialysis is the method of choice, especially if albumin is added to the peritoneal fluid to remove mycetous toxins. If toxicity is induced by *Amanita muscaria,* atropine is effective in neutralizing the muscarine effects of poisonous mushrooms.

Drugs

Drug-induced acute oliguric renal failure is a by-product of man's ever-increasing exposure to a vast array of noxious chemicals and drugs that result from industrial and medical progress.* The kidney, with its numerous enzyme systems, its rich blood supply, and its complex, superior excretory function, is especially vulnerable to the adverse effects of drugs. In my experience, approximately 20 to 25% of all patients with acute oliguria have renal failure induced by chemicals or drugs. Other clinical syndromes of drug-induced nephropathy include the nephrotic syndrome,[944,967,979] chronic renal failure,[1154] tubular disorders, and acute hemorrhagic glomerulonephritis.[945]

In general, drugs induce renal damage through any one of or a combination of many pathopharmacologic mechanisms. Of these, the nephrotoxicity mechanism is the most common and is dose-related; in general, excessively large doses are used. Drugs such as methicillin, penicillin, phenylbutazone,[720] sulfonamide,[376,689] diphenylhydantoin (Dilantin),[539] phenindione[48] and meralluride (Mercuhydrin)[804a] produce acute oliguric renal failure when administered in either the usual dosages or in very small amounts. Hypersensitivity to these drugs can produce acute renal failure. There are also metabolic,[320] mechanical, and secondary mechanisms that produce the disease; the latter are usually caused by drug-induced hemolytic anemia.

The tetracyclines may produce prerenal azotemia through a metabolic mechanism, such as their antianabolic action on the proximal tubules.[355,412] This is reflected by proteinuria, amino-aciduria, phosphaturia, hypokalemia,[407] a low plasma urate, and acidosis. Tetracycline may undergo spontaneous degradation during storage, especially under warm and moist conditions. Anhydrotetracycline and epianhydrotetracycline are the nephrotoxic degradation products that produce the Fanconi syndrome.[405,477] Kunin's table on drug half-life in acute renal failure should serve as a guide to all physicians who treat patients with acute oliguria (Table 3-2).

In addition to classification according to the pathopharmacologic mechanism, nephrotoxic drugs (Table 4-4) can be classified according to the site of morphologic damage. Finally, drug-induced acute renal failure can be classified therapeutically—for example, antibiotics and chemotherapeutic agents, diuretic agents, radiologic contrast media, and so on. In this section I will review nephrotoxic drugs by therapeutic classification and will emphasize the morphologic site of drug interaction.

Drugs interact at specific morphologic sites within the kidney to produce acute renal failure (Fig. 1-17). On a structural basis drugs interact at all four major components: the vessels, the glomeruli, the tubules, and the interstitium. Arteritis has resulted from arsenic, bismuth, diphenylhydantoin (Dilantin),[539] gold salts,[469] horse serum, iodides, penicillin, propylthiouracil, chlorathizides,[633] and

Text continued on p. 226.

---

*See references 799, 935, 1076, and 1131.

Table 4-4. Commonly used drugs that can produce acute renal failure

Drug	Morphologic site of action	Pathologic lesion produced	Pathopharmacologic mechanism of action	Other toxicity associated with renal disease
Acetazolamide (Diamox)[168,437,876]	Proximal tubules	Acute tubular necrosis	Nephrotoxicity	Agranulocytosis, thrombocytopenia, dermatitis
Acetylsalicylic acid[523]	Proximal tubules	Tubular degeneration	Nephrotoxicity	
Aminopyrine[338]	Tubules	Acute tubular necrosis	Nephrotoxicity	Hematoxicity, central nervous system, herpes labialis
Ammoniated mercury[80]	Tubules	Acute tubular necrosis	Nephrotoxicity	Dermatitis
Amphotericin B*	Proximal and distal cortical tubules	Tubular necrosis, calcium deposition	Nephrotoxicity	Anemia, fever, phlebitis, hypokalemia
Aristolochic acid	Proximal tubules	Acute tubular necrosis	Nephrotoxicity	Polyuria
Arsenic compounds	Tubules	Acute tubular necrosis	Nephrotoxicity	Dermatitis, diarrhea
Bacitracin[428]	Proximal tubules	Acute tubular necrosis	Nephrotoxicity	Dermatitis, local injection
Bishydroxycoumarin (Dicumarol)[596]	Ureteral obstruction	Hematoma	Mechanical	Hemorrhage, dermatitis
Bismuth thioglycollate (Thio-Bismol)[606,881]	Proximal tubules	Acute tubular necrosis	Nephrotoxicity	Liver damage, central nervous system damage
Bunamiodyl (Orabilex)	1. Glomeruli 2. Proximal tubules	1. Proliferative glomerulonephritis 2. Acute tubular necrosis (birefringent crystals)	1. Hypersensitivity 2. Nephrotoxicity	Hepatitis
Calcium versenate[112,917]	Tubules	Acute tubular necrosis	Nephrotoxicity	
Carbon tetrachloride[495]	Proximal tubules	Acute tubular necrosis	Nephrotoxicity	Hepatitis, bleeding

Cephaloridine[602]	Proximal tubules	Acute tubular necrosis	Nephrotoxicity	Dermatitis, anaphylaxis, eosinophilia
Chlorothiazide[4,299] (Diuril)	1. Arterioles[633] 2. Interstitium 3. Glomerulus[377]	1. Nodular necrotizing vasculitis 2. Interstitial nephritis 3. Proliferative glomerulonephritis	Sensitivity	"Allergic" purpura, thrombocytopenia, potassium depletion
Cresol	Proximal tubules	Acute tubular necrosis	Nephrotoxicity secondary to shock	Local irritation
Cyclophosphamide (Cytoxan)	Renal pelvis	Uric acid crystallization	Mechanical	Alopecia, leukopenia, hemorrhagic cystitis
Dextran[92] (Gentran)	1. Tubules 2. Glomerulus	1. Tubular lumen obstruction 2. Glomerulonephritis	1. Mechanical 2. Hypersensitivity	Anaphylactic shock
Dibenamine	Renal pelvis	Uric acid crystallization	Mechanical	
Diphenylhydantoin	1. Arteries 2. Interstitium	1. Angiitis 2. Interstitial nephritis	Hypersensitivity	Agranulocytosis, anemia, lymphadenopathy, gingiva hypertrophy, dermatitis
Epsilon-amino caproic acid (EACA Amican)	Glomeruli	Intraglomerular capillary thrombosis	Thrombosis	Hypotension
Ferrous sulfate	Tubules	Acute tubular necrosis	Secondary to shock	Gastroenteritis with hemorrhage, hepatic damage, circulatory collapse
Gentamicin	Tubular	Acute tubular necrosis	Nephrotoxicity	Ototoxicity
Gold salts;[469] gold sodium thiosulfate (Sodium aurothiomalate)	Tubules	Acute tubular necrosis (Metabolic inclusion bodies)	Nephrotoxicity	Dermatitis, polyneuritis, bone marrow depression, hepatic damage
Horse serum	Glomeruli	Glomerulonephritis	Hypersensitivity	

*See references 86, 186, 577, 919, 952, and 1060.

Table 4-4. Commonly used drugs that can produce acute renal failure—cont'd

Drug	Morphologic site of action	Pathologic lesion produced	Pathopharmacologic mechanism of action	Other toxicity associated with renal disease
Hydralazine[10,11] (Apresoline)	Glomeruli	Glomerulonephritis	Hypersensitivity	1. Hypotension 2. Features of systemic lupus erythematosus 3. Polyneuritis 4. Knee and ankle itching
Hydrochlorothiazide[633] (Hydrodiuril)	1. Arterioles 2. Tubules	1. Necrotizing angiitis 2. Tubular necrosis	1. Hypersensitivity 2. Reduced blood pressure	Agranulocytosis, thrombocytopenic purpura, potassium depletion
Iodine[106] (Iodoform iodides)	Arteries	Necrotizing angiitis	Hypersensitivity	Corrosion of mucous membrane, fever, dermatitis, eosinophilia, anaphylactic shock
Iopanoic acid (Telepaque)	Arteries	Glomerulonephritis and necrotizing angiitis	Hypersensitivity	Eosinophilia
Kanamycin sulfate[102,656] (Kantrex)	Proximal tubules	Acute tubular necrosis	Nephrotoxicity	Ototoxicity, eosinophilia
Mechlorethamine[926] (Mustargen)	Renal pelvis	Uric acid crystallization	Mechanical	Bone marrow depression
Methylglucamine diatrizoate (Retrografin)	Ureters	Ureteral edema	Mechanical	
Meglumine and sodium diatrizoate (Hypaque)	Proximal tubules	Acute tubular necrosis	Nephrotoxicity	Dermatologic lesions
Merbaphen[1038] (Novasurol)	Renal tubules	Acute tubular necrosis	Nephrotoxicity	

Meralluride[217] (Mercuhydrin)	1. Cortical tubules 2. Interstitium	1. Acute tubular necrosis 2. Acute interstitial nephritis	1. Nephrotoxicity 2. Hypersensitivity	Nephrotic syndrome,[929] fever, agranulocytosis, dermatitis, eosinophilia
6-Mercaptopurine[217] (Purinethol)	Renal pelvis	Uric acid crystallization	Mechanical	Jaundice, bone marrow depression, alopecia
Methicillin[148,359,546]	Interstitium	Acute interstitial nephritis	Hypersensitivity	Nephrotic syndrome, fever, agranulocytosis, dermatitis, eosinophilia
Methylsergide maleate	Ureters	Retroperitoneal ureteral fibrosis	Hypersensitivity	Vascular constriction, dermatitis, eosinophilia
Neomycin sulfate[336]	Proximal tubules	Tubular necrosis	Nephrotoxicity	Neurotoxicity, ototoxicity
Nitrofurantoin (Furadantin)	Interstitium	Interstitial nephritis	Hypersensitivity	Dermatitis, pulmonary infiltration, neurotoxicity
Nitrogen mustard[611,926] (Mechlorethamine)	Renal pelvis	Uric acid crystallization	Mechanical	Bone marrow depression, dermatitis
Ortho-novum[762]	Tubular	Acute tubular necrosis	Secondary	Pulmonary embolism
Para-aminosalicylic acid†	Proximal tubules	Acute tubular necrosis	Nephrotoxicity	Dermatitis, acute hemolytic anemia[724]
Parathion	Proximal tubules	Acute tubular necrosis	Nephrotoxicity	Neurologic
Penicillin[82]	1. Proximal tubules; 2. Glomerular	1. Acute tubular necrosis 2. Proliferative glomerulonephritis	1. Secondary to shock 2. Hypersensitivity	Anaphylactic shock Dermatitis
Pertussis vaccine[110]	Arterioles	Vasculitis (bilateral cortical necrosis)	Hypersensitivity	Local dermatitis
Phenacetin	Interstitium	Acute interstitial nephritis	Hypersensitivity	Eosinophilia, chronic interstitial nephritis[920,921]

†See references 145, 294, 487, 701, and 857.

Table 4-4. Commonly used drugs that can produce acute renal failure—cont'd

Drug	Morphologic site of action	Pathologic lesion produced	Pathopharmacologic mechanism of action	Other toxicity associated with renal disease
Phenindione[43,53] (Hedulin)	Interstitium	Acute interstitial nephritis	Hypersensitivity	Eosinophilia, ulcerative colitis
Phenylbutazone[324a,700,720] (Butazolidine)	1. Glomerulus 2. Proximal tubules 3. Interstitium	1. Thrombotic thrombocytopenic purpura[324a] 2. Acute tubular necrosis[700] 3. Acute interstitial nephritis	1. Hypersensitivity 2. Nephrotoxicity 3. Hypersensitivity	1. Thrombocytopenia 2. Hemolysis 3. Nephrotic syndrome[779]
Hexadimethrine (Polybrene)[491]	Proximal tubules	Acute tubular necrosis	Nephrotoxicity	
Polymyxin-B[83]	1. Tubules 2. Interstitium	1. Acute tubular necrosis 2. Interstitial nephritis	1. Nephrotoxicity 2. Hypersensitivity	Neurotoxicity
Potassium bromate[326] (Toni neutralizing solution)[1114]	Tubules	Acute tubular necrosis (calcium deposits)	Nephrotoxicity	
Procainamide[60] (Pronestyl)	Glomeruli	Lupus glomerulonephritis	Hypersensitivity	
Quinine sulfate	Proximal tubules	Acute tubular necrosis	Secondary to hemolysis	Thrombocytopenia, gastro-intestinal upset
Renacidin[639]	Tubules	Acute tubular necrosis	Nephrotoxicity	
Salicylates‡[38,302,465,478,728,958,980,1027]	Proximal tubules	Acute tubular necrosis	Secondary to shock	Hypokalemia[933]
Sodium acetrizoate (Urokon)	1. Proximal tubules 2. Renal arteries	1. Acute tubular necrosis 2. Renal artery thrombosis	1. Nephrotoxicity 2. Hypersensitivity	Vasodilatation, hypotension
Sodium bismuth tartare[313]	Tubules	Acute tubular necrosis	Nephrotoxicity	
Sodium chlorate	Tubules	Acute tubular necrosis	Nephrotoxicity	
Sodium colistimethate[345] (Coly-mycin)	Proximal tubules	Acute tubular necrosis	Nephrotoxicity	Neurologic

Sodium methicillin (Staph-cillin, Dimocillin-RT)	Interstitium	Hypersensitivity, interstitial nephritis	Hypersensitivity	Dermatitis, eosinophilia
Streptomycin[755]	Proximal tubules	Tubular necrosis	Nephrotoxicity	Vestibulitis[532]
Sulfadiazine[143,533]	Proximal tubules	Acute tubular necrosis	Nephrotoxicity	Hemolytic anemia, dermatitis, drug fever, agranulocytosis
Sulfamerazine[616]	Renal pelvis	Nephron obstruction	Obstructive	Dermatitis
Sulfathiazole[95,240,767] (Sulfasuxidine)	Glomeruli	Glomerulonephritis	Sensitivity	Dermatitis (exfoliation dermatitis)
Sulfonamides[158,400]	1. Glomeruli 2. Intrarenal arteries	1. Glomerulonephritis 2. Polyarteritis nodosa	1. Hypersensitivity 2. Hypersensitivity	Dermatitis, agranulocytosis, drug fever, hemolytic anemia[1020]
Tetracycline[209] (Tetrex, Achromycin)	Proximal tubules	Mild tubular degeneration	Nephrotoxicity	Brown-teeth, hepatitis, renal tubular acidosis,[1118] Fanconi syndrome[405]
Thiourea	Renal pelvis	Uric acid crystallization	Mechanical	Bone marrow depression, gastro-intestinal, hypothermia, tinnitus
Trichloroethylene (Trilene)	Glomeruli	Glomerulonephritis	Sensitivity	Cardiac dysrhythmia
Triethylene melamine[647]	Renal pelvis, ureter	Uric acid crystallization	Mechanical	Bone marrow depression
Typhoid vaccine	Cortical tubules, cortex	Acute tubular necrosis, renal cortical necrosis	Anaphylactic shock	Local reactions
Urethan[7,87,378]	Tubules	Acute tubular necrosis	Nephrotoxicity	Hepatic necrosis, bone marrow depression
Vitamin D	Interstitium	Interstitial nephritis	Metabolic	Metastatic calcification
Zoxazolamine[226,659]	Renal pelvis	Obstruction	Mechanical	

‡See references 38, 302, 465, 478, 728, 958, 980, and 1027.

sulfonamides. Glomerulonephritis has followed hydralazine,[10,11] bunamiodyl (Orabilex), phenylbutazone,[324a] and sulfonamides.[314] Acute tubular necrosis has followed a large variety of drugs. These include amphotericin B,[86,186] aristolochic acid,[806] bacitracin, colistin,[345] ferrous sulfate,[599] kanamycin,[101] meralluride (Mercuhydrin), neomycin,[336] bunamiodyl (Orabilex), para-aminosalicylic acid,[101] penicillin, phenylbutazone,[700] quinine sulfate, salicylates, and sodium acetrizoate (Urokon).

Acute interstitial nephritis and subsequent acute renal failure have followed treatment with meralluride (Mercuhydrin),[804a] methicillin,[806] nitrofurantoin,[806] penicillin, phenacetin,[28] phenindione,[48] polymyxin B,[83] sulfonamides,[400] diphenylhydantoin (Dilantin),[539] and phenylbutazone.

In the section to follow, drug-induced acute oliguric renal failure will be discussed according to drug groups.

Radiologic contrast media

The essential ingredient in all absorbable radiologic contrast media is iodine. Individuals sensitive to iodine in any form may have mild to severe hypersensitivity reactions to contrast media. When inorganic iodine was used, such as sodium iodide in a concentration of 80 to 100%, numerous hypersensitivity reactions occurred. These varied from iodine mumps, dermatologic lesions, and anaphylactic shock to fatal acute oliguric renal failure.[100] Although contrast media containing organic iodides are safer than those containing inorganic iodides, the former have been implicated in a steady flow of reports of severe nephrotoxicity.[574]

Physicians depend on radiologic contrast media for diagnosis of biliary diseases, vascular diseases, and diseases of the kidneys and genitourinary tract. These agents are usually administered orally to evaluate the biliary tract, intravenously to evaluate the arterial circulation and the kidneys, and by retrograde injections into the renal pelvis to evaluate the upper genitourinary tract.[19,103,574]

Cholecystographic medium. In 1924, Graham and Cole introduced oral cholecystography using tetrabromophenolphthalein.[459] Iodine is the essential component of all absorbable contrast media used in roentgenography. Because of individual sensitivity to iodine, a significant number of allergic reactions occur. This was especially noted following the introduction of 100% sodium iodide in 1929.[312] The use of organic iodide preparation has reduced the number of hypersensitivity reactions; however, sporadic reports have been made regarding nephrotoxicity of the cholecystographic medium. When the patient has delayed excretion of the contrast material because of biliary disease, an increased load of a potentially nephrotoxic agent is presented to the kidney.[127]

The use of the oral contrast media iopanoic acid (Telepaque)[370,409,915] and bunamiodyl (Orabilex)[453,738,916] has resulted in acute renal failure. Bunamiodyl in a double oral dose is more prone to induce acute renal failure.[916] This may be explained by the fact that bunamiodyl has an iodine content of 57% and is more completely absorbed from the gut than other cholecystographic material. Because of a local alteration of pH within the nephron, an enhancing dissociation to inorganic iodine occurs. The cholecystographic media are physiochemically similar to the sulfonamides in that both groups of compounds are weak acids and the solubility of each increases in direct proportion to increases in pH. This may explain the crystalluria of bunamiodyl. The nephrotoxicity is further enhanced by the relatively dehydrated state of the patient prior to the roentgenographic procedure.[832] The inorganic iodine may produce a hypersensitive mechanism in inducing acute oliguric renal failure.[575,625] Such a hypersensitivity mechanism is illustrated by the following case presentation.

A nephrotoxic mechanism of bunamiodyl produces an acute tubular necrosis.[994] Deposits of birefringent green-brown crystals can be found at the base of the tubular epithelial cells. In addition, bunamiodyl produces hepatic lesions, which are usually caused by an acute reactive hepatitis. Bunamiodyl has been withdrawn from the drug market by the United States Food and Drug Administration because of its nephrotoxicity. Acute renal failure induced by other cholecystographic material is rare, but I have observed the nephrotoxic effects of bunamiodyl.

CASE PRESENTATION

M. B., a 36-year-old mother of five children, developed nausea and pain in the right upper quadrant. A cholecystogram was ordered by her physician. On May 8, 1961, while she was on fluid restriction, bunamiodyl (Orabilex) was given. Because there was no gallbladder filling, a double dose of bunamiodyl was given and the study was repeated. The next day she had complete anuria and was found to have fever and leukocytosis. (Her hospital course is plotted in Fig. 2-48.) Hemodialysis was done on the eleventh day of anuria when the BUN was 190 mg per 100 ml. Intravenous Solu-Cortef (2.0 gm daily) was given for 5 days. Later, 200 mg of prednisone was given daily She started diuresis on the seventeenth day. A percutaneous renal biopsy was done on the twenty-fifth day and again later, following recovery of acute oliguric renal failure, at 3½ and 16 months (Figs. 2-50 and 2-51). The initial renal biopsy study revealed a severe sensitivity proliferative glomerulonephritis with healing tubular necrosis and tubular regeneration (Fig. 2-49). Subsequent renal biopsy studies revealed that the glomeruli returned to normal but that a residual interstitial fibrosis developed.

Comment. The morphologic lesions of hypersensitivity glomerulonephritis justified the use of high dosages of adrenocortical steroids. Without steroid treatment it was believed that recovery might not occur. The hypersensitive reaction may have occurred through the following mechanism. Iodine was drawn to protein and therefore combined with glomerular capillary endothelial cell protein to produce a delayed hypersensitivity. This resulted in a glomerulonephritis similar to that observed in patients with poison oak sensitivity glomerulonephritis.

Over the past 5 years, twenty-six patients were reported to have developed acute renal failure following administration of bunamiodyl.[1126] Most of these patients were given a double dose. The nephrotoxic lesion of acute tubular necrosis was the common morphologic lesion reported. Although mild glomerular lesions were reported, severe hypersensitivity glomerulonephritis was rare.

To evaluate the urinary excretion of cholecystographic media, studies were done in healthy individuals. Telepaque was excreted 36% in the urine and 62% in the feces. Tyropouric acid was excreted 50% in the urine and 50% in the feces.[831]

However, bunamiodyl was excreted 70% in the urine. This large amount could be further concentrated within the tubular lumen to reach a toxic level and could subsequently result in tubular necrosis. In a single dose (4.5 gm), sodium bunamiodyl produced significant depression of the creatinine clearance in four of seven patients. One of the four developed a transitory oliguria. When bunamiodyl was given to jaundiced dogs with a ligated common bile duct, a marked diffuse tubular degeneration was noted. Intravenous cholangiography has produced a relapse of malaria.[476]

Aortography. Nephrotoxicity was the most significant complication in 13,207 patients[752] following abdominal aortograms.[670,698] Twelve patients of this group died in acute oliguric renal failure, and twenty-seven had reversible nephrotoxicity. Fatal acute renal failure following translumbar aortography has appeared in numerous reports.[22,946] Proteinuria, cylindruria, pyuria, hematuria, and progressive azotemia and impaired renal function persisted for months, even after recovery from acute oliguric renal failure.[331,332,718]

Crawford and associates reported thirty-one patients who had aortographic nephrotoxicity.[244] Twenty percent died in acute oliguric renal failure. Schreiner and Maher reported that three of nine patients with renal injury died; a series of 300 aortograms had been done. The morphologic lesions involved the glomeruli and tubules; acute damage was associated with interstitial hemorrhage.

The use of transfemoral aortography appears to be safer than the translumbar technique,[57,884] but the former is not without hazard.[218,628] Sodium acetrizoate in a 70% solution appears to be the least nephrotoxic of the current group of contrast media.[892] The patient's safety can be further protected by not repeating the injection on the same day.

Pyelographic medium. Retrograde and intravenous pyelograms are frequently implicated in reports of nephrotoxicity; nephrotoxicity due to cholecystograms is quite rare.

Retrograde pyelography. Since 1897, retrograde pyelography has been used in studying genitourinary tract disease. The first report of reversible acute oliguric renal failure of 2 days' duration was made by Morten in 1923.[797] The patient developed oliguria following bilateral retrograde pyelography that utilized sodium bromide as a contrast medium. In 1939, Quinby and Austen described four patients who developed a reversible acute oliguric renal failure within 24 hours of a retrograde and intravenous pyelogram using sodium iodohippurate and sodium methiodal.[900] In addition to the risk of hypersensitivity reactions, retrograde pyelography carries a principal risk of infection.[12]

In 1945, Eskelund reported a patient who developed papillary necrosis following bilateral retrograde pyelography using 10 ml of 25% sodium iodohippurate.[350] The papillary necrosis probably resulted from local irritation caused by the hypotonic solution of sodium iodohippurate. It is also possible that the contrast medium entered the papillary ductules with subsequent obstruction caused by epithelial necrosis. Others[559] have described patients with temporary anuria caused by hydronephrosis or papillary necrosis following retrograde pyelography.[389]

Sirota and Narins attributed oliguria and rapidly progressive azotemia following retrograde pyelography to edematous obstruction of the ureteral orifices.[1017] In three patients they found bullous edema of both ureteral orifices on cystoscopy. They attributed the edema to idiosyncratic reactions from an unusual sensitivity of the bladder and ureteral mucosa to trauma, to the formaldehyde used in sterilization of the catheters, or to the pyelographic contrast medium. Harrow and Sloane reported a patient with acute anuria caused by bilateral edematous obstruction of the ureteral orifices following retrograde catheterization without injection of contrast medium.[520]

Grieve and Lowe attributed anuria to interstitial edema following severe pyelotubular backflow.[470] In my experience, renal interstitial edema has accompanied acute anuria in two patients following use of methylglucamine diatrizoate (Retrografin). Both required peritoneal dialysis before recovery. Retrografin is a 30% solution of methylglucamine diatrizoate with neomycin sulfate added. A 60 or 70% solution of methylglucamine of diatrizoate (Renografin) is used for intravenous pyelography and arteriography.

Epstein and associates reported a patient who developed anuria following retrograde pyelography with 30 ml of a 50% solution of methylglucamine diatrizoate.[347] Repeat ureteral catheterization failed to exclude parenchymal renal disease. The patient did not undergo a spontaneous diuresis as expected. It was very likely that the patient was hypersensitive to the nephrotoxic antibiotic (neomycin) and that the antibiotic recirculated and produced intrinsic renal disease.

Intravenous pyelography. Intravenous urography results in fewer complications than does arteriography because a less concentrated contrast material is used and because of the admixture of the media with blood. Pendergrass and associates reported thirty-one patients who died out of 3,800,000 patients who had intravenous pyelograms.[871,871a] Twenty-five deaths occurred immediately after the intravenous injection of the contrast medium. The patients usually died in anaphylactic shock, from cardiac arrest, or from drug sensitivity. Three patients died as a result of acute oliguric renal failure.

Perillie and Conn focused attention on the potential danger of intravenous pyelography in patients with multiple myeloma.[874] Acute oliguric renal failure occurred in five patients with plasma cell myeloma following intravenous pyelography.[70,373,823] Dehydration appears to predispose patients with multiple myeloma to acute oliguric renal failure.[166] The pathogenesis of pyelogram-induced acute oliguric renal failure in patients with multiple myeloma is related to precipitations of concentrated urinary proteins and contrast media within the tubular lumen. The sudden blockage of a large percentage of the renal tubules may result in sudden suppression of urine flow. The combination of Bence Jones protein in a concentrated urine and dehydration induced by purgatives leads to protein precipitation within the lumen of the nephron.[70] In all reported cases the diagnosis of multiple myeloma was not made before the intravenous pyelogram and the subsequent development of acute renal failure. I suggest that all efforts should be made to exclude multiple myeloma before pyelography is done.[626] Once the diagnosis of multiple myeloma is made, the patient should be adequately hydrated before intravenous pyelography is done.

Antibiotics and chemotherapeutic agents

Antibiotics and chemotherapeutic agents have become indispensable in the treatment of urinary tract infection as well as in the treatment of systemic and local infections. As these agents become more extensively used, their adverse side effects and nephrotoxicity become more apparent.[418,1040] In the presence of underlying renal disease it may be difficult to recognize nephrotoxicity of a specific antibiotic.[634] Moreover, when antibiotics are used in combination with other antibiotics or with chemotherapeutic agents their exact nephrotoxic effect as well as the specific agent of the adverse reaction may be impossible to determine.[74] I have not observed nephrotoxicity caused by chloramphenicol or erythromycin.

Sulfonamides. Damage to the kidney is the most serious and frequent complication of sulfonamide treatment.[158,1092,1101] Sulfonamides were the first effective chemotherapeutic agents to have nephrotoxic properties.[443,1124] The incidence of renal abnormalities varies considerably and depends in a great part on the solubility of sulfonamides.[314,322] Acute oliguric renal failure has been induced by sulfonamide treatment of parenchymal lesions[767,817] and of obstructive uropathy caused by sulfonamide crystallization[616] of the unchanged drug or of its acetyl derivative within the renal pelvis.[95,533] The method of prevention of sulfonamide obstructive uropathy is the preferential use of a more soluble sulfonamide, adequate hydration, and alkalinization of the urine with sodium bicarbonate. Obstructive uropathy caused by the low solubility of sulfonamides is more frequently observed than are the parenchymal lesion of tubular necrosis, focal granulomatous interstitial lesions, diffuse interstitial nephritis, hypersensitivity glomerulonephritis, and acute hypersensitivity arteritis.

Several hundred patients with renal failure caused by sulfonamide crystallization have been reported.[888] The most frequent sulfonamides implicated were sulfapyridine, sulfathiazole, and sulfadiazine.[143] The solubility of sulfonamides depends on a number of factors that include the drug concentration, state of dehydration, urinary pH, and renal function.[950] Sulfadiazine is the most dangerous.[1140] Sulfadimidine and sulfisoxazole form more soluble crystals and are less hazardous.[713,1146] The finding of sulfonamide crystals in the urine leads the physician to suspect acute sulfonamide crystallization within the renal pelvis. The method of treatment is retrograde catheterization of the ureters and lavage of the renal pelvis with warm alkalinized solution (10% $NaHCO_3$).

Acute tubular necrosis can occur with or without sulfonamide crystallization.

The tubular lumina are plugged with amorphous debris containing erythrocytes, leukocytes, hemoglobin casts, and crystals. When sulfonamides induce a hypersensitivity renal lesion, one of three sites is involved. In some hypersensitivity reactions the intrarenal arteries were involved with angiitis or with polyarteritis nodosa. In a second type of hypersensitivity reaction the glomeruli were involved with hypersensitivity glomerulonephritis.[400] The third site for sulfonamide-induced hypersensitivity reaction was the renal interstitium. Acute interstitial nephritis was the more common interstitial lesion and was similar to a Councilman acute interstitial nephritis.[242] A focal interstitial granulomatous interstitial nephritis was a less common interstitial lesion.

Polymyxin B. The polymyxins A, B, C, D, and E are a group of closely related cyclic polypeptides. Polymyxin B is an antibiotic composed of amino acids and a fatty acid. It is active against a variety of gram-negative bacilli.[167] These include *Pseudomonas, Escherichia, Klebsiella, Aerobacter, Salmonella, Shigella,* and *Hemophilus* species.[969] Polymyxin B is antibacterially more active than polymyxin E. Nephrotoxicity of polymyxin is dose-related.[802,1147] Following administration of polymyxin B sulfate, proteinuria, epithelial cells, and casts appear in the urine and azotemia develops.[583] In the presence of normal renal function the nephrotoxicity is neglibible at 2 mg/kg body weight per day.

Beirne and colleagues reported a 44-year-old male who developed an acute oliguric renal failure caused by acute interstitial nephritis.[83] Polymyxin B sulfate seemed the most capable of several antecedent agents. The patient had an eosinophilia of 25% but had no dermatologic lesion. The patient gradually recovered when polymyxin B was withdrawn. A renal biopsy study done on the second day of oliguria revealed a Councilman type of acute interstitial nephritis.

Colistin methanesulfonate. Colistin, which differs from polymyxin B only by the absence of a single amino acid, is known to be identical with polymyxin E.[583] Because of this close structural relationship colistin shares some of the nephrotoxic potential of polymyxin B. Colistin is an antibiotic produced by the soil bacterium *Bacillus polymyxa var. garyphalus.* Its antibacterial activity is against a number of gram-negative bacteria.

Toxicity studies in animals have demonstrated that colistin produces impaired renal function and renal lesions.[1173] Partial to complete necrosis of the proximal tubules was found on histologic examination.[612] The effect of intramuscular colistin on renal function in man is unpredictable. Healthy individuals and patients with chronic pyelonephritis and other forms of renal disease have received the drug without significant changes in urinalysis or BUN.[558,880] In other patients with azotemia further elevation of BUN has occurred. Oliguria developed in a 5-year-old child who received an accidental overdose of colistin (37.7 mg/kg body weight per day for 2 days and 9.4 mg/kg body weight per day for 3 more days). When colistin was discontinued renal function returned to normal.

I have reported acute oliguric renal failure in four patients following treatment with colistin administered intramuscularly.[348] Three patients were given dosages greater than 5 mg/kg body weight per day, and they died in uremia (Table 4-5). The lesions of acute tubular necrosis were found in the kidneys (Fig. 4-13). A fourth patient developed oliguria after a dosage of 5 mg/kg body weight per day, but he recovered and survived. Randall reported a patient with acute oliguria caused by acute tubular necrosis after being treated for 9 days with intramus-

Table 4-5. Clinical data on patients with acute renal failure following treatment with colistin

Age (yr)/ sex	Colistin dosage (mg/kg/ day)	Duration of colistin treatment (days)	Total colistin dose (gm)	BUN (mg/100 ml) Before colistin	After colistin*	Preexisting renal disease	Outcome
1. 75/F	6.3	3	1.3	9	79 (6)	Mild nephrosclerosis	Died
2. 41/F	6.3	12	3.3	12	158 (12)	Severe benign nephrosclerosis	Diuresis began, patient died
3. 74/M	5.3	4	1.2	39	144 (8)	Chronic pyeloneph- ritis	Died
4. 68/F	5.0	3	0.9	17.4	150 (7)	No morphology available	Diuresis and recovery

*Figures in parentheses indicate number of days after starting sodium colistimethate.

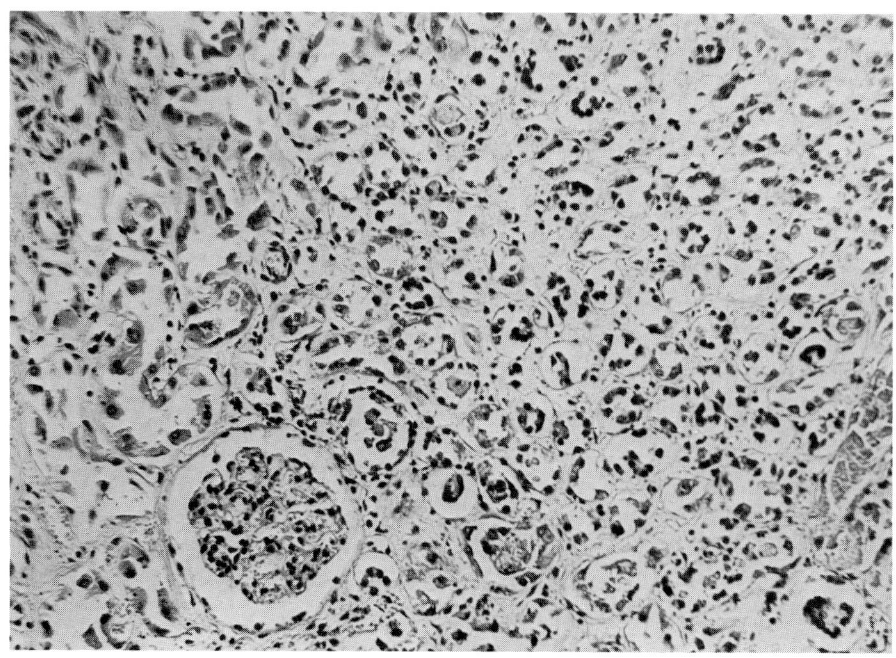

Fig. 4-13. Acute tubular necrosis from colistin. This microphotograph illustrates the renal tissue at autopsy of patient described in Fig. 4-14. The striking finding was an acute tubular necrosis as noted in the microphotograph. The tubules were separated by diffuse interstitial edema. (H&E ×210.)

cular colistin (6.3 mg/kg body weight per day).[904] Recovery followed 4 weeks of hemodialysis. Acute oliguric renal failure caused by colistin and its dose relationship is discussed in the following case presentation.

CASE PRESENTATION

A. H., a 75-year-old obese woman, was admitted to Presbyterian–St. Luke's Hospital for treatment of a fracture of the femur. On admission the urinalysis was normal and the BUN was 9 mg per 100 ml (Fig. 4-14). On the third hospital day the head of the femur was replaced by a prosthesis. Low-grade fever was noted during the postoperative period. A small diffuse opacity of the right middle lobe of the lung was seen on the x-ray film. On the fifth postoperative day treatment with tetracycline administered orally was initiated (2 gm daily) and continued for 6 days. The temperature became normal by the third day of treatment.

Less than 10,000 colonies of *Proteus* per cubic centimeter were found in each of two urine cultures taken before tetracycline was given. On the basis of disk sensitivity studies of the organism, tetracycline administration was stopped. Sodium colistimethate, 150 mg, was given intramuscularly three times daily (6.3 mg/kg body weight per day). Oliguria was noted after the fourth injection of the drug. No hypotensive episodes had been noted during hospitalization. A total of 3,000 ml of fluids was given on the first day of oliguria, and there was no increase in urinary output. Urinalysis revealed a specific gravity of 1.011 and proteinuria (1+). A total of 1,350 mg of sodium colistimethate had been given before the drug was discontinued and treatment for acute renal failure was initiated. Despite fluid restriction, adequate caloric intake and treatment with cationic-exchange resins, clinical symptoms of uremia appeared 5 days after sodium colistimethate had been started. The BUN was 79 mg per 100 ml, the serum creatinine was 11.7 mg per 100 ml, and the serum potassium was 7.8 mEq/L. She died 20 minutes after hemodialysis was begun on the sixth day following the first injection of colistin.

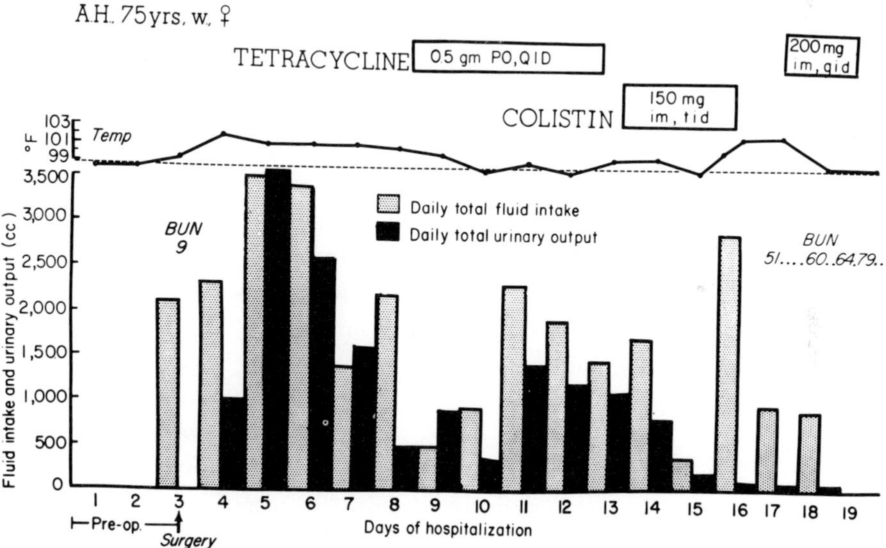

Fig. 4-14. The hospital course of a patient with colistin-induced acute renal failure. A 75-year-old woman entered the hospital with a fracture of the femur neck. On her thirteenth hospital day she was given colistin (150 mg three times a day) for 3 days. On the fifteenth day she had oliguria and her BUN rose to 79 mg per 100 ml. She died while undergoing hemodialysis.

Morphologic findings. Acute tubular necrosis of cortical convolutions of tubules and collecting tubules was found at autopsy (Fig. 4-13). There was regeneration of the tubular lining epithelium with mitotic figures, the tubular lumina were filled with casts and debris, the interstitial tissue was edematous and infiltrated with lymphocytes, and a mild nephrosclerosis was noted. The pathologic diagnosis was acute tubular necrosis.

Comment. Colistin was given in excess of the recommended dosage of 5 mg/kg body weight per day. It is recognized that the serum level and potential toxicity of colistin are highly dependent upon the renal clearance of the drug and that dosage should be based upon the glomerular filtration rate. Patients with impaired renal function should receive proportionately reduced dosages of colistin.[1154] Patients receiving treatment with this drug should have frequent urinalysis, BUN or creatinine determinations, and urinary output measurements. Colistin treatment should be discontinued promptly at the first indication of serious renal affliction.

Although the mechanism of colistin nephrotoxicity is unknown, it may be related to the ability of the drug to disrupt the integrity of certain cell membranes,[359a] probably by acting as a cationic detergent that destroys the cellular osmotic barrier, combines with polyphosphates, and thus allows leakage of substances essential to cell function. Such an action is therapeutically valuable when limited to the cell wall of various bacteria but may be harmful if human renal tubular cells exposed to high concentrations of the drug share this susceptibility. In this respect colistin nephrotoxicity may resemble that of amphotericin B; the latter also disrupts cell membranes, but does so by binding to sterols rather than to polyphosphates. Mammalian cell membranes contain sterols, and amphotericin B[186] has been shown to damage both tissue cells in culture and human red blood cells in vitro.[1124a] Although not proved, it is conceivable that human renal tubular cells may be damaged in like manner by high luminal concentrations of the drug.

Streptomycin. Streptomycin is an antibiotic that was discovered in 1944 by Schatz, Bugie, and Waksman in cultures of the actinomycete *Streptomyces grieseus.*[960] Streptomycin, a carbohydrate derivative, is N-methyl-L-glucosaminido-streptosidostreptidine. It has a wide spectrum of antibacterial activity.[551] Streptomycin, vancomycin, kanamycin, and neomycin have several features in common. They are relatively strong organic bases that cross cell membranes very slowly; therefore, they are poorly absorbed from the gut.[532] They are almost entirely distributed in the extracellular fluid and are excreted mainly in the urine.[1123] In addition, all four antibiotics have ototoxicity. The nephrotoxicity is increased in patients in whom there is a reduction of glomerular filtration rate. If these antibiotics are used in combination, their nephrotoxicity is greatly increased.

In individuals with normal renal function approximately 70% of parenterally injected streptomycin is excreted unchanged in the urine within 24 hours. In patients with renal insufficiency, less than 2% of an injected dose of streptomycin is excreted in the urine. Vestibular damage caused by streptomycin is frequent in patients with severe renal failure. Dialysis has been useful in the removal of streptomycin in the treatment of neurotoxicity and nephrotoxicity.

During the course of treatment with streptomycin, proteinuria and cylinduria may occasionally occur. McDermott reported a patient with acute oliguric renal failure caused by acute tubular necrosis following a daily dosage of 4 gm of streptomycin.[755]

Kanamycin. The nephrotoxicity of kanamycin has been described in numerous reports whenever its clinical application was mentioned.[646,1148] Kanamycin nephrotoxicity was related neither to dose level nor to duration of treatment but occurred more frequently in elderly patients.[102,1133] Kanamycin nephrotoxicity occurred in doses of 20 to 50 mg/kg body weight per day and was clinically evident by mild proteinuria, nitrogen retention, microscopic hematuria, and fine granular casts in the urinary sediment. In approximately 10% of patients treated with kanamycin there was azotemia. Severe tubular necrosis was reported by Kleeman and Maxwell.[634] In general, nephrotoxicity was reversible when kanamycin administration was stopped.

Kuntz noted oliguria in eight patients out of ten receiving kanamycin.[656] Schriener and Maher observed acute tubular necrosis in two patients following treatment with kanamycin.[979] One of these patients died in uremia.

Ototoxicity is the most common toxic effect of kanamycin;[963] it is likely to occur in patients with renal insufficiency or dehydration. When kanamycin is given to patients with anuria or oliguria or to a diabetic patient with nephropathy, it is imperative to reduce the dose by careful calculation of the dose and to give kanamycin in "spread out" doses. (A recommended kanamycin dosage is 0.5 gm every 3 or 4 days.) Approximately 29 to 63% of the injected dose of kanamycin can be removed by effective peritoneal dialysis. In an anuric patient, approximately 30% of kanamycin can be removed by hemodialysis in an 8-hour period.

During peritoneal dialysis, however, 25 mg of kanamycin can be given safely daily. The morphologic change due to kanamycin nephrotoxicity is always seen in proximal tubules of the kidney. When acute oliguric renal failure occurs, it is the result of acute tubular necrosis. When administration of kanamycin is stopped, diuresis follows within 5 days and renal function usually returns to normal within 2 months.

Bacitracin. Bacitracin is a polypeptide antibiotic produced by the Tracy 1 strain of *Bacillus subtilis.*[991] Bacitracin has proved to be highly effective against gram-positive cocci and organisms that cause gas gangrene. Its chemical use is limited to topical application and local infiltration. Transitory urinary abnormalities of proteinuria, cylinduria, azotemia, and occasional oliguria were noted in nearly all reported patients. Bacitracin is very nephrotoxic and produces both proximal and distal tubular necrosis.

Genkins, Uhr, and Bryer reported a 57-year-old housewife with prior normal renal function.[428] She developed a fatal acute oliguric renal failure following five divided doses of 50,000 units daily of bacitracin. On the third day of bacitracin treatment she developed proteinuria, oliguria, and azotemia. She died on the tenth day after intramuscular bacitracin treatment. Acute tubular necrosis was found at autopsy.

Neomycin. Neomycin is an antibiotic discovered by Waksman and Lechevalier. It is derived from the metabolic products of *Streptomyces fradiae.* Neomycin is primarily a topical antibiotic and is used for its local antibacterial action within the lumen of the gut.[607,1109] It is extremely nephrotoxic and damages the eighth cranial nerve.[830,893] Although the drug is poorly absorbed it crosses the peritoneal cavity much more readily. Therefore, renal damage can occur when neomycin is administered into the peritoneal cavity.

Emmerson and Pryse-Davies[345a] found neomycin to be very nephrotoxic and to cause severe proximal tubular necrosis.[336] Randall reported four patients who suffered adverse effects from injections of 4, 6, 8, and 72 gm of neomycin, respectively.[904] Two patients developed deafness. One patient developed acute oliguric renal failure, and one subsequently had permanent renal insufficiency. Hemodialysis and peritoneal dialysis removed large amounts of neomycin, and mannitol prevented acute renal failure in two patients. Hemodialysis rapidly reduced serum neomycin concentration in two patients, while mannitol diuresis removed significant amounts in another. Peritoneal dialysis was the least effective of all methods.

Penicillin. Penicillin induces acute oliguria through a hypersensitivity mechanism.[82] Dehydration was a possible contributing factor in two infants with abnormal renal function. When acute oliguria occurs, it is usually associated with dermatologic lesions and eosinophilia.[1153]

Randall reported acute oliguric renal failure caused by hypersensitivity manifestations of ampicillin, oxacillin, oral penicillin, and intramuscular penicillin G.[904] Two patients died. One was a 24-year-old student who received oral penicillin; he developed clinical features of the hemolytic uremic syndrome Necrotizing arteriolitis was found at autopsy. The other patient had a marked acute interstitial nephritis characterized by interstitial cellular infiltrates of plasma cells. Penicillinase may be helpful in treatment of acute renal insufficiency caused by penicillin hypersensitivity.[1093]

Methicillin. Methicillin (Staphcillin) does not differ in its sensitizing potential from other penicillins.[171] The clinical hypersensitivity features of methicillin are dermatologic lesions, nephropathy, and eosinophilia. During the past few years, methicillin-induced nephropathy has been reported by several individuals. The clinical manifestations of renal disease were proteinuria, hematuria, dysuria, and azotemia with or without oliguria. Nephropathy usually appeared between 7 to 21 days after treatment was begun; in most instances, it subsided within 24 to 48 hours after cessation of treatment with methicillin.

Hewitt and associates reported three men, aged 34, 43, and 57 years, who developed proteinuria, hematuria, pyuria, and eosinophilia following treatment with methicillin for a staphylococcal septicemia.[546] These patients had previous reactions to penicillin. All patients made a complete recovery after methicillin was stopped. Allen and associates reported twenty-two patients who were treated with methicillin for a staphylococcal septicemia.[15] During the second week of treatment, a syndrome resembling glomerulonephritis occurred in two patients (aged 50 and 67 years). The nephropathy was characterized by oliguria, microscopic hematuria, proteinuria, hyaline casts, and transient azotemia. These two patients had BUN levels that reached 79 mg and 140 mg per 100 ml, respectively. Both patients received methicillin for 3 weeks and both eventually recovered. Although the authors attributed these renal findings to a nephrotoxic feature of the staphylococcal infection, it appears that the nephropathy was most likely drug-induced.

Lany and associates reported three patients, aged 32, 42, and 51 years, who developed proteinuria and hematuria; only one had mild azotemia.[667] After administration of methicillin was discontinued, all made a complete recovery. Grattan reported a 5-year-old boy who had had cystic fibrosis of the pancreas since infancy.[462] The boy developed recurrent attacks of pneumonia and received treatment with methicillin. During his second, third, and fourth treatments with methicillin, he developed dysuria and gross hematuria. These renal abnormalities appeared 5 to 7 days after each treatment period with methicillin. The abnormal renal findings subsided completely within 12 to 24 hours after administration of methicillin was discontinued. The BUN level was slightly elevated (30 mg per 100 ml) and the creatinine clearance was mildly impaired; on subsequent follow-up evaluations, both were normal. The boy developed progressive pulmonary disease and died. At autopsy his kidneys appeared grossly normal; light microscopy study revealed no evidence of inflammatory or degenerative processes involving either the glomeruli or the tubules.

Feigin and Fiascone reported a boy, 2½ years old, who had a lung abscess.[359] They treated him with intravenous methicillin—a total dose of 250 mg/kg body weight was given for 3 days. From the fourth day 750 mg was given intramuscularly every 6 hours. On the twenty-third day he developed hematuria and proteinuria, which subsided promptly once treatment with methicillin was stopped. Later the BUN and creatinine clearance were normal. The authors observed transient mild eosinophilia preceding the renal abnormalities. The eosinophilia subsided as the urinary findings returned to normal. They suggested that eosinophilia may be an early clinical sign revealing hypersensitivity disorders induced by methicillin.

Schrier and others reported a 42-year-old woman who had rheumatic valvular heart disease that was complicated by pneumonia.[984] She developed acute glomerulitis following treatment with methicillin for 6 days. Marked azotemia, proteinuria, and a large number of erythrocyte casts were noted. Glomerulitis was accompanied by a maculopapular rash, a transient thrombocytopenia, and an eosinophilia. The patient eventually recovered, only to be readmitted 1 month later for a similar complaint. This was preceded by treatment with chloramphenicol for pulmonary symptoms without any skin rash or urinary abnormalities.

Patients with methicillin-induced nephropathy had additional manifestations of hypersensitivity.[148] The most common was an eosinophilia. In some patients thrombocytopenia was observed. Hypersensitivity dermatologic lesions were noted; they included hemorrhagic bullae, urticaria, maculopapular lesions, purpura with petechiae, and exfoliative dermatitis. None of these reported patients with methicillin-induced nephropathy had a renal biopsy study. In general, knowledge regarding the overall morphologic renal changes is insufficient. The complete reversibility of methicillin-induced nephropathy, together with other allergic manifestations, suggests that a pathopharmocologic mechanism of hypersensitivity occurs.

Histologic abnormalities of the kidney include an acute interstitial nephritis with or without tubular damage.[148] This interstitial nephritis is characterized by cellular infiltrates of eosinophils, plasma cells, and small lymphocytes. Adrenocortical steroids have been effective in resolving this drug-induced lesion.

Tetracycline. Tetracycline, a so-called broad-spectrum antibiotic, is produced by several *Streptomyces* species. The tetracyclines produce changes in nitrogen metabolism.[355] The tetracyclines are not usually nephrotoxic agents. However, if storage degeneration occurs they may produce proximal tubular damage.[263] Chemical deterioration is more likely to occur if the drug is improperly stored under moist or warm conditions. Anhydrotetracycline and epianhydrotetracycline are the nephrotoxic products. The formation of these products is accomplished by temperature elevation, high humidity, and reduced pH. They are especially likely to occur when citric acid is added to tetracycline. However, tetracycline preparations containing lactose are less likely to degenerate into nephrotoxic products.

The tetracyclines are concentrated in the liver, the teeth, and the bones and are excreted through the kidneys and bile. Death has resulted from severe hepatic and pancreatic damage with excessive intravenous doses of tetracycline. Aged or degenerated tetracycline produces a reversible Fanconi syndrome[405,1008] associated with polyuria, proteinuria, renal glycosuria, phosphaturia, aminoaciduria,[156] acidosis, hypokalemia, and a low plasma urate. In general, tetracycline-induced Fanconi syndrome is slowly reversible once the drug is discontinued.[477]

Acute nonoliguric renal failure has been reported by Solomon, Galloway, and Patterson.[1031] They gave 2 gm of tetracycline daily and observed an increase in BUN from 63 mg to 161 mg per 100 ml. Tetracycline toxicity is also directly related to existing renal insufficiency.[1064] Large doses of oxytetracycline have produced azotemia. Prerenal azotemia may be induced by a negative nitrogen balance that produces anorexia, nausea, vomiting, and death. Nephrogenic diabetes insipidus has been induced by dimethylchlorotetracycline.[209]

Para-aminosalicylic acid. Para-aminosalicylic acid (PAS) is highly active in inhibiting the growth of tubercle bacilli in vitro. The most common hypersensitivity complication of PAS treatment is hepatitis. A reactive hepatitis induced by PAS has been associated with fever, rash, pruritis, conjunctivitis, hemolytic anemia,[724] and eosinophilia. Renal involvement[487] due to PAS was uncommon and was usually confined to patients who had hepatitis.[294] Inasmuch as PAS is an organic acid, it requires a fixed cation to accompany its excretion;[701] therefore, hypokalemia can occur as well as an acidosis in children.[145]

Owen reported a 31-year-old Irishman with pulmonary tuberculosis receiving treatment with calcium PAS for 83 days without mishap.[857] After 35 days of sodium PAS treatment he developed fever, a pink vesicular rash, massive proteinuria, and acute oliguria without hepatitis. The BUN reached 245 mg per 100 ml and spontaneously fell to normal. The patient made a rapid and complete recovery from acute renal failure.

Cephaloridine. Cephaloridine is a semisynthetic derivative of cephalosporin C. Its antibacterial activity is against many gram-positive and gram-negative bacteria. Adverse reactions of cephaloridine occurred in 35% of seventy-six patients. In general, they were minor reactions and included allergic phenomena, phlebitis at infusion sites, transient leukopenia, and gastrointestinal symptoms. More serious reactions include acute renal failure, Coombs positive hemolytic anemia, superinfections, and anaphylaxis. For example, cephaloridine produced anaphylaxis in a nurse who prepared an injection of the drug.[360]

Renal damage caused by cephaloridine appears to be a result of a nephrotoxic mechanism. The drug has been localized by autoradiographic studies to the renomedullary interstitium and proximal tubular cells.[254] Cephaloridine is accumulative and dose-related. In large doses it produces a severe nephropathy, while in low doses it produces proteinuria, hematuria, and cylindruria.[602] When the drug is discontinued urinary abnormalities disappear.

Cephaloridine has produced hypersensitivity reactions such as urticaria, eosinophilia, drug fever, and Coombs positive hemolytic anemia. Antibiotics such as ampicillin and polymyxin B have produced a hypersensitivity acute interstitial nephritis. I predict that cephaloridine will also produce an acute (hypersensitivity) interstitial nephritis and subsequent acute oliguric renal failure.

Diuretic agents

In the majority of instances the kidney responds favorably to diuretic agents with a prompt diuresis. However, the kidney also becomes the target of untoward effects of diuretic agents. It is not unlikely that acute oliguric renal failure developed in patients following treatment with meralluride (Mercuhydrin), acetazolamide,[268] the thiazides, and aristolochic acid.

Mercurial diuretic agent. Calomel (mercurous chloride) was the active diuretic in the famous "Guy's Hospital Pill" (calomel, digitalis, and squill). The diuretic effects of organic mercurial were first discovered as a side effect in patients receiving antisyphilitic treatment. The primary action of the mercurial diuretic agents is their ability to inhibit sulphydryl-containing enzyme systems that normally supply energy for sodium reabsorption. Immediate fatal reactions to mercurial diuretic agents are rare;[517] when they do occur they are related to anaphylactic shock. Hypersensitivity reactions induced by mercurial diuretics include generalized pruritus, urticaria, exfoliative dermatitis, and asthma. Most organic

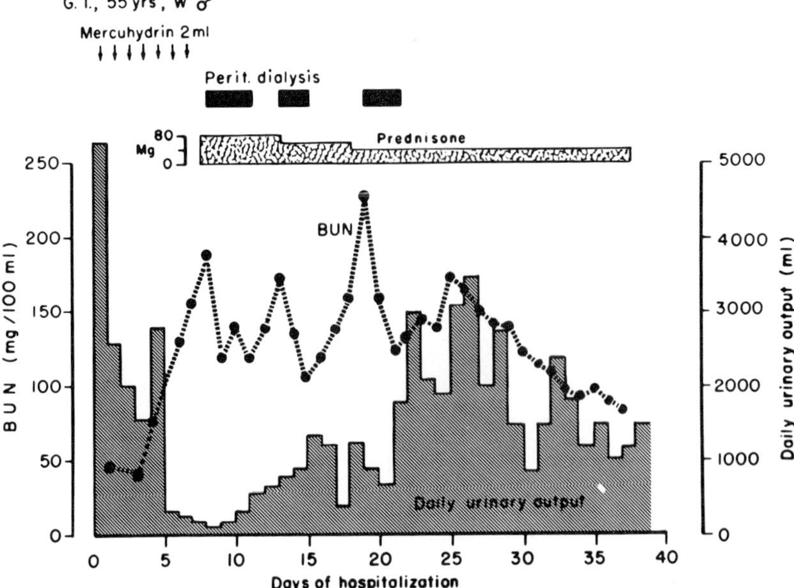

Fig. 4-15. Hospital course of patient with meralluride induced acute interstitial nephritis. A 55-year-old truck driver entered the hospital with congestive heart failure. He received meralluride (Mercuhydrin) (2 ml daily) for 7 days and developed fever, exfoliative dermatitis, eosinophilia, and acute renal failure. Peritoneal dialysis was done at three intervals. Predisone was given and a step-wise diuresis followed. Acute interstitial nephritis was found on study of his renal tissue.

mercurials are rapidly excreted by active renal tubular secretion bound with cysteine.[480] Mercurial diuretic agents produce acute oliguric renal failure from acute tubular necrosis.[75,1108] Schreiner and Maher believe that organic mercurials are slowly converted to inorganic mercury secondary to abnormal renal retention by the kidneys.

Meralluride-induced acute oliguric renal failure has developed as the result of acute tubular necrosis.[339] This is probably the result of a nephrotoxicity mechanism. Acute oliguric renal failure, exfoliative dermatitis, fever, and eosinophilia have sometimes followed several injections of meralluride (Fig. 4-15). Adrenocortical steroids were used to reverse this condition. This hypersensitivity reaction produces an acute interstitial nephritis (Fig. 4-16). There have been a few reports of patients developing nephritis following meralluride treatment.[184] The morphologic lesion was tubular degeneration associated with interstitial nephritis (Fig. 4-17).

Thiazide diuretic agents. The thiazides were discovered as a by-product of a search for diuretic agents similar in structure to acetazolamide. In 1958, chlorothiazide was introduced as a potent oral diuretic agent. In a short time numerous other thiazides were found. The untoward effects of the thiazide diuretic agents are potassium deficiency, aggravation of preexisting diabetes mellitus, aggravation

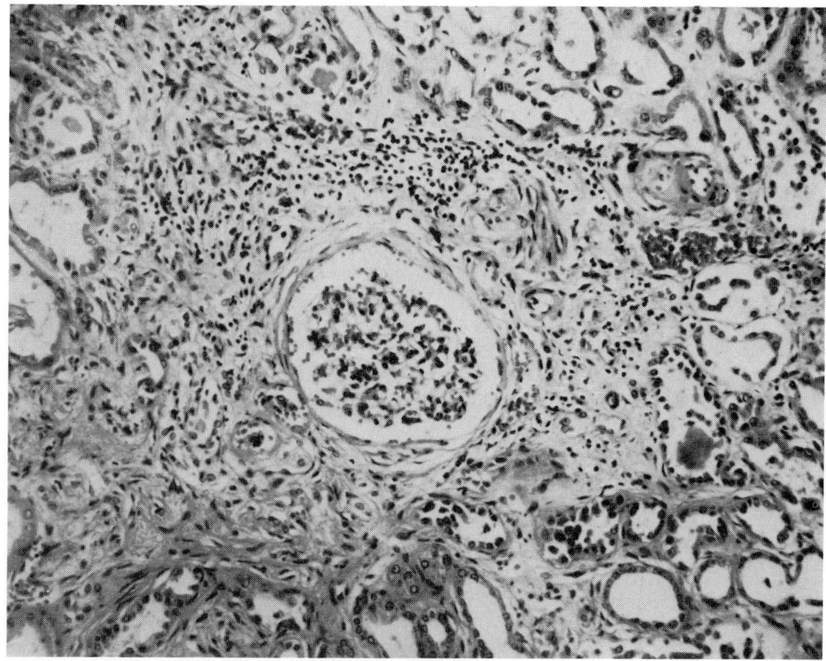

Fig. 4-16. Councilman acute interstitial nephritis. This microphotograph illustrates the kidney findings of acute interstitial nephritis. A 54-year-old truck driver developed acute oliguric renal failure following daily injections of meralluride. He had fever, exfoliative dermatitis, and eosinophilia (16%). The striking morphologic finding was a diffusely edematous interstitium with cellular infiltrates of plasma cells, eosinophils, and small lymphocytes. (H&E ×320.)

of gout, and blood dyscrasias.[999] The latter include leukopenia, thrombocytopenic purpura, and aplastic anemia.

Thiazide diuretic agents cause acute oliguric renal failure in two ways. The first is: chlorothiazide and hydrochlorothiazide produce acute renal necrotizing angiitis, glomerulonephritis with interstitial nephritis, and acute tubular necrosis.[4] These lesions produce acute renal parenchymal damage, which causes acute oliguric renal failure.

Kjellbo observed a patient who had acute necrotizing angiitis simultaneously in the skin and kidney.[633] His patient was a 62-year-old mildly hypertensive woman who developed fever, right kidney pain, gross hematuria, proteinuria, and azotemia. Renal biopsy study revealed interstitial granulomatous inflammatory nodules enclosing necrotic arterioles. The glomeruli appeared normal. The granulomas were composed of lymphocytes, histiocytes, plasma cells, and neutrophilic leukocytes.

Fitzgerald reported a patient who had fatal glomerulonephritis with interstitial nephritis complicating "allergic purpura" caused by chlorothiazide.[377] Abry and Cavusoglu reported a patient with fatal acute oliguric renal failure caused by

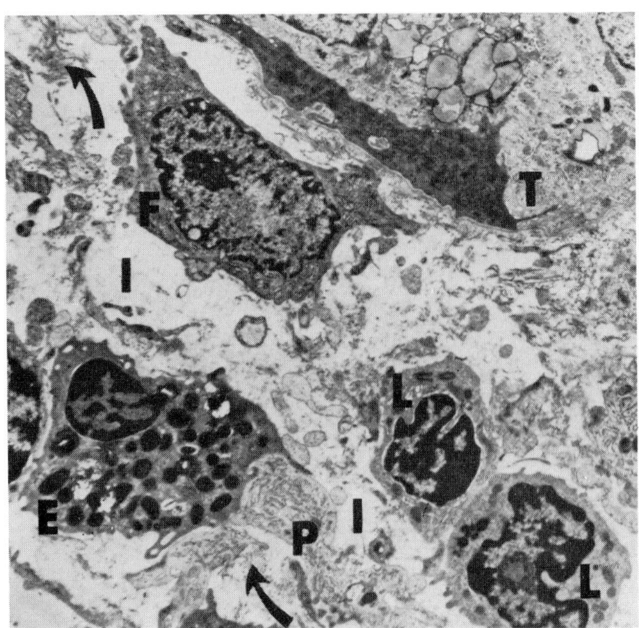

Fig. 4-17. Drug-induced acute interstitial nephritis. This electron microphotograph illustrates acute interstitial nephritis. An abnormal proximal tubule (T) is seen at right top. The interstitium (I) is edematous and contains loosely packed bundles of collagen fibers (arrows). An eosinophil (E) with its dark granules is seen at the bottom left. Its villus projections are interlocked with a portion of a plasma cell (P). A large fibroblast (F) is seen adjacent to the tubule. Two small lymphocytes (L) are seen at the lower right. (×4,700.)

acute tubular necrosis following chlorothiazide treatment.[4] Elwood encountered a patient with coexisting thrombocytopenic purpura and acute oliguric renal failure following chlorothiazide treatment.[345]

The second mechanism of acute oliguric renal failure is the more common. Thiazides induce acute oliguric renal failure by a gradual and chronic reduction in the effective circulating blood volume; this reduction is associated with severe hyponatremia.[999] Treatment consists of fluid and sodium chloride replacement. The physician must be very careful so that he does not excessively expand the blood volume and precipitate the primary illness, especially if the condition is congestive heart failure.

Aristolochic acid. Aristolochic acid has been used experimentally as a diuretic agent and as an anticancer drug. It has produced renal damage in horses, rabbits, rats, and mice; it can abolish the antidiuretic effect of vasopressin in rabbits and is therefore thought to have diuretic properties. Peters and Hedwall intensively studied the effects of aristolochic acid toxicity in rats. They found that a single injection of 30 mg/kg body weight of the drug induces reversible renal failure associated with a decrease in glomerular filtration rate and a BUN and creatinine increase. Maximum polyuria occurred on the eighth day. Their data reveal a decrease in the permeability of the collecting ducts and proximal tubules to urea.

I have observed two entirely opposite effects of aristolochic acid. In one patient it produced a tremendous diuresis, and in the other patient it resulted in a severe acute tubular necrosis with fatal acute oliguric renal failure.

Diuretic effect. The profound diuretic effect of aristolochic acid is discussed in the following case presentation.

CASE PRESENTATION

A. W., a 57-year-old cachectic Negro male, had a resection of a rectal carcinoma in January, 1959. He was admitted to the hospital on January 26, 1962, with severe pain over the lumbosacral area caused by metastatic lesion. Initially he received a course of 5-fluorouracil with slight relief of back pain.

On March 3, 1962, he was given 4 mg daily of intravenous aristolochic acid. A total dose of 1,069 mg was given (Fig. 4-18). His last dose of aristolochic acid (120 mg) was given on April 25, 1962. His fluid intake and urinary output increased. Four days after aristolochic acid was stopped his daily urinary output was 7,400 ml, and it reached a peak of 18.5 liters 5 days later. This was not controlled by injections of either chlorothiazide or the antidiuretic hormone. This fluid and electrolyte balance was maintained by oral and intravenous fluid supplements. He tolerated this very well; the diuresis subsided gradually over a 3-week period.

Acute tubular necrosis. Fatal acute tubular necrosis caused by aristolochic acid is discussed in the following case presentation.

CASE PRESENTATION

A 53-year-old white female had a radical mastectomy in December, 1957, for carcinoma of her left breast. Metastases developed in her right breast, regional lymph nodes, and lungs. She was treated with radiation, 5-fluorouracil, and bilateral oophorectomy and adrenalectomy. She

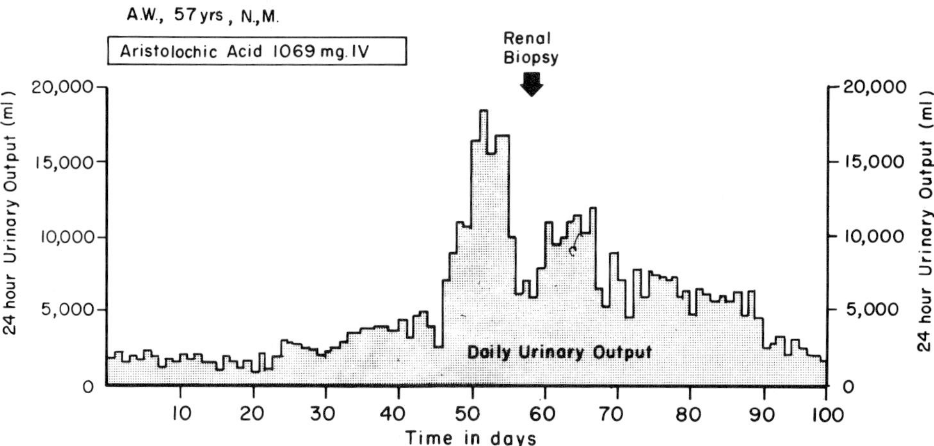

Fig. 4-18. Hospital course of patient with massive polyuria following treatment with aristolochic acid. This chart illustrates the hospital course of patient aged 57 years. He was given intravenous aristolochic acid as an experimental drug for metastatic rectal adenocarcinoma. Four days after aristolochic acid was stopped the daily urinary output exceeded 7,000 ml and reached 18.5 liters 6 days later. A percutaneous renal biopsy was taken 2 days after the peak diuresis.

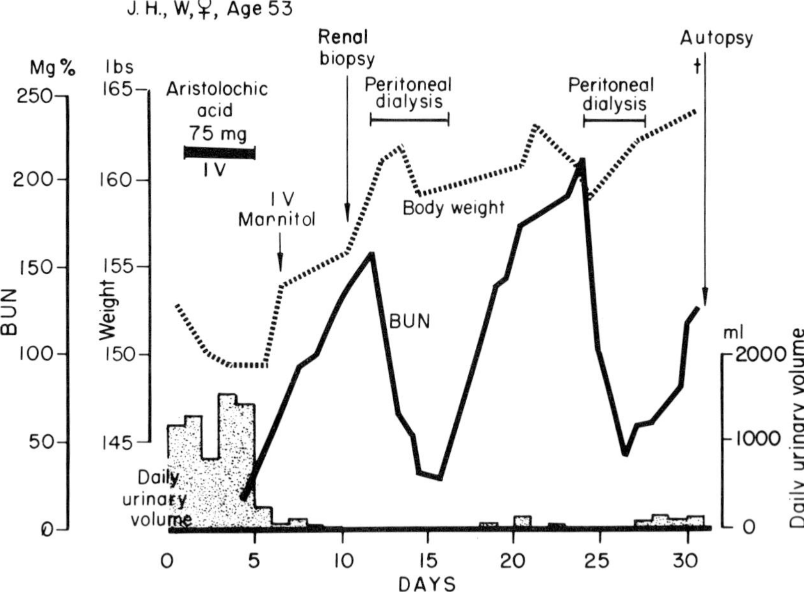

Fig. 4-19. The hospital course of patient with fatal acute renal failure from aristolochic acid. A 53-year-old woman with metastatic adenocarcinoma of the breast was given aristolochic acid as antimalignancy therapy. Four days later she had acute oliguria, which required treatment with peritoneal dialysis. A percutaneous renal biopsy study revealed severe acute tubular necrosis. On the thirty-first hospital day she died.

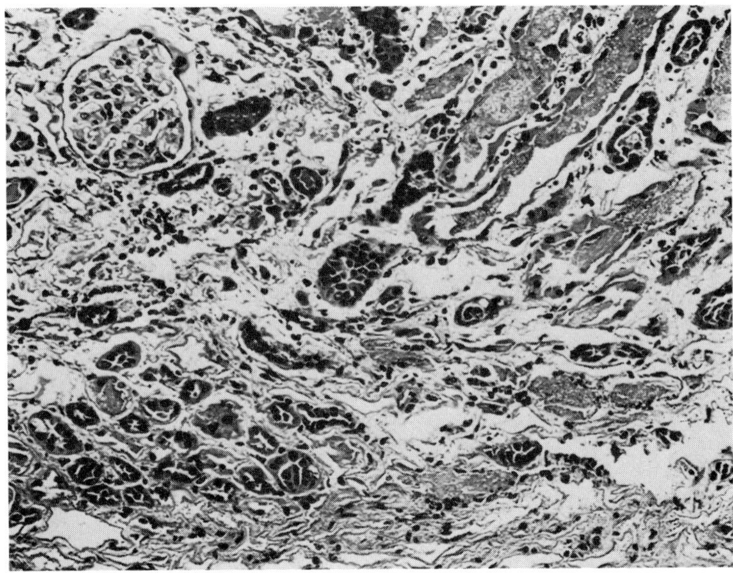

Fig. 4-20. Aristolochic acid–induced acute tubular necrosis. Renal biopsy was obtained from patient described in Fig. 4-19. There was a severe acute tubular necrosis. Many tubules were necrotic down to the tubular basement membrane with complete dissolution of the cytoplasm. The interstitium was edematous and the glomeruli were normal. (×140.)

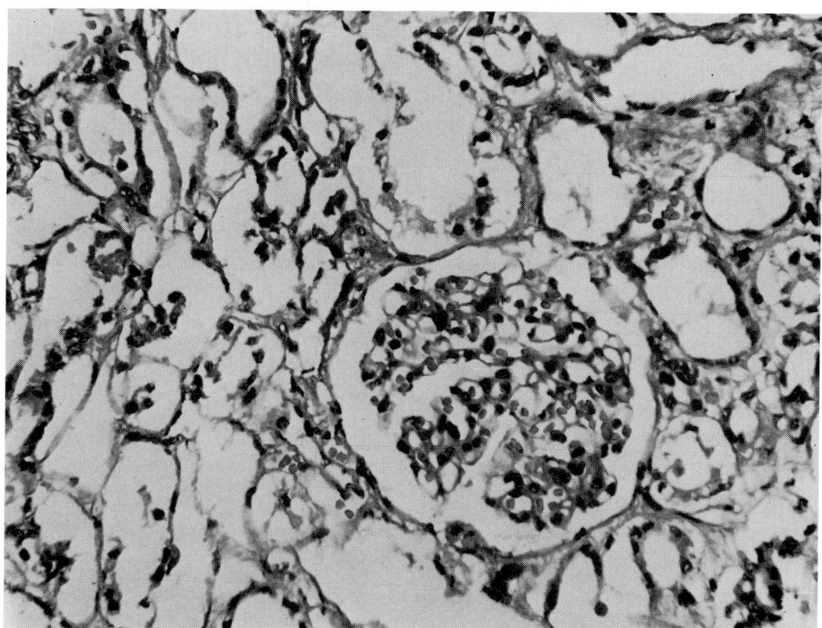

Fig. 4-21. Fatal acute tubular necrosis induced by aristolochic acid. This microphotograph illustrates the kidney at autopsy of patient described in Fig. 4-19. With a rare exception, all tubules had necrosed down to the tubular basement membrane. This would explain the complete anuria and the reason for tubules' failure to regenerate. (H&E ×250.)

was again admitted to hospital in a near terminal state on May 5, 1962 (Fig. 4-19). Serum electrolytes were normal and the BUN was 24 mg per 100 ml. On the next day the patient was started on a course of aristolochic acid, given in intravenous doses of 75 mg daily. Four days later she had oliguria, and aristolochic acid therapy was discontinued. A percutaneous renal biopsy was performed and revealed severe tubular necrosis (Fig. 4-20). The patient remained oliguric and expired June 6, 1962. At autopsy massive renal tubular necrosis was found (Fig. 4-21).

Anticoagulants

Bishydroxycoumarin (Dicumarol) and phenindione (Hedulin) have been implicated as possible causes of acute oliguric renal failure.

Bishydroxycoumarin. In 1941, Butt and Allen[187] at the Mayo Clinic and Meyer and associates at the University of Wisconsin introduced bishydroxycoumarin as an anticoagulant into clinical medicine. Doses in the therapeutic range have produced nausea, vomiting, and diarrhea, and excessive doses cause bleeding. In general, painless gross hematuria is the first evidence of toxicity. This bleeding may arise from the kidney and in some patients is followed by renal pain, ureteral colic, and gross hematuria. Ureteral obstruction has followed blood clots within the ureters.

In one patient retroperitoneal hematoma dissected down around the urinary bladder to produce an external ureteral obstruction and acute oliguria.[596]

Phenindione. Phenindione is known as phenylindanedion (P.I.D.), Danilone, Hedulin, and Eridone. It has been used as a short-acting anticoagulant, for it is rapidly absorbed from the gut and is rapidly excreted by the kidney. Phenindione interfers with the liver synthesis of prothrombin. Proteinuria is commonly observed during the first day of phenindione treatment. Heavy proteinuria has resulted in the nephrotic syndrome.[1059]

Six patients with severe and significant renal damage caused by phenindione have been reported by Brooks and Calleja. Four patients developed acute oliguric renal failure, one had the nephrotic syndrome, and the sixth had a heavy proteinuria.[48,413] The other clinical features were fever, skin rash, jaundice, and eosinophilia.[153] The histologic renal abnormality in the patients with oliguria was an acute diffuse interstitial nephritis characterized by interstitial infiltrates of plasma cells, eosinophils, and small lymphocytes; in addition, there were interstitial fibrosis and intimal fibrosis of the interlobular artery. The glomeruli were usually normal. Adrenocortical steroids were beneficial in reversing the acute interstitial nephritis caused by phenindione hypersensitivity.

Calcium versenate

Calcium versenate is a synthetic, water-soluble polyamino acid (calcium disodium ethylenediamine tetraacetic acid). It is an organic chelating agent that is used in the treatment of heavy metal poisonings.

In 1957, Vogt and Cottier reported a 38-year-old man with chronic lead poisoning.[1102] He was treated with 600 mg/kg body weight of calcium versenate daily for 4 days (ten times the average dose). Acute anuria developed on the fifth day, and he died on the sixth day. Acute tubular necrosis was found with dilated proximal tubular epithelial cells.

In 1957, Moeschlin described two patients who were treated for lead intoxication with calcium versenate.[784] Both died in uremia caused by acute oliguric renal failure. Acute tubular necrosis was found at autopsy.

In 1958, Weinig and Schwerd described acute renal failure associated with a bleeding tendency in a 59-year-old factory worker who received 3 gm of calcium versenate.[1121] Acute tubular necrosis and dilated proximal tubules were found at autopsy.

In 1960, Reuber and Bradley reported a 1-year-old girl who had lead intoxication.[917] The child was treated with calcium versenate in a dose of 1 gm (125 mg/kg body weight) daily; the subcutaneous dose was given for 3 days. She developed acute oliguric renal failure 12 days after the first injection and died 4 days later. Acute tubular necrosis and dilated proximal tubules were found at autopsy.

I again emphasize the important need not to exceed the recommended dosage of calcium versenate of 75 mg/kg body weight. Moreover, the physician should carefully screen the patient for kidney disease before administering calcium versenate.

Dextran

Low molecular weight dextran (Dextran-60, Gentran) has a molecular weight of 40,000.[427] It passes through the glomerular membrane. It is used in clinical medicine as a short-term flow improver in small blood vessels and as a "plasma volume expander."[106,340,747] The high urinary concentration of dextran creates a urine of high viscosity.[550] An increase in blood clotting time has occurred in a substantial number of individuals receiving dextran. Adverse reactions to dextran originate as hypersensitivity and include urticaria, angioneurotic edema, bronchospasm, and severe anaphylactic shock. Hypersensitivity glomerulonephritis caused by Arthus's phenomenon and acute oliguric renal failure are two renal conditions induced by dextran.[635,1075]

Hypersensitivity mechanism. Dextran is a potent antigen with a molecular weight similar to that of many antigens. It may be given by injection without any reaction. However, subsequent injections of dextran such as iron-dextran can precipitate an immunologic reaction leading to acute renal failure.

The following patient was studied by Drs. Victor Pollak and Robert M. Kark. An acute renal failure was induced through an immunologic reaction to dextran.

CASE PRESENTATION

M. W., a 40-year-old Negro female, was admitted to Research and Educational Hospital because of intermittent diarrhea of 8 years' duration. Physical examination revealed that the lower abdomen was slightly distended with flatus. She had a hypochromic microcytic anemia with decreased bone marrow iron stores. Occult blood was found in the stool. Findings from proctoscopy and intestinal tract x-ray studies were normal, and no cause for the diarrhea and gastrointestinal occult blood loss was found. Intramuscular injections of iron-dextran (Imferon) were given. A reticulocytosis up to 5% followed, and the hematocrit returned to normal by the twenty-second hospital day. An oral lactose tolerance test was performed; there was no rise in blood glucose levels.

She was given 500 ml of 6% dextran in normal saline. Five hours later she had a rectal temperature of 103° F. The next day the oral temperature rose to 104° F; that temperature persisted for 3 days. Four days after the initial febrile reaction the patient complained of pain in the buttock where the iron-dextran had been injected. On examination a swollen indurated mass was noted. Several days later another site of iron-dextran injection, the opposite buttock, became swollen and tender. Biopsy study of the initial site revealed perivascular infiltration and iron macrophages.

Nine days after the febrile reaction there was hematuria, massive proteinuria, and oliguria. Diuresis occurred 14 days later; the BUN was 23 mg/100 ml. Erythrocyte casts were found in the urinary sediment. Percutaneous renal biopsy was done on April 8, and the study revealed an acute proliferative glomerulonephritis (Fig. 4-22). Epithelial humps on the glomerular basement membrane were seen by electron microscopy. They were similar to those described in poststreptococcal glomerulonephritis. A dose of 60 mg daily of prednisone was started. The patient became afebrile. Proteinuria and hematuria diminished. However, the proteinuria persisted in the range of 2 to 4 gm/day; the red cells in the urine diminished but had not cleared after 3 months. The initially depressed creatinine clearance was at this time 65 ml/minute. The patient was followed in the renal outpatient department. She was being given 7.5 mg of prednisone per day; this dose suppressed the proteinuria.

Comment. Iron-dextran injectable (intramuscularly) is a stable complex of ferric hydroxide and dextran in 0.9% sodium chloride solution. Dextran is known as a potent antigen.[594] In man, the injection of such small amounts as 1 mg can lead to the development of precipitins and

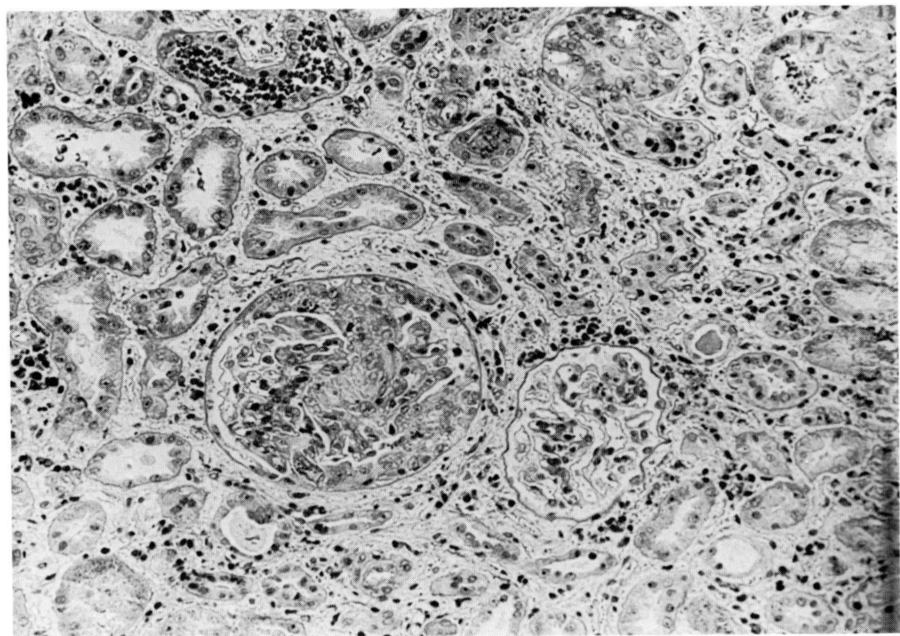

Fig. 4-22. Proliferative glomerulonephritis caused by dextran. Dextran induced a severe proliferative glomerulonephritis with epithelial crescents in a woman previously injected with iron dextran. The tubules appeared normal but erythrocytes were seen within the lumen. The interstitium was edematous and contained collagen fibers. Adrenocortical steroids were effective in resolving the clinical features of hematuria, proteinuria, and oliguria. Electron microscopic study revealed epithelial humps on the lamina densa. This finding suggested a reaction of soluble antigen-antibody complex disease with excess antigen. (H&E ×180.)

cutaneous erythema and wheal reactions. Dextran is a polysacchride with a molecular weight similar to that of many antigens.

The patient developed Arthus's phenomenon of perivasculitis at the site of previous iron-dextran injections. A serum sickness immunologic reaction occurred at 9 days, which is sooner than a serum sickness reaction occurs. The morphologic renal lesions of humps on the epithelial side of the glomerular basement membrane support a soluble antigen-antibody complex in an excess antigen reaction. The clinical improvement following the administration of adrenocortical steroids supports the immunologic aspects of this reaction.

Tubular obstructive mechanism. Acute oliguric renal failure induced by low molecular weight dextran has produced two distinct renal lesions. The first was observed by Morgan and colleagues in three hydrated patients with acute oliguria following dextran infusion.[793] They did renal biopsy studies on each patient and found grossly swollen tubular cells crammed with a foamy material. The distended cells completely occluded the tubular lumen. Special stains revealed large quantities of dextran within the tubules but none in the tubular lumen.

The second lesion occurred in dehydrated patients given dextran.[736] Acute oliguric renal failure was associated with the finding of dextran casts obstructing the tubular lumen.[835] Once within the tubular lumen, the dextran becomes concentrated and a highly viscous urine is formed; this results from the proximal tubular reabsorption of electrolytes and water.[37] The highly concentrated viscous dextran urine forms tubular casts. The massive obstruction within nephrons results in no urine flow and subsequent acute oliguric renal failure. Mannitol infusions (20% solution) have been effective in initiating a diuresis.[92]

Ferrous sulfate

The ingestion by children of large doses of ferrous sulfate frequently produces iron poisoning. The mortality rate in a large series of children with iron poisoning was approximately 50%. Acute oliguric renal failure occurred as a result of acute tubular necrosis.[599] This renal lesion may be related to gastrointestinal tract damage.[1023]

Aminopyrine

Aminopyrine is a closely related compound to antipyrine and to phenylbutazone. It is used clinically as an analgesic and an antipyretic, is rapidly and virtually completely absorbed from the gut, and is demethylated in the liver.

The toxic effect of aminopyrine is a severe and often fatal agranulocytosis. It can cause herpes labialis and angioneurotic edema in hypersensitive individuals. Eknoyan and Matson reported a 37-year-old woman who developed acute oliguric renal failure.[338]Although she did manifest renal damage following a brief course of treatment with amphotericin B, a marked decrease in renal function occurred coincident with aminopyrine administration. Recovery occurred after aminopyrine was discontinued. There was a dramatic decrease in renal function coincident with a second course of aminopyrine ingestion. The patient died in uremia. Unfortunately, no autopsy was done.

Phenylbutazone

Phenylbutazone (Butazolidin) is a congener of aminopyrine and can induce damage to the skin, lungs, heart, liver, bone marrow, adrenal glands, and gut.[827] Phenylbutazone has produced both acute nonoliguric renal failure and acute oliguric renal failure.[159,421,1150]

Richardson and Alderfer reported a 43-year-old executive who developed acute nonoliguric renal failure after taking 2.2 gm of phenylbutazone for 6 days.[925] The patient had severe hyponatremia (sodium, 96 mEq/L) and acidosis (CO_2, 14 mM/L). After massive sodium repletion the patient recovered. Approximately 8 days after the onset of renal failure, findings from a renal biopsy study were normal.

Phenylbutazone-induced acute oliguric renal failure results from three distinct morphologic lesions. These include acute tubular necrosis,[962] acute interstitial nephritis, and TTP. Lipsett and Goldman reported a patient with reversible acute oliguric renal failure following treatment with phenylbutazone.[700] A renal biopsy study done on the fifth day of oliguria revealed acute tubular necrosis.

Herrmann, Hopefeld, and Berning reported a patient with fatal acute oliguric renal failure caused by treatment with phenylbutazone.[544] An acute interstitial nephritis was found at autopsy. Dunea and colleagues reported a 44-year-old housewife who was treated with phenylbutazone, 600 mg daily for 3 days; this treatment was followed by acute anuria and jaundice.[324a] She remained anuric until her death 30 days after the onset of her illness. A renal biopsy study performed during the third week of her illness revealed TTP associated with a hemolytic anemia. In vitro phenylbutazone was found to be the antigen to produce a positive Coombs test; the Coombs test became negative after treatment with adrenocortical steroids.

Bismuth compounds

Bismuth compounds have induced nephrotoxicity through repeated intramuscular injections, rectal suppositories, accidental ingestion, and idiosyncrasies to heavy metals. The proximal renal tubules are the organs most sensitive to injury.

Although the large number of bismuth compounds formerly available to physicians has been greatly reduced, bismuth compounds have been used extensively in the treatment of syphilis,[81] oral infections such as Vincent's gingivostomatitis, and gastroenteritis. Although bismuth compounds have been used in the treatment of verrucae, they have no known beneficial value when so used.

The toxicity of bismuth compounds is directly related to the rapidity of absorption. Approximately 90% of the absorbed dose of a soluble bismuth salt is excreted by the kidneys. Bismuth tends to concentrate in renal tissue to amounts five times that in the liver. Therefore, damage to the kidney occurs. Proximal tubular necrosis and intranuclear inclusion bodies are frequently observed in bismuth nephropathy. In addition to kidney damage, these compounds have produced gut, liver, and central nervous system damage. Acute oliguric renal failure was the chief cause of death in patients poisoned with bismuth.

Robinson and Wong believe that bismuth compounds are the second most common cause of nephrotoxicity in children.[934] In 1932, Beerman reviewed the literature and found twenty-two patients with fatal bismuth toxicity. Barnett[58] described four patients and Weinstein[1122] added eleven children with fatal poisoning caused by bismuth-containing suppositories. Dowd had three patients who died from bismuth toxicity; two had acute renal failure.[313] McClendon reported two children who received a single injection of bismuth thioglycollate (Thio-bismol) for Vincent's gingivostomatitis.[753] Both recovered from prolonged acute oliguria. In 1946, Boyette reported a child who died in acute oliguric renal failure 13 days after injection of bismuth.[141] Although the child had an excellent diuresis, he suddenly died. At autopsy widespread tubular degeneration was found. Other patients with bismuth thioglycollate intoxication were reported by Petersilge[881] and by Karelitz and associates.[606]

Chamberlain and Franks reported a 9-year-old schoolgirl with acute oliguric renal failure following an intramuscular injection of 3 gm of bismuth thioglycollate.[211] She was treated with BAL and recovered. The efficacy of BAL treatment was questioned by the authors. In general, bismuth thioglycollate has produced death in approximately 50% of all patients with bismuth toxicity. Bismuth tartrate has produced the nephrotic syndrome in a patient with rheumatoid arthritis. Czerwinski and Ginn found that ingestion of 1.5 gm of bismuth compounds produced the Fanconi syndrome with reversible renal insufficiency.[255]

ACUTE OLIGURIC RENAL FAILURE IN OBSTETRICS

Acute oliguric renal failure is one of the most serious complications of pregnancy.[841,1024,1025] It occurs in approximately 15 to 25% of all patients with acute renal failure treated at renal dialysis centers. Acute oliguric renal failure occurs in a greater proportion, both during pregnancy and in the immediate postpartum period, than is generally appreciated.[949]

The incidence of acute renal failure in pregnancy varies from 1 in 1,400 to 1 in 5,000 pregnancies; the condition results from a variety of causes. Acute oliguria is frequently transitory, lasting a few hours or at most a few days. When oliguria or anuria is severe or prolonged, it usually reflects a grave complication of pregnancy.[276,417]

Acute renal failure in the obstetric patient can be divided into three main groups, each group having a distinct prognosis (see outline). Group 1 contains patients in whom renal failure developed in the first half of pregnancy.[174] Acute oliguria is usually associated with induced abortion and is complicated by sepsis. Group 2 contains patients in whom acute renal failure occurs late in pregnancy; the condition is usually associated with massive uterine hemorrhage. Group 3 contains patients in whom renal failure developes in the postpartum period; the condition is usually associated with eclampsia and preeclampsia.

Acute oliguric renal failure due to obstetric complications

I. First trimester
    A. Septic abortion
        1. Gram-negative endotoxemia
        2. *Clostridium perfringens*
    B. Abortifacients (quinine sulfate, creosol, soap)
    C. Blood transfusions

II. Second and third trimester
    A. Abruptio placentae
    B. Intrauterine sepsis
    C. Shock
    D. Hemorrhage
    E. Blood transfusions
    F. Abdominal pregnancy
    G. Eclampsia
    H. Operative trauma
    I. Uterine rupture
    J. Acute pyelonephritis
    K. Amniotic fluid embolism

III. Postpartum
    A. Eclampsia-preeclampsia
    B. Drug-induced
    C. Hemorrhage
    D. Blood transfusions
    E. Thrombotic thrombocytopenic purpura
    F. Lupus nephritis
    G. Endotoxemic shock
    H. Generalized Shwartzman reaction
    I. Sickle cell disease
    J. Acute poststreptococcal glomerulonephritis

Acute renal failure in the first trimester

Approximately one-half of the women who develop acute renal failure during pregnancy develop it during the first trimester, usually in the eighth to thirteenth week. Acute renal failure results from direct interference with pregnancy. It occurs after an induced abortion, usually under the most adverse conditions outside of hospitals. Only a single instance of acute renal failure has been reported after a therapeutic abortion within a hospital. The patient was markedly depressed. An abortion was induced in her by inserting UTUS paste into her uterus at 16 weeks and by later curetting the uterus.

Acute renal failure is frequently associated with a subsequent infection. In some patients acute renal failure occurs following use of quinine sulfate as an abortifacient, following a soap and water douche, or following forceful injection of soap solution into the cervix. Finally, oliguria follows hypotension that results from blood loss and hypovolemia. Intrauterine damage, nephrotoxicity, hemolytic anemia, chemical abortifacients, and sepsis each may singly produce acute renal failure or may do so collectively.

Infection

Overwhelming infection is the leading cause of death and originates from retained uterine secundine, which serves as the foci for infection. In some patients the portal of entry is either a perforated uterus or the fallopian tubes. Sepsis initiated within the pelvis subsequently results in either a focal or a diffuse peritonitis with the adverse sequel of acute renal failure.

The leading infecting organisms are *Clostridium perfringens* and *Staphylococcus pyogenes*. The presence of clostridia should be suspected in any pregnant or postpartum patient with hemoglobinuria, jaundice, hemolytic anemia, muscle pain, and high fever. Because of the adverse condition of the induced abortion, the infection may be present for several days before the patient seeks medical aid. The women usually have excessive uterine bleeding for prolonged periods and may be in shock.

Fever, leukocytosis, and local pelvic inflammation are common clinical findings in these patients. In a high percentage of women, cultures taken by high vaginal swabs have the best chance of growing *Clostridium welchii*. The prevalence of these organisms in the vagina may be the result of unhygienic methods used in the abortion, or the organisms may have been present in the vagina prior to abortion. Therefore, the presence of *Clostridium welchii* may not necessarily be invasive. However, the presence of clostridia in necrotic uterine tissue is most likely invasive. When I encounter a pregnant woman with acute renal failure, I take high vaginal swabs and then institute treatment with large doses of penicillin or ampicillin. Surgical curettage should not be done when acute renal failure occurs since the procedure may disseminate a previously localized infection or may result in uterine perforations. Local abscesses should be drained. In a rare situation, a transabdominal hysterectomy to remove necrotic tissue may be a life-saving method of treatment.

Intravascular hemolysis

Ingestion of quinine sulfate as an abortifacient has produced acute renal failure; it results from an immunohemolytic anemia with subsequent hemoglobinuria.[664] Liquid soap and water douches or forcible injection into the vagina have both produced acute renal failure through massive hemolysis, through peritonitis, or directly as a nephrotoxin. When soft soap is used by women as a douche in concentrations greater than a 5% aqueous solution it gains entrance into the maternal circulation via disrupted maternal sinuses.

Nephrotoxic cresol saponified solutions have induced abortion and have resulted in peritonitis and acute renal failure. Cresol, a coal tar derivative, is an active protoplasmic poison; it is similar to phenol in toxicity and action.[451] When absorbed it is extremely nephrotoxic and produces severe acute tubular necrosis. The most common morphologic renal lesion found in the first trimester is an acute tubular necrosis. The tubular abnormalities vary from normal and mild tubular changes to severe tubular necrosis. Bilateral renal cortical necrosis is rare; when it does occur it is usually fatal. This lesion can be patchy in distribution or it can be very severe and diffuse.

Acute renal failure in the second two trimesters

Acute renal failure occurring late in pregnancy has a greater mortality rate and is associated with an irreversible renal lesion such as bilateral renal cortical necrosis. The onset of oliguria occurs at approximately the twenty-seventh week, with a peak occurrence between the thirty-sixth and thirty-eighth weeks.

Late in pregnancy acute renal failure results from preeclampsia, from a concealed accidental antepartum hemorrhage, or from acute pyelonephritis or hypotension resulting from hemorrhage with or without hypofibrinogenemia.

Preeclampsia-eclampsia

When acute renal failure occurs in the fourth to second week prior to term, the patient is usually a primiparous woman whose condition is complicated by eclampsia or preeclampsia.[467] Such a patient has no antecedent history or physical or laboratory findings suggestive of diabetes mellitus, pyelonephritis, or glomerular or cardiovascular hypertensive renal diseases. There is a reduced urinary output, but it may suddenly become anuric prior to convulsions. The course of oliguria is usually prolonged and may extend to several weeks. It is quite possible that glomerular lesions of eclampsia lead to tissue ischemia and even infarction without evidence of hypotension or anemia. This morphologic lesion as described by Pollak and associates involves the glomeruli with endothelial cell edema.[889] The narrowing of the glomerular capillary lumen may result in renal ischemia and subsequent oliguria.[764] The associated tubular lesions may be slight and vary from mild to severe tubular necrosis.

Uterine hemorrhage

Acute renal failure caused by uterine hemorrhage has occurred in multiparous women 30 years of age or older. It results from interplacental apoplexy with subsequent abruptio placentae or a concealed retroplacental hemorrhage. In many women, abruptio placentae is associated with eclampsia. Afribrinogenemia is a common finding in these patients and contributes to the massive blood loss. Many of these women develop intrauterine hemorrhage (Couvelaire uterus).

Bilateral renal cortical necrosis is believed to develop early in the course of abruptio placentae and not as a consequence of ischemia resulting from the anemia or hemorrhagic shock. It is an infrequent complication of severe abruptio placentae and leads to a grave prognosis. Initially the patient has hematuria but later develops complete anuria. She remains oliguric or anuric for many weeks. The diagnosis of bilateral renal cortical necrosis was formerly believed to have a fatal prognosis, but clinicopathologic study has changed this belief.

In 1927, Crook reported a 29-year-old postpartum woman who recovered from anuria.[247] He obtained a renal biopsy at the time he decapsulated the kidneys. Cortical necrosis was found on morphologic study. Subsequently, Gormsen and colleagues[450] and Muehrcke and associates[805a] reported renal biopsy studies of women who survived acute renal cortical necrosis. Currently, eighteen patients surviving cortical necrosis have been reported. Riff and associates reported a 26-year-old housewife who made a partial recovery after 49 days of oliguria.[930] They stress the need to sustain life by continuing dialysis in spite of renal biopsy evidence of cortical necrosis. Their patient had died suddenly several months before the patient's case presentation was published.

Concealed hemorrhage may be severe and may be initially overlooked until hypotension occurs. Bleeding may be present for a time before a physician is consulted. The blood loss may be greatly underestimated, and the clinical state of shock may be mild even though the blood volume is markedly depleted. The prompt replacement of blood in these patients may prevent the progression of renal abnormalities to renal cortical necrosis.

Pyelonephritis

In normal pregnancy there is dilatation of the ureters, pelvis, and calyces; this dilatation is associated with a decreased amplitude of ureteral peristaltic waves occurring about the third month. Thus, during the last four months of pregnancy a marked structural trauma occurs to the urinary bladder and ureters. These functional and morphologic alterations greatly predispose the urinary tract to infection.

Pyelonephritis is the most frequent and most important complication of pregnancy. Kass has emphasized the value of doing quantitative colony count cultures of clear voided urine. He and his co-workers related a count of 10^5 organisms per ml as significant bacteriuria. If untreated, subsequent pyelonephritis will develop and may be most severe.[610]

Kincaid-Smith found an increased incidence of prematurity, fetal loss, and preclampsia in women with a significant bacteriuria of 10^4 bacteria per ml. In pyelographic studies of women with bacteruria, she found alteration and deformity such as papillary necrosis or a congenital anomaly.

The symptoms of chills, fever, renal pain, urinary frequency, and dysuria are indicative of renal infection. In some pregnant women with pyelonephritis, the disorder is stubbornly antibiotic-resistant. Acute pyelonephritis can progress to intrarenal abscess. I have seen one pregnant woman who developed acute renal failure and a fulminating renal infection with abscess formation. Unfortunately, the abscess ruptured into the peritoneal cavity and caused the deaths of baby and mother.

Fulminating pyelonephritis of pregnancy often leads to septicemia with gram-negative endotoxic shock and subsequent acute oliguric renal failure. Management is very difficult and the prognosis is usually very poor.

Circulatory collapse

Acute circulatory collapse can produce oliguria from renal circulatory failure. The renal impairment is purely functional with no apparent structural changes. In the majority of patients, diuresis usually occurs once circulatory collapse has been effectively treated. If diuresis does not occur, 25 gm of a 20% solution of mannitol should be rapidly infused.

The dividing line between patients with acute renal circulatory failure and mild tubular necrosis is not clearly differentiated. If circulatory collapse is prolonged, acute tubular necrosis or renal cortical necrosis may ensue. I studied women in the postpartum period with so-called acute tubular necrosis. Renal biopsy studies revealed renal lesions that varied from apparently normal-appearing tubules to severe acute tubular necrosis and complete renal cortical necrosis. In some patients the tubular lesions were superimposed on the eclamptic lesion of pregnancy.

Patients with mild tubular lesions had oliguria for less than 1 week. Following recovery from acute renal failure, correlative clinical and pathologic studies revealed complete functional and structural resolution.

Acute renal failure in the postpartum period

Acute renal failure in the postpartum period can result from eclampsia, acute necrotizing arteriolitis, lupus nephritis, and generalized Shwartzman phenomena,[573] or it can be associated with fatty liver of pregnancy.[795]

Preeclampsia-eclampsia

Postpartum acute renal failure caused by eclampsia can occur as a result of focal deposits of fibrin in the glomeruli. It has occurred up to 2 weeks postpartum. The patients become anemic and have jaundice caused by a microangiopathic hemolytic anemia. Bleeding tendencies are noted. These occur in the skin as purpura, from the uterus as vaginal bleeding, and from the gastrointestinal tract. Although in this postpartum period coagulation factors such as factors V, VII, IX, and XI may be within the normal range, they are relatively low since they are usually elevated in the normal postpartum period.

Since 1913, McKay has repeatedly presented evidence that acute tubular necrosis as well as acute renal cortical necrosis can result from intravascular thrombosis.[757-760] The mechanism for this is an initial degeneration of the labyrinth and giant cell trophoblasts of the placenta. Focal deposits of fibrin accumulate in the maternal spaces, and extension of parauterine thrombosis follows. Later, intravascular thrombosis of microemboli to the renal arterioles and subsequent extension of the thrombosis to the glomerular capillaries occur. Other extensions can be disseminated to other organs, such as the lungs, and to muscle.

Acute necrotizing arteriolitis

Acute necrotizing arteriolitis can delay the onset of acute oliguric renal failure. It occurs 2 to 3 weeks postpartum and without a precipitating obstetric complication.

Wagoner, Holley, and Johnson have reported three patients with delayed postpartum acute renal failure caused by acute necrotizing arteriolitis.[1107] The blood pressure was normal during acute oliguric renal failure. Funduscopic examination revealed no abnormality, or the retinal arterioles were narrowed. The patients died despite intensive medical management with dialysis.

At autopsy, the abnormal findings are discovered primarily in the kidneys. The interlobular arteries and afferent arterioles have marked, laminated internal fibrosis with focal fibrinoid necrosis. Some glomeruli may be entirely infarcted. These vascular lesions are similar to the renal vascular changes found in primary malignant nephrosclerosis. A renal biopsy study would be helpful in making the diagnosis while the patient is still alive.

Generalized Shwartzman reaction

Recurrent episodes of acute pyelonephritis with gram-negative bacteria can produce a generalized Shwartzman reaction, which is initiated by bacterial endotoxin. Bacterial endotoxins render the blood hypercoagulable and result in a slow deposition of fibrin in aggregates and later small thrombi that interfere with blood flow to a key organ. If the kidneys are the target organs, acute renal failure develops. Thomas and associates found that endotoxin-induced hypercoagulability resembles hypercoagulable states induced by the activities of the Hegeman factor (factor XII). Others believe that endotoxin produces an increase in platelet factor III and is responsible for the increased conversion of fibrinogen to fibrin.[1035] Moreover, Gans and associates described changes in most or all of the factors following systemic endotoxemia.[415] Infections by a gram-negative bacillus, usually *E. coli,* produce intravascular formation of fibrin. Injections of endotoxins have produced these lesions in experimental animals.

The generalized Shwartzman reaction is discussed in detail on pp. 192.

THE HEPATORENAL SYNDROME

The term "hepatorenal syndrome" was first coined by Helwig and Schulz in 1932.[535] The syndrome has been used to describe a variety of clinical conditions characterized by a concomitant dysfunction of both the liver and kidney. These include (1) infections such as Weil's disease, general sepsis, hemorrhagic fever, and yellow fever, (2) drugs, chemicals, and biologicals such as phenurone, anesthetic agents,[968] carbon tetrachloride,[280,429] and mushrooms, and (3) generalized disease processes such as systemic lupus erythematosus, eclampsia, shock, and fever therapy. Sherlock has questioned the hepatorenal syndrome as a specific entity. She maintains that it pertains to a large group of patients with liver disease or biliary tract disease who develop acute renal failure following shock. The review and critical analysis of the hepatorenal syndrome by Lassen and Thomsen has helped clarify this disorder.[671] They exclude such causative factors as toxic agents and vasodepressor substances released by the liver. Furthermore, they conclude that the concept of a specific hepatorenal syndrome is illogical. Therefore, the term should be used only in a descriptive sense and without implication of a causal relationship.

The hepatorenal syndrome has two specific components. One is associated with jaundice and biliary tract disease,[204] the other with advanced cirrhosis of the liver. The patient's final outcome is very much affected by the efficiency of treatment directed toward renal failure as well as toward the primary illness.

Biliary or gallbladder disease

Acute oliguric renal failure appears to be associated with surgical procedures and disease of the biliary tract and liver. This hepatorenal syndrome is characterized by high fever, rigors, shock, and acute oliguric renal failure in a jaundiced patient following gallbladder or biliary surgery.[579,695,909] The incidence of the hepatorenal syndrome in jaundiced patients with biliary tract disease was found to be approximately 12 to 14% of all causes of acute renal failure.[411]

The precipitating factor is frequently a gram-negative septicemia or an overwhelming infection that follows gallbladder and biliary tract surgery or that occurs in patients with cholecystitis.[500] This type of surgery should be regarded as not "clean surgery." This was implied in numerous clinical bacteriologic studies related to the bile and gallbladder. For example, Pyrtek and Bartus found pathogenic bacteria in thirty-three of one hundred patients studied.[899] Edlund and associates cultured the bile and gallbladder wall aerobically and anaerobically in 296 patients who had biliary surgery. In patients with acute cholecystitis, approximately 75% of the cultures were positive; the majority were aerobic organisms. In patients with chronic cholelithiasis without common duct stones, approximately 50% had positive cultures; the majority were anaerobic bacteria. When common duct calculi were present, over 90% of the patients had positive cultures; anaerobic bacteria were found in approximately 33%.

I have observed the hepatorenal syndrome precipitated by *Clostridium welchii* infection complicating biliary tract surgery; oliguria occurred within hours after surgery. The patient had a rapid pulse rate, normal temperature, wound pain, and a terror of impending death. In spite of massive dosages of intravenous penicillin and adrenocortical steroids, the patient died. *C. welchii* infections complicating biliary surgery were reported by Pyrtek and Bartus.[899] They described the surgical wound as whitish and tense. The wound was tender, and a study of the wound exudate revealed gram-positive rods with leukocytes. They pointed out that the wound may trap air in various tissue planes. Later the wound became bronzed, crepitant, and gangrenous. *E. coli* and anaerobic streptococcus were found with the saprophytic *C. welchii.*

Patients with gallbladder disease who develop acute renal failure following administration of oral or intravenous contrast media should not be included with those who have the hepatorenal syndrome. The contrast material is retained and produces nephrotoxicity; in some patients it produces hepatotoxicity.

Treatment of the hepatorenal syndrome should be directed toward supporting the central venous pressure, recognizing and treating shock and water and electrolyte imbalance, and administering intravenous antibiotics to eliminate the septicemia as well as the local infection.[709] Often the causative factors are septicemia, subphrenic abscesses, and bile peritonitis. Large dosages of adrenocortical steroids are given intravenously to neutralize the endotoxin. If *C. welchii* infection is present, antitoxin and massive quantities of penicillin should be given, and adequate wound debridement should be performed.

The morphologic abnormality found in patients with acute renal failure following biliary or liver conditions is tubular damage varying from mild to severe tubular necrosis.[122] The interstitium becomes secondarily edematous, as occurs in other kidneys involved with acute tubular necrosis. So-called bile casts may be found in the tubular lumen. Bilateral renal cortical necrosis has been found in some patients. Animal experimentation has helped to clarify the susceptibility of the jaundiced patient to acute oliguria. These investigations have shown that elevated serum bilirubin levels predispose the tubules to damage by endotoxin or to anoxic shock. This observation may shed light on the pathogenesis of acute renal failure in a jaundiced patient.

The mortality rate of patients with the hepatorenal syndrome associated with biliary disease is approximately 83% in patients who are not radically operated on or are inoperative. On the other hand, patients who have benign biliary tract disease and radical surgery have a mortality rate of approximately 26%.

Advanced cirrhosis of liver

The second major clinical condition of the hepatorenal syndrome is the sudden or gradual occurrence of oliguria in patients with advanced decompensated cirrhosis of the liver and portal hypertension.[140] They may develop impaired renal function characterized by scanty concentrated urine or by impaired concentrating ability. They have a low glomerular filtration rate and azotemia. These findings may follow paracentesis and may not be associated with hepatic coma. These functional abnormalities may or may not be associated with morphologic renal abnormalities.

In 1685, John Brown recorded the association and distortions of body fluids with liver disease.[155] Over 150 years later, Richard Bright called attention to the association of liver disease in patients with kidney disease.[150] In 1863, Austin Flint made specific reference to the frequency of oliguria in patients with liver cirrhosis and hydroperitoneum,[383] and this was reemphasized by Gilbert and Lereboull in 1901.[431] Since then the development of oliguria in patients with decompensated cirrhosis has captured the interest of numerous physicians. The condition has resulted from dehydration, diuretic agents, electrolyte imbalance following abdominal paracentesis, gastrointestinal hemorrhage, pancreatitis, bacterial toxemia, hypoglycemia, and other complications.

The main factor controlling the excretion of water in decompensated cirrhotic patients is the decreased renal excretion of sodium.[530] Although increase in antidiuretic hormone may play a role in limiting water excretion, it is not the outstanding factor.[1009] Papper suggested that a decrease in effective extracellular volume is the important stimulus to the kidney to retain sodium and water.[861-863] The reduced extracellular volume was probably secondary to the accumulation of ascites and the trapping of fluid in the enlarged portal veins and lymphatic vessels.

Numerous morphologic renal abnormalities have been reported in patients with the hepatorenal syndrome associated with decompensation of liver cirrhosis.[50] These findings include glomerular lesions such as glomerulosclerosis, tubular lesions varying from very mild degeneration to severe necrosis, and interstitial lesions varying from edema to fibrosis. Bloodworth and Sommers more specifically described glomerular lesions in patients with liver cirrhosis.[122] They noted that the glomerular stroma was thickened by a PAS positive fibrillar substance. They found an increased number of both epithelial and endothelial cells. Some glomeruli were bloodless and contained lipid-containing cells.

Treatment is prevention of the hepatorenal syndrome and in general is directed toward correction of the abnormalities that produced the hepatic coma.[591] This includes the correction of electrolyte abnormalities such as severe potassium deficiency, control of water abnormalities, administration of antibiotics to reduce the gastrointestinal bacterial flora, and in some patients administration of adrenocortical steroids, especially if there is gamma globulin elevation in serum. Once the patient becomes edematous and the serum sodium level drops below 118 mEq/L, the so-called sick-cell syndrome is present and the "siren of death" is said to have been sounded.[988] Recovery depends on the success in treating the portal-systemic encephalopathy.

The prognosis is extremely poor when oliguria develops in association with severe cirrhosis. In many series the mortality rate may approach 100%. When a patient with severe hepatocellular disease caused by viral hepatitis develops acute renal failure he almost certainly will die. Several systemic disorders have produced both hepatic parenchymal failure and renal disorder. I observed membranous glomerulonephritis in a patient with liver cirrhosis following splenorenal shunt. The morphologic findings were similar to the renal lesion in myxedema[300] and to the membranous glomerulonephritis observed in patients with renal vein occlusion (Fig. 2-39, *B*).

LESIONS OF THE BRAIN

Brain lesions have been known to affect renal function. Proteinuria was noted in patients with grand mal epilepsy, subarachnoid hemorrhage, and brain tumors. In 1933, Schmidt reported transient oliguria in patients with increased intracranial pressure caused by brain tumors. Impaired tubular function occurred in patients with cerebral concussions following electroshock therapy.[356]

Steinmetz and Kiley reported four patients with acute cerebral insults accompanied by loss of consciousness and followed by acute renal failure.[1043] At autopsy, acute tubular necrosis was found to be associated with degenerative changes in the cerebral cortex, the cerebellum, and the basal ganglia, and to a lesser degree in the hypothalmus. The pathogenesis of acute tubular necrosis is believed to be based on renal ischemia closely related to the visceral brain.

PHEOCHROMOCYTOMA

Acute oliguric renal failure associated with pheochromocytoma is rare.[205] It may be caused by hypotension following a hypertensive crisis. The sustained production of norepinephrine may cause the blood vessels to become increasingly insensitive to the pressor action of norepinephrine. When norepinephrine production or release is stopped, the sympathetic tree of the blood vessels seems to be absent. Acute tubular necrosis is the morphologic lesion associated with pheochromocytoma-induced acute renal failure.

CADAVER KIDNEY TRANSPLANT

Postmortem ischemia of cadaver kidney transplants may induce acute tubular necrosis with subsequent delay in function, or a damaged organ may cause failure of function. If the latter occurs, the recipient of a homograft cadaver kidney may require dialysis to maintain homeostasis until renal function returns.

If a patient develops oliguria with hematuria immediately following transplantation of a cadaver kidney, one must suspect that a vascular infarction has occurred. Moreover, persistent hematuria and anuria may indicate that the underlying renal damage is extensive, such as renal infarction or cortical necrosis.

The occurrence of delayed oliguria after a functioning renal homograft reflects a severe rejection of the transplanted kidney. Percutaneous renal biopsy can differentiate the effects of acute ischemia, acute rejection, and acute infection. The diagnosis of rejection requires serial sections and detailed examination of the renal morphology; otherwise, the diagnosis may be missed.

If absolute anuria occurs, one must suspect the possibility of ureteral stenosis or intraabdominal spillage of urine during ureteral rejection.

EPIDEMIC HEMORRHAGIC FEVER

Epidemic hemorrhagic fever was first described by the Russians, who encountered it in Far Eastern Siberia. They knew the disease as "epidemic hemorrhagic nephroso-nephritis" or "Far Eastern hemorrhagic fever." The Japanese military physicians encountered the disease in Manchuria and Korea. They referred to it as "epidemic hemorrhagic fever." During the Korean War in June, 1951, American and United Nations military physicians encountered an acute febrile illness characterized by prostration, vomiting, hemorrhagic manifestation, shock, proteinuria, and acute oliguric renal failure. After consulting the Russian and Japanese medical literature, this disease process was identified as acute epidemic hemorrhagic fever. A comprehensive symposium on epidemic hemorrhagic fever was published in a series of excellent reviews.*

In Korea the majority of patients were troops of front line units serving in terrain composed of heavy growth of grass and brush and infested by a large rodent population. The illness had a distinct seasonal trend; a spring outbreak began in April, reached its peak in June, declined in July and August. The fall outbreak began in late September and declined in November.

Although there were considerable variations in the clinical course, it was divided into four general phases—febrile, hypotensive, acute oliguric, and diuretic. Oliguria was proportionate to the severity of the disease; there was a rapid increase in BUN. Acidosis was rarely severe. Gross hematuria, proteinuria, either isothenuria or hyposthenuria, purpura, and gastrointestinal bleeding were the most striking features.

The patient rapidly improved after diuresis occurred. Although the BUN increased for the first 3 days of diuresis, it rapidly returned to normal. Hematuria and proteinuria disappeared and hyposthenuria appeared during diuresis. Early in the Korean War the mortality rate was 10%; later it dropped to 5%. Death during oliguria resulted from a combination of pulmonary edema and bronchopneumonia. In the diuretic phase death was usually the result of pulmonary complications.

The kidneys were enlarged with a prominent pale gray to yellowish brown surface, while the medulla was congested and dark red. Microscopically, there was striking congestion of the renomedullary area. The collecting ducts and Henle's loops were compressed and distorted. Tubular necrosis and tubular regeneration were noted. Hemoglobin casts filled the tubular lumen.[848]

Antibiotics and adrenocortical steroids had no beneficial effect to the patient with epidemic hemorrhagic fever. In general, excellent nursing care was the essential part of the patient's management, and treatment was usually supportive. Strict attention was given to the basic principles in treating patients with acute oliguria. Repeat hemodialysis and careful fluid and electrolyte balance were the outstanding factors in reducing the mortality rate.

---

*See references 430, 714, 947, and 1003.

Chapter 5

Management of the patients with acute oliguric renal failure

The management of patients with acute oliguric renal failure requires the detailed coordinated efforts of a team of physicians (nephrologist, internist, urologist, surgeon, and house officer), nurses, dialysis technicians, and other paramedical personnel.* Optimal success in the management of patients with acute oliguric renal failure can be attained only in large dialysis centers or poison control centers,[580] where patients with acute renal failure are treated frequently rather than occasionally.[344,774,1050]

Within a renal center, patients with acute oliguric renal failure can best be managed in the intensive care unit where strict methods of environmental asepsis must be enforced. The urinary output, blood pressure, central venous pressure, and cardiac rate and rhythm should be continuously monitored. Daily observations should be made of patients' body weight, intake of fluids, urinary specific gravity and output, serum electrolytes—such as potassium, sodium, and chloride—blood CO_2 combining power, and BUN.[1069]

Excellence in conservative treatment is the fundamental principle in the management of patients with acute oliguric renal failure.[12] Treatment must be directed toward prevention and minimization of the adverse effects of metabolic derangement caused by acute renal failure.[588] The principal effort should be directed toward correction of the primary or precipitating disorder and toward reestablishment of adequate blood flow to the kidneys. Shock should be controlled, the circulating blood volume must be restored, necrotic tissue should be debrided, hemorrhage should be controlled, and infections must be eliminated.

Conservative management can be supplemented by dialysis but can never be replaced by it.[151,731] The basic management of patients with acute oliguric renal failure is directed toward maintenance of fluid and electrolyte balance and toward prevention of acidosis. Hypersensitivity states should be recognized and

---

*See references 673, 773, 839, 986, and 1028.

effectively treated with adrenal corticosteroids. The use of early and frequent dialysis produces marked generalized improvement in the patient and may reduce the complications associated with acute oliguric renal failure.* Meticulous attention to every detail leads to decreased patient morbidity and mortality and lessens the period needed for rehabilitation.[557,711]

HISTORIC OLDER METHODS IN MANAGEMENT OF ACUTE RENAL FAILURE

Once parenchymal damage occurs to the kidney, infiltration of the splanchnic nerves with local analgesic agents, spinal anesthesia, short wave diathermy, and decapsulation of the kidney are ineffective and bring no benefit to the patient.[142,911] These methods are mentioned for their historic interest and will not be discussed further.

The treatment of patients with acute oliguria by exchange whole blood transfusion either with fresh whole blood or cross-circulation transfusions with a healthy individual has interested physicians since the 1940's.[265,324,1029] I found exchange whole blood transfusions to be extremely valuable adjuvants to conservative treatment of patients with oliguria caused by a nondialyzable nephrotoxic substance, especially a substance not dialyzed by crossing either the peritoneal membrane or the hemodialyzer membrane. For example, the use of whole blood transfusions can remove large quantities of arsine-hemoglobin complexes from the patient. In addition, the exchange transfusion can return the red blood cell mass to normal.

My exchange transfusion technique is to remove 500 ml of blood from the patient and transfuse 500 ml of fresh whole blood. In the adult the procedure is repeated for at least twenty exchanges. Care must be taken in performing an exchange transfusion, for an excess amount of sodium citrate may cause a serious sodium overload and may result in pulmonary edema. Moreover, the citrate may provoke hypocalcemia and an associated alkalosis. Therefore, calcium ions must be replaced by intravenous infusion of calcium chloride. This procedure is of particular value to patients with severe hemolysis, especially oliguric patients with severe shock caused by acute intravascular hemolysis. Exchange fresh whole blood transfusions produce a striking improvement in such patients. This improvement probably results from correction of the circulating red cell mass, the blood volume, the serum potassium level, and perhaps the metabolic acidosis.[342]

FLUID AND ELECTROLYTE BALANCE

Over the years, the most common immediate cause of death in patients with acute oliguria has been excessive water overloading, and the next most common cause has been potassium intoxication. Therefore, fluid balance and potassium balance are of the greatest importance in treatment of patients with acute oliguric renal failure.

---

*See references 20, 32, 33, and 329.

Fluid balance

Lack of knowledge regarding fluid balance in patients with acute oliguric renal failure was the greatest single factor responsible for the high mortality rate of patients suffering from this disorder.[414]

Schreiner and Berman emphasized that overhydration during oliguria is usually caused by two factors. The first is the physician's delayed recognition of the acute oliguric failure, and the second is the physician's failure to appreciate the large amount of endogenous water produced by the metabolism of food and body tissue.[975] In patients with acute renal failure, therefore, water intake must be sharply restricted.

In calculating water balance, water released by the endogenous oxidation of fats and protein must be considered. For example, a 70 kg patient on a 100 gm carbohydrate diet may metabolize approximately 70 gm of protein and 300 gm of fat. This caloric intake liberates 425 ml of water. In general, 400 ml of fluid should be administered to replace the insensible water loss. Added to the fluid requirements, additional fluid should be given equal to the previous day's output. This fluid replacement includes the fluid volume of gastric suction, vomitus, urine, wound drainage, and so on.

When possible, fluid should be given by mouth. The physician must consider the additional fluid required by the febrile patient. For each rise in body temperature of 1° F, a 10% increase adjustment is made in the insensible water loss. The best guides to estimating fluid balance are daily body weight, serum sodium levels, and central venous pressure recordings. When properly managed, the patient with acute oliguria is expected to have a daily weight loss between 0.3 and 0.7 kg. During oliguria any weight gain reflects fluid retention. In the absence of vomiting or diarrhea decrease in serum sodium results from excessive fluid retention. The central venous pressure is a sensitive indication of excessive fluid retention. This method aids in managing severe hypovolemia. Finally, fluid excess can also be evaluated by the clinical findings of dyspnea, tachycardia, pulmonary edema, distended neck veins, and peripheral edema.

Potassium balance

In patients with acute renal failure, potassium intoxication is the leading biochemical cause of death. Protein catabolism results in the release of cellular potassium into body fluids. The rate of cellular potassium release is increased in patients with devitalized tissue as a result of trauma, intravascular hemolysis, burns, and infections. Moreover, the metabolic acidosis of acute oliguric renal failure encourages potassium to accumulate in the extracellular space.

Although total body potassium may not change, the potassium in the extracellular space does increase. This results from the usual daily catabolism of protein and fat, a shift of potassium from intracellular to extracellular space because of metabolic acidosis, mobilization of glycogen stores—most of the available body glycogen is utilized within 24 hours—and potassium release from devitalized tissues and hemolyzed erythrocytes.

In battle casualties, the rapidity of the catabolic response is increased; after 5 or 6 days of oliguria the serum potassium may reach a level of 9 mEq/L. A rapid and out-of-proportion (to the increase in BUN) rise in serum potassium, serum phosphate, or serum creatinine serves as a diagnostic aid in detection of the presence of devitalized tissues. Loss of potassium from the gastrointestinal tract by gastric suction, vomiting, or diarrhea leads to decrease in serum potassium levels. Such a decrease may be beneficial to the patient, especially if serum sodium levels are maintained and acidosis is corrected.

The electrocardiographic changes usually attributed to serum potassium excess are the summation of several factors. These include the serum potassium concentration, hydrogen ion concentration, serum calcium, serum magnesium, and serum sodium. Continuous cardiac monitoring has been most useful in detecting myocardial irritability. Various cardiac dysrhythmias, bradycardia, muscle paresis or paralysis, and loss of deep tendon reflexes may reflect potassium intoxication.

Potassium intoxication requires immediate and emergency treatment. When both acidosis and hyperkalemia are present, intravenous administration of sodium bicarbonate (44 to 88 mEq) is the most rapid method of decreasing the serum potassium and preventing potassium intoxication. In an emergency situation 50 to 100 ml of a 10% calcium gluconate solution or 200 ml of a 3% sodium chloride solution may be equally beneficial.[569] These measures are only temporary adjuvants until dialysis can be done. The main attempts in treating potassium intoxication should be aimed toward removing potassium from the body and not toward shifting potassium from one body space to another.[637] Such treatment can be accomplished by gastric suction, by potassium exchange resins such as sodium polystyrene sulfonate (Kayexalate) or resonium A, and by artificial dialysis.[97] A retention enema containing 20 to 60 gm of the polystyrene sulfonate resins in the sodium form should be retained in the colon for periods of 30 to 40 minutes. If used for a prolonged period, this resin may act as a dangerous sodium donor.[352] For example, as much as 60 to 180 mEq of sodium may be added to the total sodium intake.

The polystyrene sulfonate resins are not very palatable; in some patients they may lead to fecal impaction. Sodium polystyrene sulfonate, a sodium cycle resin, appears more palatable when mixed with sorbitol. Such mixing leads to rapid emptying of the gastrointestinal tract. Increasing the potassium loss from the gut by inducing diarrhea with cathartics can be dangerous, especially when other electrolytes are not replaced.[98]

Metabolic acidosis

The patient with acute oliguria cannot eliminate the daily load of hydrogen ions produced by routine metabolic processes. This inability is reflected by a fall in the blood CO_2 combining power and blood pH. In general, metabolic acidosis in acute oliguric renal failure results from the production of hydrogen ions derived from oxidation of sulfur-containing amino acids, from phosphoprotein residues, and from incompletely metabolized organic acids. When the CO_2 combining power falls below 12 mM/L, acidosis is severe, Kussmaul's respiration occurs, and the patient's life is threatened. Hypertonic (7.5%) sodium bicarbonate solution should be given to improve the severe metabolic acidosis rather than to restore the blood CO_2 combining power to normal. Molar lactate solutions are not as effective as sodium bicarbonate solutions and may aggravate lactate acidosis and result in irreversible lactate acidosis.

The airway should be kept open and assistance should be given to ventilation; this ensures an intact respiratory compensation effect. Gastric suction has removed excessive hydrogen ions and has reduced metabolic acidosis. However, caution must be taken not to remove excessive gastric hydrochloric acid; otherwise, metabolic alkalosis can occur. This altered metabolic state leads to tetany and severe mental aberrations. In a rare oliguric patient with metabolic alkalosis, dilute solutions (0.01 to 0.05N) of hydrochloric acid (10 to 50 mEq of HCl per liter of 5% dextrose solution) may be given intravenously.

Sodium balance

Hyponatremia usually results from excessive hydration with water or saline-poor solutions. Unless hyponatremia is a result of marked sodium depletion and dehydration, the physician's attempt to correct this deficiency usually results in excessive hydration and pulmonary edema. The usual treatment of hyponatremia is water restriction. Large losses of sodium from the gut because of vomiting, diarrhea, or gastric suction should be replaced with hypertonic sodium chloride solution (3 to 5%). In general, during the oliguric phase sodium intake should be restricted to 0.5 gm per day. The usual losses from sweat and from the gut do not require replacement. However, when severe and dangerous water intoxication is present, one must partially correct the low serum sodium using hypertonic (5%) saline solution. The oliguric patient with water intoxication has usually had surgery and has been given large quantities of electrolyte-deficient fluids.

Asymptomatic hyponatremia may require correction when potassium intoxication is present, especially when ECG abnormalities of hyperkalemia are noted.

The serum chloride level usually reflects the serum sodium level and the degree of metabolic acidosis. In general, hypochloremia requires no specific treatment.

Calcium and phosphorus balance

In general, electrolyte disorders of calcium or phosphorus do not require specific treatment. Hypocalcemia is rare; and when present it is rarely the cause of seizures, tetany, or muscle spasms. Therefore, one should look for other causes, such as overhydration or severe hypertension. Calcium chloride or calcium gluconate should be given intravenously when the serum calcium falls, which usually occurs following massive exchange whole blood transfusion (an urgent measure for potassium intoxication).

Meroney has recommended a daily infusion of 100 ml or more of a 10% calcium gluconate solution as a prophylactic and specific measure of treatment for potassium intoxication.[769] This regimen can be dangerous to patients receiving digitalis preparation, especially when rapid intravenous calcium replacement is given. In the presence of severe acidosis and hypocalcemia, the hypocalcemia should be corrected before the metabolic acidosis; otherwise, cardiac arrest can occur.

Hyperphosphatemia occurs late in the course of acute oliguric renal failure. Its toxic effects are not well understood.[109] I use aluminum hydroxide gels administered orally—one to two tablespoonfuls (10 to 20 ml) four times daily. This insoluble aluminum phosphate is eliminated in the gut.

NUTRITIONAL FACTORS

Sir William Osler recommended dietary measures in the management of patients with chronic renal failure.[853,855] He restricted the protein intake and permitted milk and eggs* in the diet. Borst and Bull and his colleagues stressed the importance of high-calorie, low-protein intake in the management of patients with acute renal failure.[136,137] Their regimen minimized the exogenous protein loss and had the advantage of the so-called protein-sparing action of carbohydrates. Bull fed his patients a basic diet (through a gastric tube) of 400 gm of glucose and 100 gm of peanut oil in water to a volume of 1 liter, assuming both were completely metabolized; the total water administered was 810 ml.[172] Today, this regimen is not popular among patients or nephrologists. It is a generalized rule that protein of any sort is contraindicated in patients with acute renal failure.

Nutritional factors are most important in the management of patients with acute oliguric renal failure. By using good basic nutritional principles, the physician can reduce the serious metabolic derangements of protein breakdown such as azotemia, hyperkalemia, and acidosis. High caloric mixtures (800 to 1,000 calories) of glucose and fats are especially recommended for the so-called protein-sparing actions by reducing protein catabolism.[317] These nonprotein calories are utilized for energy as they are oxidized to water and carbon dioxide. Glucose ingestion of 100 gm per day can decrease endogenous protein catabolism by 50%. Such a decrease has particular benefit to oliguric patients with an accelerated protein catabolism such as associated with trauma, burns, or severe infection.

Whenever possible the patient should be allowed a choice of oral nutrients.[641] Patients with oliguria who are maintained on dialysis should receive a diet supplying 20 to 40 gm of protein, 0.5 gm of sodium, and 2,500 calories.[608] This diet should include hard candy, sweet butter, sugar, salt-free matzos (light weight

---

*Egg has a high degree of digestibility and has a high biologic value (0.94). This is the ratio of the amount of a protein fed to the amount utilized in the synthesis of tissue protein. Therefore, the egg is often called the ideal food.

biscuits) or toast covered with copious amounts of sweet butter and jelly, chilled mixtures of Karo syrup and gingerale, and noodles or steamed rice saturated with sweet butter. Parenteral feedings with intravenous catheters should be avoided, for they predispose to septicemia and pulmonary embolism.

High-calorie artificial diets of sugar and emulsified fats are unpalatable and often lead to diarrhea, vomiting, and aspiration pneumonia.[1127] Nonprotein calories not only reduce hydrogen ions released from acid metabolites but prevent cellular destruction and release of potassium when protein is metabolized. Glucose not only decreases protein catabolism but prevents the accumulation of ketone acids, which result from incomplete oxidation of fat in the presence of inadequate calories of glucose.

The long-term administration of intravenous fats can lead to the "fat overloading syndrome." This syndrome is characterized by high fever, headaches, sore throat, anorexia, vomiting, hypoproteinemia, and thrombocytopenia. Patients may develop hepatosplenomegaly, and large numbers of foam cells are found in their bone marrow and kidneys. There appears to be no beneficial effect from the use of fat emulsions for short periods. Regardless of the dietary skills in preparing fat emulsions, they are not well tolerated by the gastrointestinal tract and result in increased vomiting, which may further complicate the condition.

When food cannot be taken by mouth, at least 100 gm of glucose should be given intravenously. Infusions of 50% glucose should be given through a plastic Introcath placed into a large arm vein. This allows rapid dilution of the hypertonic glucose solution. A very small amount of heparin and adrenal corticosteroids reduces thrombosis, infection, and inflammation. Five hundred milliliters of a 50% glucose solution should be given constantly until diuresis occurs or until hemodialysis is started.

Multivitamin supplements should be given daily. Moreover, patients undergoing prolonged peritoneal dialysis require parenteral injections of vitamin K and water-soluble vitamins including vitamin B_{12}.[513] Amino acids may be essential for wound repair. In the absence of an exogenous source, tissue protein may be broken down to supply the necessary amino acids for wound healing. Therefore, the administration of amino acid supplements may have a protein-sparing action.

It is obvious that potassium and phosphorus should be restricted in the diet. Raisins, bananas, coffee, and citrus fruits and juices should be avoided during oliguria. Losses of potassium from the gut because of vomiting, diarrhea, or gastric suction need not be replaced. Finally, the physician must not forget the high potassium content of stored blood and the high potassium content of certain antibiotics.

ANABOLIC ANDROGENS IN SUPPRESSION OF NITROGEN CATABOLISM

Norethandrolone, a "newer" anabolic androgen, is related to testosterone but it has a greater anabolic-to-androgenic ratio. Norethandrolone and testosterone were both found to suppress nitrogen catabolism by significantly decreasing protein breakdown, first in postpartum women with acute oliguric renal failure and more recently in patients of both sexes with acute oliguric renal failure from a variety of causes.[117,435]

Wolthins observed that 19-nor-andro-sterolone phenylpropionate and testosterone phenylpropionate have an equal protein-sparing effect.[1138,1138a] This effect was greater than that obtained with methyl androstenidial. Testosterone or norethandrolone can be given orally or intramuscularly in doses of 25 to 50 mg daily for the duration of the oliguric phase. No adverse side effects are noted during the short periods the agents are used. Anabolic steroids such as norethandrolone (Nilevar) and nandrolone phenpropionate (Durabolin) have also been effective in reducing protein catabolism.[117,434]

HYPERSENSITIVITY STATES

Acute oliguric renal failure caused by hypersensitivity states can result from drug-induced disorders. Interstitial nephritis,[242,734] acute glomerulonephritis,[25,289,826] TTP, polyarteritis nodosa,[115] and necrotizing angiitis are the morphologic lesions reflecting drug-induced hypersensitivity states. The numerous drugs that induce hypersensitivity renal lesions are discussed in detail on pp. 204 and 205.

Hypersensitivity states are associated with dermatologic lesions, fever, eosinophilia, neutropenia, and thrombocytopenia. Once renal biopsy study has provided a diagnosis, prompt withdrawal of the drug and intensive adrenal corticosteroid treatment are started. High doses of prednisone have been very effective in reversing the hypersensitivity state and producing a diuresis. Adrenal corticosteroids have no beneficial effect in treatment of ischemic and nephrotoxic parenchymal disease. In fact, adrenal corticosteroids can be hazardous, can aggravate uremic symptoms, and can result in dissemination of infection.

Lupus nephritis rarely results in acute oliguric renal failure. When acute oliguria develops in a patient with lupus nephritis the renal lesion is an active and fulminating proliferative glomerulonephritis. The combination of adrenal corticosteroids in high doses and so-called immunosuppressive agents—azathioprine (Imuran) or nitrogen mustard—has been helpful.[1057a] Before the steroids are started, however, care must be taken to exclude tuberculosis and fungal infections.[992] Lawrence referred to uremia as "nature's immunosuppressive device."[676]

In patients with acute renal failure caused by poststreptococcal glomerulonephritis, adrenal cortiscosteroids have produced no beneficial effect. The physician's patience with conservative treatment and, when necessary, adequate, prompt, and frequent dialysis, have been most successful in producing a remission.

A rare patient with acute renal failure caused by acute proliferative glomerulonephritis associated with epithelial crescents has been benefited by treatment with high doses of adrenal corticosteroids. In general, however, the therapeutic response has been very poor. Some patients with the hemolytic uremic syndrome have improved following treatment with intravenous heparin, with or without adrenal corticosteroids.

MANAGEMENT OF INFECTION

The common cause of death of patients with acute oliguric renal failure is complication of bacterial infections. Inflected flesh wounds are the portal of entry for septicemia and pneumonia following prolonged stasis. These complications occur in approximately one-third of all patients with acute renal failure. Prophylactic use of antibiotics should be avoided. Reverse isolation in the management of the patient prevents hospital-borne infections of gram-positive bacteria. The best prophylactic measure is to avoid the use of indwelling ureteral catheters and the use of inferior cava cannulas. If arteriovenous cannulation is used to facilitate repeated hemodialysis, daily cleansing must be scrupulously done. In my experience, early and frequent dialysis has not reduced the incidence or severity of complicating infections; however, it has provided time to bring the infection under antibiotic control.

Fever, leukocytosis with a differential cell shift to the left, and pyuria occur in patients with acute renal failure in the absence of infection. Therefore, antibiotics should be administered only after the presence of infection is proved by bacterial cultures.[610] When possible, the use of appropriate antibiotics should be determined by laboratory sensitivity studies. Antibiotics should be administered vigorously and with full knowledge of their neurotoxicity and ototoxicity.[335,348] So-called broad-spectrum antibiotics should be used with caution lest they lead to superinfections of nocardia, monilia, or fungi.[631]

When prescribing antibiotics the physician must recognize that some antibiotics are excreted by the kidneys and that others are metabolized by the liver.[460] Colistin, streptomycin, kanamycin, tetracycline,[655] and polymyxin B are excreted by the kidney; if their blood levels increase they become toxic to the central nervous system as well as extremely toxic to the kidney.[348] Ideally, the physician should obtain blood levels to monitor the dose requirement; unfortunately, this may not be possible. Chloramphenicol is metabolized by the liver and is one of the safer and more effective antibiotics used in oliguric patients with bacterial infection. Kunin studied extensively the safe and therapeutic dose levels for numerous antibiotics when administered to patients with acute renal failure[650-654] (Table 3-2).

CONGESTIVE HEART FAILURE

Congestive heart failure in the patient with acute oliguric renal failure usually results from overhydration. The use of central venous pressure monitoring has been helpful in preventing or detecting early heart failure. The rate of fluid administration can be "cut back." Excessive fluid should be removed with hypertonic dextrose solution by peritoneal dialysis or by ultra-filtration during hemodialysis with hypertonic glucose solution in the dialysate. Salt overloading and uncontrolled hypertension can also produce heart failure.

Merrill uses digitalization in any previously undigitalized patient with acute oliguric renal failure and congestive heart failure.[773] However, Johnson uses digitalization only when the congestive heart failure is caused by heart disease.[588] I use digoxin at the first clinical indication of congestive heart failure, in a dose half the digitalizing dose given to a cardiac patient. The patient with acute oliguric renal failure and acute heart failure does not respond to digitalization in the same manner as does a patient with heart failure but without acute oliguria. This response is altered by hyperkalemia, acidosis, and hypocalcemia.

Therefore, the physician should use great caution when digitalis is given intravenously, as patients with acute renal failure are more prone to develop digitalis intoxication.[6] This effect is usually caused by electrolyte imbalance and/or severe alternations in acid-base balance.

Supportive measures of oxygen therapy and the use of automatic tourniquets have been helpful. In a rare patient with heart failure and severe anemia, the slow administration of packed red blood cells has been helpful.

HYPERTENSION

When hypertension occurs in patients with acute renal failure it results from any of the following causes: sodium excess, fluid excess, or an associated fulminating glomerular or renal vascular lesion. Severe hypertensive encephalopathy is usually associated with acute glomerulonephritis, lupus glomerulonephritis, necrotizing angiitis, polyarteritis nodosa, severe benign nephrosclerosis, and renal artery occlusion.

Sodium should be restricted and fluid intake should be markedly cut back. If hypertension remains a clinical problem the use of intravenous diazoxide has been most helpful. Diazoxide should be given rapidly intravenously—300 to 600 mg in a 15% solution within 30 seconds. Care should be taken not to expose diazoxide solution to light. When diazoxide is given by slow intravenous infusion the bottle should be enclosed by a brown paper bag.

A dose of 500 mg. of methyldopa (Aldomet) given intravenously over 4 hours has reduced and controlled hypertension. I have found that the use of oral guanethidine (Ismelin) has been very effective in controlling hypertension. The starting oral dose should be 25 to 50 mg. I have found that diuretic agents such as furosemide have no effect in reducing blood pressure in patients with acute oliguric renal failure.[266]

DIALYSIS
Introduction

In general, the life and well-being of patients with acute renal failure depend on artificial dialysis.[1058,1075] Although improvement in the conservative management of patients with acute renal failure has reduced the mortality rate, artificial dialysis is fairly well established as an absolute requirement in the treatment of many patients with acute renal failure until renal function recovers.[1,315] In spite of artificial means, the mortality rate of patients with acute renal failure in general is still approximately 50%. Artificial dialysis is currently accomplished by either extracorporeal hemodialysis or peritoneal dialysis, by irrigation of some intestinal segment, or by gastric lavage. The latter is very rarely used.

Because of peritoneal dialysis and extracorporeal hemodialysis, patients with acute renal failure can be artificially kept alive and free of the major manifestations of the uremic syndrome for indefinite periods.[1135] For example, Maher, Schreiner, and Waters kept a patient with acute renal failure alive for 181 days.[735]

Life is sustained by differential transfer of solutes and water through a porous membrane, either artificial or natural, placed between the body compartment and the dialyzing fluid. In extracorporeal hemodialysis the membrane is cellophane (artificial), and in peritoneal dialysis the membrane is the inert peritoneum (natural).[898]

Peritoneal dialysis is accepted as a simple, relatively inexpensive, and effective method of treating patients with renal failure.[198] It requires less in the way of apparatus and experienced personnel than does extracorporeal hemodialysis. The technique was first used by Ganter in 1923, but it fell into disuse because of infections and technical difficulties.[446] In independent studies in 1959, Doolan and associates[308] and Maxwell and associates[749] simplified the method of peritoneal dialysis. Later, commercial prepackaged administration sets, solutions, and plastic or nylon catheters became available. Subsequently the use of peritoneal dialysis became widespread, and the need for using hemodialysis became less frequent.

History of peritoneal dialysis

The historic review and background material on peritoneal dialysis has appeared in several publications.[131,132,308]

Wegner was the first to use peritoneal lavage.[1119] He studied the effects of temperature change in the infused peritoneal solution on body temperature. His technique consisted of placing two catheters into the peritoneal cavity. The irrigating fluid continuously entered through one catheter and left through the other.

Starling, in 1894 with Tubby,[1041] and in 1895 with Leathes,[680] injected hyperosmotic solutions of saline and glucose into the peritoneal cavity and in the following few hours observed an increase in the intraabdominal fluid volume. They observed that all fluid was absorbed after 12 hours. Their studies indicated that transfer across the peritoneal membrane from one compartment to another depends on the concentration of the solute.

In 1895, Hamburger studied the peritoneal membrane of dead animals and found it to be passive in movement of solute or water.[492] In 1918, Maxcy was the first to apply intraperitoneal infusions to infants with severe gastrointestinal disturbances.[748] In 1921, Clark established the existence of an osmotic equilibrium

Table 5-1. Hemodialyzer data

Author	Type of dialyzer	Type of membrane	Dialyzing surface area (cm²)	Volume of blood (ml)	Thickness of blood layer (mm)	Blood flow (ml/min)	Dialysis flow (ml/min)	Dialysance or clearance (ml/min)	Permeability (cm/min)
Merrill, 1950[775]	Kolff-Brigham	No-jax	22,500	500-700		300	bath, 100L	225	0.0183
Lowsley, 1951[711]	Parallel flow		21,000	300		220		80	0.0050
Lunderquist, 1952[715]	Alwall	No-jax	16,600			473	bath, 85L	237	0.0339
Inouye, 1953[576]	Inouye	No-jax	9,000			140	600	47	0.006
Battezzati, 1954[76]	Battezzati	Kalle cellophane	16,250	150		150	12,000	59	0.007
Keitzer, 1954[617]	Skeggs-Leonards	Dupont 300	22,000	< 500		150 to 200	400 to 600		
Kolff and Watschinger, 1956[645]	Twin-coil		18,000	750		200	bath	140	0.0111
Anthonisen, 1956[32]	Skeggs-Leonards	Cuprophane PT 150	21,200	300	0.5	300 to 600	2,000 to 3,000	150 to 250	0.0098-0.0152
Hillenbrand, 1957[548]	Hillenbrand	No-jax	15,000	Ca. 900	1.0	250 to 360	bath, 100L	250 (Cl-)	0.0284
Kuhn, 1957[649]	Capillary system		2,800	20	0.03	240		80	0.0348
Berman and Schreiner, 1957[101]	Twin-coil	No-jax	18,000	1,215		300	bath, 100L	172	0.0142
Sartorius, 1957[955]	Twin-coil	Cellulose tubing	18,000	700		200	bath, 100L	160	0.0179
Antoine and Ducrot, 1957[33]	Kolff-Necker	No-jax	30,000			500	bath, 100L	300	0.0151
Maher and Broadbent, 1958[731]	Skeggs-Leonards	Dupont 300	20,000	500		200	800 to 1,000	150	0.0139
Taddei, 1958[1058]	Taddei-Dogliatti-Battezzati	No-jax	19,200	1,200		300	bath, 210L	189	0.0159
Kupfer and Rosenak, 1959[658]	Parallel-flow	No-jax	10,000			550		180	0.0180
MacNeill, 1959[727]	MacNeill	No-jax	20,000			300	2,000 to 3,000	135	0.0089
Michelli, 1960[780]	Battezzati-Taddei	Kalle cellophane	19,200					90	
Savino, 1960[956]	Capillary system	Cellophane 20 nm	1,800	150	0.083	250	550	125	0.0962
Kiil, 1960[621]	Parallel-flow	Cuprophane PT 150	18,000	800	0.3	800	300 to 4,000	350	0.0255
Kiil and Glover, 1962[622]	Parallel-flow	Cuprophane PT 150	21,000	800	0.2	1,000		410	0.0255
Brown and Schreiner, 1962[157]	Skeggs-Leonards	Dupont 300	9,500	375		120	bath	72	0.0116
	Skeggs-Leonards	Cuprophane PT 150	25,000	800	0.5	650	2,500	225	0.0111
Jørgensen, 1962[592]	Skeggs-Leonards	Cuprophane PT 150	38,000	1,000	0.5	650	2,500	302	0.0107
	Skeggs-Leonards	Cuprophane PT 150	43,000	1,200	0.5	878	2,500	431	0.0140
Cole, 1963[227]	Kiil (modified)	Cuprophane PT 150	9,500	300	0.1	142	2,000	70	0.0101
Miller, 1960[780b]	Twin-coil	Cuprophane PT 150	7,000	140	0.18	200 to 340		140	

between the peritoneal fluid and the circulating plasma.[218a] Two years later, Ganter produced renal failure in rabbits and guinea pigs by ureter ligation.[446] Using peritoneal lavage, he was able to significantly lengthen their survival time. In 1951, Grollman and associates extended this observation by keeping nephrectomized dogs alive up to 111 days.[474,475] Darrow and Yannet used peritoneal infusion in a study of fluid equilibrium between extracellular and intracellular spaces.[264] Their studies formed a basis for our knowledge of fluid balance between body compartments.

Intermittent peritoneal dialysis was first used in clinical medicine in 1923 when Ganter treated a woman who had uremia due to urethral obstruction caused by a uterine carcinoma.[416] He inserted a single tube into the peritoneal cavity. After a brief interval, the perfused fluid was siphoned back out through the same tube. Four years later, Heusser and Werder, by continuous peritoneal dialysis, treated three uremic patients who had acute anuria caused by mercuric chloride ($HgCl_2$) poisoning.[545] Unknown to them, they used too little fluid and treated their patients without success. However, they did observe that peritoneal dialysis caused extraction of nonprotein nitrogen, mercury, and body proteins.

Up to 1948, a total of 101 patients were treated by peritoneal dialysis. Of these, sixty-three had acute renal failure, thirty-two had chronic renal failure,* and six had poisoning. Continuous dialysis was used in seventy-five patients and intermittent in twenty-two. Thirty-one patients died of acute renal failure, while thirty-two patients survived. All thirty-two patients with chronic renal failure died. Fenn and associates used peritoneal dialysis for 26 days to treat one patient with azotemia.[361] In 1953, LeGrain and Merrill reported intermittent or short-term continuous peritoneal irrigation as an effective way of treating patients with acute renal failure.[683] The technical difficulties and high incidence of peritonitis discouraged the further clinical use of peritoneal dialysis.[786,932] In 1959, however, Doolan and associates[308] and Maxwell and associates,[749] after reexploring peritoneal dialysis, simultaneously and successfully simplified the technique and made it much safer and of greater potential for clinical application.[182,225,260] Through their improvement in techniques, widespread use of peritoneal dialysis was made practical, especially after the availability of easily inserted plastic or nylon catheters, the commercial production of sterile dialysis solutions, and the availability of simple commercial equipment to administer and withdraw the dialyzing fluids.[488]

History of extracorporeal hemodialysis

Extracorporeal hemodialysis with an artificial kidney is the most rapid method of dialyzing a patient.[715]

In 1914, Abel, Rowntree, and Turner efficiently removed salicylate from rabbits.[2] They utilized a crude device to convoy blood through colloidon and

---

*See references 1, 368, 369, 391, 401, 481, 922, and 1051.

branching glass tubes surrounded by a jacket filled with isotonic saline. Coagulation of the circulatory blood was prevented by hirudin extracted from leech heads. These investigators made their own colloidon tubes and personally extracted hirudin from leeches in their laboratory. Although they studied intermediate metabolites, they predicted the use of dialysis as a valuable form of treatment in patients with acute renal failure and of removal of toxic agents such as sodium salicylate from the body.[302] Approximately 40 years later, Doolan and associates successfully applied this observation to the care of patients with salicylate intoxication.[308]

In 1915, McGuigan and Couoheri reduced the tendency toward thrombus formation in their apparatus by making smoother inner surfaces of the tubes and by reducing the number of connections. They used this apparatus in dialyzing the intestinal membrane of various animals. In 1923, Necheles studied the functions of the intestinal mucosa and peritoneal membrane in the transfer of solutes.[829] He concluded that the peritoneal membrane was inert and that the intestine was active in transfer of various solutes. In 1926, heparin was introduced as an anticoagulant. Two years later, Haas introduced a pump between the dialyzing machine and the patient, which permitted physicians to establish an even and controlled blood flow.[485]

In 1938, Thalhimer employed a cellophane membrane with heparin in the technique of extracorporeal dialysis.[1074] His cellophane membrane fulfilled the requirement of an ideal artificial membrane. The cross-section size of each pore of the membrane was approximately 30 Angstrom units (A). Its submicroscopic size permitted the transfer of crystalloids and yet it was impermeable to serum proteins. Since then, cellophane has been used in every type of hemodialyzer.[76] Currently, two artificial kidneys are widely used—the so-called disposable twin coil and the flat plate.[34]

The method of hemodialysis had its birth during World War II. In 1943, Kolff, working under harsh conditions of the German occupation in the Netherlands, introduced to clinical medicine the first practical artificial kidney—a rotating drum apparatus.[193,639] He wound viscose cellophane tubing around a rotating drum. The lower portion of the horizontal drum was immersed in the fluid bath. The patient's blood was forced through the cellophane by the principle of an Archimedes' screw and was returned to the patient's vein by means of a pump. Although Kolff treated a series of patients with uremia, he believed that one patient with probable acute glomerulonephritis owed her life to treatment with the artificial kidney. Her BUN rose to 396 mg/100 ml and her serum potassium to 55 mg/100 ml. Eight liters of blood flowed through the kidney in 11½ hours. Her BUN dropped to 121 mg/100 ml and her serum potassium to 19 mg/100 ml.[644] From this pioneer work of Kolff stemmed the dialysis programs now carried on all over the world.[193,640,955]

In 1947, Alwall designed a stationary type of appartaus consisting of a vertical drum with an attached flattened cellophane tube supported by wire screening.[16-18]

The apparatus was immersed into a dialyzing solution that circulated around the membrane in a countercurrent direction to the blood flow. One year later, Skeggs and Leonards used an effective and ultrafiltering flat plate machine consisting of layers of flat cellophane membranes sandwiched between layers of rubber pads designed with fine surface grooves.[32,1019] These grooves indented the cellophane membrane and formed small channels, which permitted the flow of blood. On the other side of the membrane the rinsing fluid was pumped in a countercurrent direction to the blood flow and directly through small adjacent channels.

Kiil modified the flat plate dialyzer of Skeggs and Leonards.[621] He replaced the rubber mats with rigid plastic dialyzer boards and changed the flow of blood entering and leaving the cellophane sheets.[592-617] The apparatus must be put together and tested by technicians prior to use.[227] A similar plate-type dialyzer was designed by MacNeill and associates and is now commercially available.[727] Other hemodialyzers have followed[548] (Table 5-1).

In 1953, Inouye and Engelberg described the pressure-cooker artificial kidney.[576] It consisted of concentrically wound cellophane and a plastic screen immersed in a dialyzing solution within a pressure cooker. From this kidney a disposable twin-coil kidney was designed by Kolff and Watschinger.[645] They adapted the idea of winding cellophane around a fiberglass screen; first they wound it on fruit cans and later on beer cans. This apparatus was further refined and is now commercially produced as the disposable twin-coil kidney (Fig. 5-1).

The cellophane tubing is obtained from a commercial firm that manufactures it as sausage casing. The two parallel cellophane tubes are 10.8 meters long and

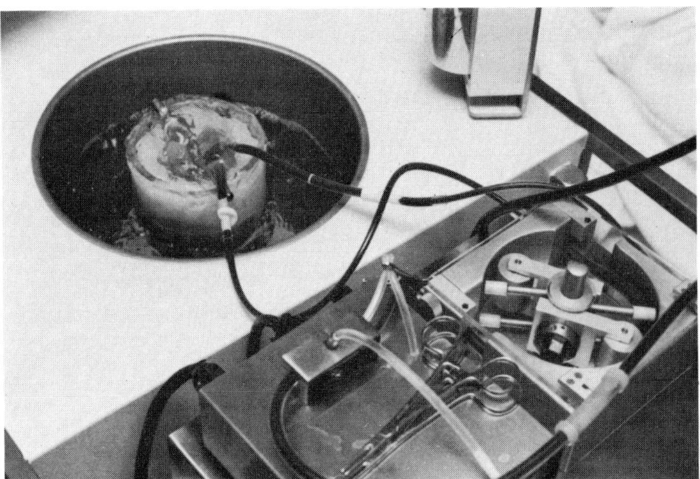

Fig. 5-1. Top view of canister containing EX-ol coil in single pass recirculating kidney. Rotary infusion pump is at right. Positive-negative pressure monitor is at center bottom. This dialyzer was used either as single unit or as part of central dialysis unit in treating patients with prolonged oliguria.

are wrapped around a central core of fiberglass screen 10.8 cm in diameter. The dialyzing area is 1.9 square meters. The coils require a priming volume of from 800 to 1,200 ml of blood. There are various types of disposable coils to meet the patient's clinical needs. The disposable twin coil kidney is a high-pressure ultra-filtrating unit that requires a pump to propel the blood through the high resistances of the tubing. Because of ultrafiltration,[101] fluids must be given to patients with normal hydration or underhydration once hemodialysis is completed. Because of the inexpensive prepackaging and sterile availability of the disposable cellophane twin coils and plastic units, this artificial kidney has gained widespread popularity. The unit can be easily assembled and is ready for use within an hour. A total of 6 hours is usually required for a satisfactory dialysis.

The disposable twin coil kidney has several disadvantages.[775,777,972] The unit requires priming with blood and thus exposes the patient to hazards of blood transfusions such as hemorrhage, reactions, and hepatitis. The use of a blood pump increases the possibility of spontaneous blood leaks. Unless a hemoglobin detector is used, close and constant attention is required to detect blood in the bath and sudden pressure changes in the system. Repeated bath changes are needed to prevent bacterial growth and to maintain the solute concentration. In view of the undesirable factors, the disposable twin coil kidney is still the most popular artificial kidney used in the United States[157,956] (Fig. 5-1).

An inexpensive minicoil artificial kidney is simple to set up and requires close attention only when the bath water is being changed.[678] However, it has a relatively low efficiency and is not suitable for patients with a high catabolic rate

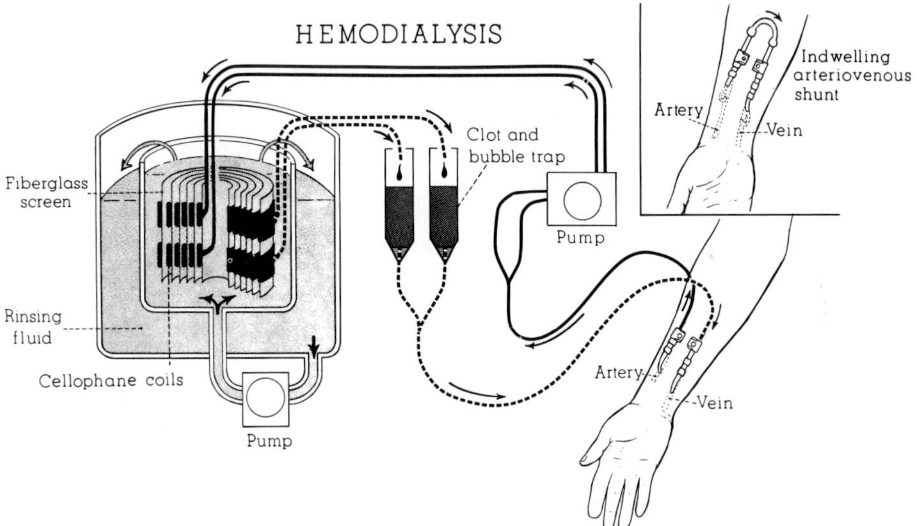

Fig. 5-2. Use of A-V shunt and hemodialysis. Teflon cannulas are within the right radial artery and a wrist vein. A pump conveys arterial blood into the twin coils. There the blood is dialyzed and recirculated through a trap for clots and bubbles. The blood is then returned through a wrist vein. This method facilitates a rapid and effective dialysis in the "prophylactic" use of extracorporeal hemodialysis.

producing 40 to 50 mg/100 ml rise of urea a day. A compact capillary kidney may prove to be most successful.[649]

When an experienced physician and adequate dialyzing and laboratory facilities are available, daily prophylactic hemodialysis as used by Teschan is an effective means of preventing uremia in the severely catabolic patient.[1073] To simplify the technique of continuous dialysis, Scribner and associates utilized indwelling silastic Teflon cannulas[819,982] (Fig. 5-2). First, the cannulas are inserted into the radial artery and into a wrist vein through a subcutaneous tunnel so that they emerge from the skin through a tight-fitting puncture wound.

This technique permits a single cannulation of vessels at the onset of treatment and simplifies further dialysis.[397] There is no need for anticoagulation, and the risk of infection is reduced by the skin tunnel and puncture wound. A special fitting connects the arterial cannula directly to the venous cannula, thus creating an arteriovenous fistula. Shunts have remained in position for more than 18 months. Shaldon and associates use percutaneous femoral venous catheterization when attaching a patient to the dialyzer.[1000] I have found this technique to be very effective.

Complications

When peritoneal dialysis was first used, complications of pulmonary edema, cerebral edema, and circulatory collapse resulted from inadequate knowledge of fluid balance and electrolyte shifts.[1046] Development of solutions (7% glucose) hyperosmotic to plasma overcame the problems of overhydration. Infection of the peritoneum, as it was early in the use of peritoneal dialysis, is still the prime complication, especially in patients undergoing prolonged dialysis for acute renal failure. Initially, peritonitis prevented the widespread acceptance of peritoneal dialysis. Peritonitis appears to occur more frequently when hyperosmotic solutions (7% dextrose solutions) are used. This can be explained by the transmural migration of bacteria through the wall of the gastrointestinal tract, especially when the gut is made more permeable because of uremia. Once infection occurs, the peritoneal fluid should be cultured and appropriate antibiotic treatment should be started. Oral neomycin has been given to reduce the bacterial flora and to reduce the occurrence of peritonitis.

Cardiac dysrhythmia has occurred when electrolytes are removed too rapidly; it is more likely to occur with hemodialysis than with peritoneal dialysis. The use of electronic equipment to monitor patients undergoing dialysis may help to detect dysrhythmia and to institute effective treatment early. Herniation of the small intestine into the puncture site rarely occurs when the catheter is removed. I observed one patient who developed intestinal obstruction after the catheter was removed. During surgery the obstructed bowel was resected without morbidity to the patient. Perforation of the gut has followed peritoneal catheter insertion.[1014a]

An unusual complication of dialysis is the disequilibrium syndrome characterized by headaches, confusion, muscle twitching, and convulsions. This syndrome of disturbed cerebral function can occur during extracorporeal hemodialysis. One can prevent and lessen these symptoms by slowing the rate of dialysis.

In prolonged dialysis due to removal of excessive nutrients such as amino acids, protein, and vitamins (fat- and water-soluble) such as vitamin K and vitamin B_{12}, the following nutritional deficiencies can occur: hypoproteinemia, marked prolongation of the prothrombin time, and megaloblastic anemia.

Transitory leukopenia and thrombocytopenia occur as a result of trapping of both platelets and leukocytes by the cellophane membrane. Other complications include excessive bleeding when heparin is used, drop in blood pressure caused by distention of cellophane membrane by blood, clotting and leaks in the cellophane membranes, and aspiration pneumonia caused by vomiting. Hepatitis is a complication of extracorporeal hemodialysis that occurs in members of the renal unit such as physicians, nurses, and technicians.[115,931]

It is very dangerous for an untrained physician to use peritoneal dialysis; therefore, a short training period in a renal unit is strongly recommended.

Indications

The foremost purpose of dialysis is to maintain the life and the well-being of the patient until his kidney function is restored.* The purpose is the same, whether peritoneal dialysis[488] or hemodialysis is contemplated.[811] There is no absolute contraindication for the use of peritoneal dialysis. It can be used within 24 hours of abdominal surgery and in the presence of bacterial peritonitis.[131] I have used it in the presence of hemoperitoneum following laceration of the liver. The type and method of dialysis depends on the facilities available to the physician caring for the patient. Indications for dialysis should not be rigid and, above all, dialysis should not be postponed until all other measures have failed.[812] Specifically, the indications should meet the clinical requirements of each individual patient and therefore they are usually numerous and broad. Peritoneal dialysis is simpler and more effective to use in children than is hemodialysis.[1055]

Initially, the prime indication for dialysis was uremic coma or the effects of uremia on the central nervous system. Improvement in the safety of hemodialysis followed increased knowledge of the conservative management of patients with acute renal failure. Hemodialysis is now used much earlier in the course of renal failure and much more frequently. Eventually daily prophylactic dialysis became popular for treating all the adverse effects of the uremic syndrome. The early use of artificial dialysis not only increases the patient's mobility, but it also helps in fighting infection, preventing pneumonia, promoting wound healing, and preventing thrombosis.

The indications for dialysis of patients with acute renal failure are usually based

---

*See references 131, 684, 772, and 780.

on the deterioration of either the patient's clinical state or his blood biochemistry. The clinical criteria usually include progressive muscle twitching, mental aberrations, pulmonary edema, abdominal distention, cardiac dysrhythmia, and persistent vomiting.

Teschan and associates advocate the concept of daily prophylactic dialysis to reduce the ill effects and to prevent the complications of uremia.[1026,1073] Salisbury recommends hemodialysis on the sixth day of "severe" oliguria, regardless of clinical and biochemical abnormalities.[951] If the patient has severe oliguria and dialysis is not to be performed until the sixth day, he could die while awaiting dialysis.

When the rise in BUN was under 30 mg/100 ml per day, Parson found that the course of acute renal failure was relatively benign and that recovery was complete.[867] In general, such patients usually have low catabolic rates and are usually free of infection or trauma; therefore, the indications for dialysis in these patients are greatly reduced and they are usually managed conservatively.

Patients with acute renal failure associated with burns, fever, trauma, or infection usually have an early modified increased catabolic rate. There is a marked daily increase in BUN, serum creatinine, and serum phosphate and a decrease in blood CO_2 combining power.

The biochemical criteria for dialysis used by Kolff are a BUN level of 140 to 190 mg/100 ml, a serum potassium level exceeding 7 mEq/L, and a serum bicarbonate level of less than 12 mEq/L. Although the serum potassium level can be controlled by conservative means, it may produce either cardiac abnormalities or clinical deterioration, which will require dialysis. When potassium intoxication is present, it is the prime biochemical indication for dialysis. When muscle damage is excessive, as seen in combat casualties, hyperkalemia occurs early, frequently, and rapidly. In combat casualties with acute renal failure, daily prophylactic dialysis may well be the treatment of choice.

Technique of peritoneal dialysis

With slight modification, the technique of peritoneal dialysis described is that of Maxwell and associates.[749] The procedure is done in a private room provided for the patient. Strict aseptic techniques are employed, including sterile bedding and reverse isolation techniques. The patient is given a sedative of secobarbital and is placed in the supine position; his urinary bladder is emptied. The finding of a filled urinary bladder has occasionally embarrassed a nephrologist. The abdomen is prepared by washing with surgical soap and water; surface hairs are shaved off. The skin is cleaned with 2% tincture of iodine and is washed with 70% alcohol.

Although any site on the anterior abdominal wall can be used, a small bistoury incision is usually made in the linea alba, a third of the distance from the umbilicus to the synthesis pubis. In obese patients the site is the thin abdominal wall in the left lower abdominal quadrant. Approximately 2 liters of dialysis solution* at body temperature containing 10 mg of heparin is infused into the peritoneal cavity through a 15-gauge hypodermic needle. This distends the abdomen. A No. 17 bore trocar is aimed perpendicular to the floor and is introduced with a twisting action through the skin incision into the peritoneal cavity. After entering the abdominal cavity, the trocar tip is aimed toward the left pelvic area. The obturator is removed and a special rigid No. 17 French multihole nylon or plastic catheter 9 to 11 inches long is passed through the trocar. The trocar stylus is slipped over the plastic cannula, which is directed deep into the peritoneal cavity and toward the pelvis, either to the right or left of the lumbar paravertebral sulcus. Resistance to cannula insertions can be caused by adhesions, the bowel, or a persistent urachus. The cannula should be partially withdrawn and aimed slightly laterally. If there is still difficulty in the insertion of the cannula, then another site should be chosen. If the catheter protrudes beyond 2 inches external to the abdominal wall, the excessive length can be cut off. The outer end of the plastic cannula is attached to the Y-tubing of the dialysis-infusion-drainage set. A purse-string suture around the catheter usually decreases leakage of fluid and prevents hemorrhage.

Barry and associates developed a conduit with an internal balloon and an external Teflon attachment to anchor the device intraperitoneally and to seal the tract from leakage.[69] A plastic disk is placed over the cannula to secure over the wound externally. Although the cannula can be inserted through a trocar, it is safer to surgically introduce it under direct vision.

After 20 to 30 minutes, the fluid is drained by a siphon effect. The color of the withdrawn fluid should be observed. I have detected rupture of the urinary bladder by finding urine in the peritoneal fluid. Two liters of fluid warmed to body temperature are infused through fresh tubing into the peritoneal cavity. Commercially available peritoneal dialysis solution contains 1.5% glucose to make the osmolality 372 mOsm/L (Table 5-2). Because hyperkalemia is a main indication for peritoneal dialysis, potassium is omitted. In patients with overhydration, edema, or water intoxication, solution containing 7% glucose (70 gm/liter) is used. When hyperkalemia is not a problem, 8 mEq of potassium choride is added to one of the two liters of infused fluid.

If the catheter is properly placed, gravity drainage is a rapid and steady stream of fluid entering the peritoneal cavity. If the infusion process requires longer than 15 to 20 minutes, the catheter is poorly placed and should be repositioned as the inserted portion may be covered by omentum or may be occluded by blood. This will occur in about 10 to 15% of cases. A tight pressure dressing is applied to secure the catheter from pulling out of the cavity.

The fluid is drained through the outflow tubing in a closed system. It is usually clear and colorless. It may be opalescent or colored, varying from yellow to green

---

*Administration data: Solutions and catheters are manufactured by Abbott Laboratories, Chicago, Illinois, by Travenol Laboratories, Inc., Morton Grove, Illinois, and by McGaw and Cutter Laboratories, Inc., Berkeley, California.

Table 5-2. Chemical constituents of potassium-free peritoneal dialysis solution containing 1.5% glucose

Solute	mEq/L	mOsm/L
Sodium	140.4	140.4
Chloride	101.0	101.0
Calcium	3.5	1.7
Magnesium	1.5	1.0
Lactate	44.5	44.5
Glucose	15 gm/liter	83.0
Total	291.5	372.0

to grossly bloody. Opalescence is usually caused by the presence of polymorphonuclear leukocytes, which are present as the result of chemical irritation of the peritoneal cavity by the irrigating fluid. Once this irritation occurs, there is a more effective peritoneal dialysis.

A yellow fluid is seen in bacterial infection. It may follow the intravenous administration of multivitamins or tetracycline. Green peritoneal fluid usually reflects hemorrhage, including local trauma, pressure of the cannula on a small vessel, excessive heparinization, and hypoprothrombinemia resulting from prolonged removal of vitamin K by dialysis. If a catheter must be changed, a new catheter can be passed through the same abdominal hole.

The exact measurement of influx and drainage of fluids is necessary to maintain precise fluid balance. This represents a cycle of fluid exchange. A careful record is kept of the precise amount of fluid inserted and removed during each exchange. The exact time, exact volume of fluid, the amounts of drugs, and the vital signs should all be recorded. Exchanges in peritoneal dialysis are repeated continuously for 48 hours. Eighty to one hundred liters could be used in a single dialysis. I may change the Y-tubing every four exchanges. In 48 hours of effective peritoneal dialysis one can accomplish the same removal of urea and other substances as[733] is accomplished by hemodialysis in 6 hours.

Other methods of dialysis and treatment

In addition to extracorporeal hemodialysis and peritoneal dialysis, nerve deinnervation,[493] intestinal lavage, exchange transfusions, pulmonary lavage, thoracic duct lymph drainage, and gastrodialysis have all been used. Although these procedures gained enthusiasm from numerous investigators, they are far from approaching the potential effectiveness of extracorporeal hemodialysis or peritoneal dialysis.

The irrigation of the intestine with a gastic tube and the rectum with a rectal tube is very unpleasant to the patient.[743] The excessive loss of electrolytes and fluids presents unusual complications.

In 1958, Scribner and associates used gastrodialysis in the treatment of patients with acute renal failure.[742,983] The removal of substances other than potassium and hydrochloric acid is limited. The use of nasogastric tubes in critically ill patients leads to vomiting and secondary bronchopneumonia.

The perfusion of an isolated segment of jejunum was used by Twiss and Kolff[1090] and was further evaluated by Schloerb.[964] The operation increases the risk to a critically ill patient who will have to await healing of the surgical wound before perfusion can be started. Hemorrhage, edema, and intussusception of the gut are complications of isolated jejunum lavage. In general, methods of lavaging the gut fall short of the practical value to the patient with acute renal failure.

DIURETIC PHASE

Individually or in combination, the complications of the diuretic phase have been reported as severe dehydration, sodium depletion, and hypokalemia.[196,288] These complications are not striking and are easily treated. During the first few days of the diuretic phase the urinary concentration of sodium and potassium remains constant, and serum levels of potassium and urea nitrogen may increase. The latter is commonly noted in patients with prolonged oliguria. If uremic symptoms occur during early active diuresis, a supplemental dialysis will greatly improve the patient's condition.

Oral or intravenous fluids should be given every 6 to 8 hours, depending on the urinary output. This method of fluid replacement prevents dehydration. Blood transfusions are rarely needed during the diuretic phase—an exception to this rule is the need to replace blood lost by active hemorrhage.

During the diuretic phase anorexia subsides and oral feedings can be started. Foods and fluids should be given orally. When potassium supplements are required, oral nutrients containing potassium should be encouraged. These include bananas, raisins, fruit juices, oranges, and meats. The patient in the diuretic phase loses the excess fluid accumulated during the oliguric phase.

Early patient mobilization prevents hypostatic pneumonia, pulmonary emboli, and decubitus ulcer and leads to earlier rehabilitation of the patient. Active ambulation and nutritional rehabilitation are the prime factors to consider in restoration of the patient to a useful and productive life. A very rare patient may survive acute oliguric renal failure without regaining sufficient renal function to sustain life. Such a patient has acute oliguric renal failure caused by bilateral renal cortical necrosis or by acute progressive proliferative glomerulonephritis. The patient should be carefully evaluated regarding his clinical and psychiatric status; such evaluation aids in selection of the patient either for a chronic hemodialysis program or for a renal transplant.[531,629] Siliconized rubber–Teflon cannulas are inserted into an artery and a vein to form an A-V shunt. Chronic hemodialysis aids in nutritional rehabilitation and prepares the patient for an eventual renal transplant (Fig. 5-2).

Intense comprehensive management of the patient recovering from renal failure must be interdigitated with active and progressive physical rehabilitation to restore him as a useful member to his family, his community, and his employer.

References

1. Abbott, W. E., and Shea, P.: The treatment of temporary renal insufficiency by peritoneal lavage, Amer. J. Med. Sci. **211**:312, 1946.
2. Abel, J. J., Rowntree, L. G., and Turner, B. B.: On the removal of diffusible substances from the circulating blood of living animals by dialysis, J. Pharm. **5**:275, 1914.
3. Aboulker, P., Paraf, P., Derot, M., and Lassner, J.: Une observation d'anurie apres resection transuretrale de la prostate, J. Urol. Med. Chir. **62**:173, 1956.
4. Abry, J., and Cavusoglu, M.: Fatal tubular necrosis during chlorothiazide administration, New York State J. Med. **60**:1638, 1960.
5. Abul-Haj, S. K., Ewald, R. A., and Kazyak, L.: Fatal mushroom poisoning: report of case confirmed by toxicologic analysis of tissue, New Eng. J. Med. **269**:223, 1963.
6. Ackerman, G. L.: Doherty, J. E., and Flanigan, W. J.: Peritoneal dialysis and hemodialysis of tritiated Digoxin, Ann. Intern. Med. **67**:718, 1967.
7. Adams, F. D.: Reversible uremia with hypercalcemia due to vitamin D intoxication, New Eng. J. Med. **244**:590, 1951.
8. Addis, T.: Glomerular nephritis: diagnosis and treatment, New York, 1949, The Macmillan Company.
9. Addison, T.: On the disorders of the brain connected with diseased kidneys, Guy's Hospital Reports **4**:1, 1839.
10. Alarcon-Segovia, D., Wakim, K. G., Worthington, J. W., and Ward, L. E.: Clinical and experimental studies on the hydralazine syndrome and its relationship to systemic lupus erythematosus, Medicine **46**:1, 1967.
11. Alarcon-Segovia, D., Worthington, J. W., Ward, L. E., and Wakim, K. G.: Lupus diathesis and hydralazine syndrome, New Eng. J. Med. **272**:462, 1965.
12. Alfrey, A. C., Rottschafer, O. W., and Hutt, M. P.: Acute parenchymal dysfunction with acute anuria induced by retrograde pyelography, Arch. Intern. Med. **119**:214, 1967.
13. Allebach, H. K. B., and McPhee, W. R.: Carbone tetrachloride poisoning, Missouri Med. **50**:106, 1953.
14. Allen, A. C.: The kidney: medical and surgical diseases, New York, 1951, Grune & Stratton, Inc.
15. Allen, J. D., Roberts, C. E., Jr., and Kirby, W. M.: Staphylococcal septicemia treated with methicillin; report of 22 cases, New Eng. J. Med. **266**:111, 1962.
16. Alwall, N.: On artificial kidney. I. Apparatus for dialysis of blood in vivo, Acta. Med. Scand. **128**:317, 1947.
17. Alwall, N.: On renal failure complicating surgical diseases (laparotomy etc.), with special regard to conservative treatment, and the need for the artificial kidney (dialyser, ultrafilter) in rational renal therapy, Acta. Chir. Scand. **108**:95, 1954.

18. Alwall, N.: Treatment of electrolyte-fluid retention by ultrafiltration of the blood in vivo, London, 1954, The Kidney Ciba Foundation Symposium.

19. Alwall, N., Erlandson, P., and Tornberg, A.: The clinical course of renal failure occurring after intravenous urography and/or retrograde pyelography: casuistics of 11 cases (including 7 deaths), Acta. Med. Scand. **152**:163, 1955.

20. Alwall, N., Erlandson, P., Nyman, M., and Tornberg, A.: On the artificial kidney. XXXI. Casuistics of a further 26 cases of acute renal failure with anuria or severe oliguria (urine output less than 300 ml daily) for 4-40 days treated conservatively and on vital indication, with dialysis (26 cases) and ultrafiltration (1 case) of the blood in vivo and peritoneal irrigation (1 case), Acta. Med. Scand. **152**:353, 1955.

21. Alwall, N., Erlandson, P., Tornberg, A., Fajers, C., and Loell, H.: Two cases of acute glomerulonephritis with severe oliguria or anuria for 75 days, Acta. Med. Scand. **161**:85, 1958.

22. Alwall, N., Johnsson, S., Tornberg, A., and Werkol, L.: Acute renal failure following angiography, especially the risk of repeated examination, revealed by 8 cases (2 deaths), Acta. Chir. Scand. **109**:11, 1955.

23. Alwall, N., Lunderquist, A., and Olson, O.: Studies on electrolyte-fluid retention. I. Uremic lung-fluid lung?: on pathogenesis and therapy; (a preliminary report), Acta. Med. Scand. **146**:157, 1953.

24. Alwall, N., and Tornberg, A.: Casuistics of 11 cases of acute tubular nephritis (lower nephron nephrosis etc.), with anuria or severe oliguria of 5-11 days duration, treated conservatively, Acta. Med. Scand. **147**:11, 1953.

25. Anderson, A., and Kolff, W. J.: Artificial kidney in the treatment of uremia associated with acute glomerulonephritis (with a note on regional heparinization), Ann. Intern. Med. **51**:478, 1959.

26. Andre, R., Dreyfus, B., and Salmon, C.: Incidents et accidents de la transfusion sanguine, Paris, 1956, Masson et Cie, Ed.

27. Andre, R., Dreyfus, B., and Taleb, N.: Les accidents renaux de la transfusion sanguine, Scm. Hop. Paris **28**:214, 1952.

28. Angervall, L., Lehmann, L., and Lincoln, K.: On the effect of phenacetin and NAPA (N-acetyl-p-aminophenol) on the development of bacterial interstitial nephritis in the rat, Acta. Path. and Microbiol. Scand., suppl. **154**:61, 1962.

29. Angervall, L., Lehmann, L., and Lincoln, K.: Induction of interstitial nephritis in rats fed phenacetin and NAPA (N-acetyl-p-aminophenol), Acta. Path. and Microbiol. Scand. **54**:274, 1962.

30. Angervall, L., Lehmann, L., and Lincoln, K.: On action of NAPA (N-acetyl-p-aminophenol) on the induction of interstitial nephritis in rats, Acta. Path. and Microbiol. Scand. **54**:283, 1962.

31. Anson, M. L., and Mirsky, A. E.: Protein coagulation and its reversal: the preparation of insoluble globin, soluble globin, and heme, J. Gen. Physiol. **13**:469, 1930.

32. Anthonisen, P., Brun, C., Crone, C., Lassen, N. A., Munck, O., and Thomsen, A. C.: Clinical experience with the Skeggs-Leonards type of artificial kidney, Lancet **2**:1277, 1956.

33. Antoine, B., and Ducrot, H.: La pratique d'ud rein artificiel, Vie Med. **38**:9, 1957.

34. Antoine, B., Ducrot, H., Michielsen, P., and Dormont, J.: L'efficacite d'un appareil de dialyse extra-corporeale: analyse de quelques facteurs mecaniques, Revue Med. de Liege **13**:78, 1958.

35. Armstrong, D., and Myers, W. P. L.: Renal failure incident to reticulum cell sarcoma of the kidneys, Ann. Intern. Med. **65**:109, 1965.

36. Arnold, J. W.: Reversible renal shutdown secondary to necrotizing renal papillitis, Northwest Med. **63**:168, 1964.

37. Arturson, G., Granath, K., Thorn, L., and Wallenius, G.: Renal excretion of low-molecular-weight Dextran, Acta. Clin. Scand. **127**:543, 1964.

38. Ashworth, C. T., and McKenig, J. F.: Hemorrhagic complications with death probably from salicylate therapy; a report of two cases, J.A.M.A. **126**:806, 1944.

39. Atik, M., Manale, B., and Pearson, J.: Prevention of acute renal failure, J.A.M.A. **183**:455, 1963.

40. Atkinson, R. M., Caisey, J. D., Currie, J. P., Middleton, T. R., Pratt, D. A. H., Sharpe, H. M., and Tomich, E. G.: Subacute toxicity of cephaloridine to various species, Toxicology and Applied Pharmacology **8**:407, 1966.

41. Atlas, D. H., and Gaberman, P.: Reversible renal insufficiency: diagnosis and treatment, Baltimore, 1958, The Williams & Wilkins Co.

42. Aye, R. C.: Renal papillary necrosis, Diabetes **3**:124, 1954.

42a. Bacon, S. K.: Rupture of urinary bladder: clinical analysis of 147 cases in the past 10 years, J. Urol. **49**:432, 1943.

43. Badenoch, A. W., and Darmady, E. M.: The effects of temporary occlusion of the renal artery in rabbits and its relationship to traumatic uraemia, J. Path. Bact. **59**:79, 1947.

44. Baggenstoss, A. H.: The pancreas in uremia; a histopathologic study, Amer. J. Path. **24**:1003, 1948.

45. Baines, A. D.: Cell renewal following dichromate induced renal tubular necrosis, Amer. J. Path. **47**:851, 1965.

46. Baird, R. J., Firor, W. B., and Barr, H. W. K.: Protection of renal function during surgery of the abdominal aorta, Canad. Med. Assn. J. **89**:705, 1963.

47. Baker, A. B., and Knutson, J.: Psychiatric aspects of uremia, Amer. J. Psychiat. **102**:683, 1946.

48. Baker, S. B., De, C., and Williams, R. T.: Acute interstitial nephritis due to drug sensitivity, Brit. Med. J. **1**:1655, 1963.

49. Baker, S. L., and Dodds, E. C.: Obstruction of the renal tubules during the excretion of haemolglobin, Brit. J. Med. Path. **6**:247, 1925.

50. Baldus, W. P., Feichter, R. N., and Summerskill, W. H. J.: The kidney in cirrhosis, Ann. Intern. Med. **60**:353, 1964.

51. Balint, P.: Le flux sanguin renal au cours de l'hypotension et de l'hypovolemie experimentales. In Ier Congrès Int. Nephrologie, Genève-Evian, 1960, Bale, Karger, Ed.

52. Balslov, J. T., and Jorgensen, H. E.: A survey of 489 patients with acute anuric renal insufficiency: causes, treatment, complications and mortality, Amer. J. Med. **34**:753, 1963.

53. Bandler, C. G., and Killian, J. A.: Blood determination of ammonia and sulphur, as factors in uremia of urinary obstructions, J. Urol. **29**:337, 1933.

54. Barden, R. P., and Cooper, D. A.: The roentgen appearance of the chest in diseases affecting the peripheral vascular system of the lungs; conditions associated with increased vascular permeability, Radiology **51**:44, 1948.

55. Barie, E.: De la stomatite uremique, Arch. Gen. Med. **2**:415, 1889.

56. Barlas, G. M., and Kolff, W. J.: Transfusion reactions and their treatment, especially with the artificial kidney, J.A.M.A. **169**:67, 1959.

57. Barnes, B. A., Shaw, R. S., Leaf, A., and Linton, R. R.: Oliguria following diagnostic translumbar aortography, New Eng. J. Med. **252**:1113, 1955.

58. Barnett, R. N.: Reactions to Bismuth compound, J.A.M.A. **135**:28, 1947.

59. Barry, A. P., Carmody, M., Woodcock, J. A., O'Dwyer, W. F., Walsh, A., and Doyle, G.: Renal failure unit, obstetrical and gynecological admissions, J. Obstet; Gynoec. Brit. Comm. **71**:899, 1964.

60. Barry, K. G.: Post-traumatic renal shutdown in humans: its prevention and treatment by the intravenous infusion of mannitol, Milit. Med. **128**:224, 1963.

61. Barry, K. G., and Berman, A. R.: Mannitol infusion. III. The acute effect of the intravenous infusion of mannitol on blood and plasma volumes, New Eng. J. Med. **264**:1085, 1961.

62. Barry, K. G., Brooks, M. H., and Hano, J. E.: The prevention of acute renal failure. In Brest, A. N., and Moyer, J. H.: Renal failure, Philadelphia, 1967, J. B. Lippincott Co.

63. Barry, K. G., Cohen, A., Knochel, J. P., Whelan, T. J., Beisel, W. R., Vargas, C. A.,

and LeBlanc, P. C.: Mannitol infusion. II. The prevention of acute functional renal failure during resection of an aneurysm of the abdominal aorta, New Eng. J. Med. **264**:967, 1961.

64. Barry, K. G., Cohen, A., and LeBlanc, P.: Mannitolization. I. The prevention and therapy of oliguria associated with cross-clamping of the abdominal aorta, Surgery **50**:335, 1961.

65. Barry, K. G., and Crosby, W. G.: Prevention and treatment of renal failure following transfusion reactions, Transfusion **3**:35, 1963.

66. Barry, K. G., Doberneck, R. C., McCormick, G. J., and Berman, A.: Kinetics of mannitol in man. In Mazzer, R. I., editor: Mannitol Symposium, Washington, 1962, Walter Reed Army Institute of Research.

67. Barry, K. G., Hunter, R. H., Davis, T. E., and Crosby, W. H.: Acute uric acid nephropathy, Arch. Intern. Med. **111**:452, 1963.

68. Barry, K. G., and Malloy, J. P.: Oliguric renal failure: evaluation and therapy by the intravenous infusion of mannitol, J.A.M.A. **179**:510, 1962.

69. Barry, K. G., Shambaugh, G. E., Goler, D., and Matthews, F. E.: A new flexible cannula and seal to provide prolonged access to the peritoneal cavity for dialysis, Trans. Amer. Soc. Artif. Intern. Organs. **9**:105, 1963.

70. Bartels, E. D., Brun, G. C., Gammeltoft, A., and Gjorup, P. A.: Acute anuria following intravenous pyelography in a patient with myelomatosis, Acta. Med. Scand. **150**:297, 1954.

71. Bass, H. E., Greenberg, D., Singer, E., and Miller, M. A.: Pulmonary changes in uremia, J.A.M.A. **148**:724, 1952.

72. Bass, H. E., and Singer, E.: Pulmonary changes in uremia, J.A.M.A. **144**:819, 1950.

73. Basset, S. H.: Nitrogen and fluid balance in treatment of acute uremia by peritoneal lavage, Arch. Intern. Med. **80**:616, 1947.

74. Bateman, J. C., Barberio, J. R., Grice, P., Klopp, C. T., and Pierpont, H.: Fatal complications of intensive antibiotic therapy in patients with neoplastic disease, Arch. Intern. Med. **90**:763, 1952.

75. Batson, R., and Peterson, J. C.: Acute mercury poisoning: treatment with B.A.L., and in anuric states with continuous peritoneal lavage, Ann. Intern. Med. **29**:278, 1948.

76. Battezzati, M., Taddei, C., and Ramoino, L.: Criteri per valutare il rendimento del rene artificiale, Min. Med. **3**:1624, 1954.

76a. Baxter, C. R., Zedlitz, W. H., and Shikes, G. T.: High output acute renal failure complicating traumatic injury, J. Trauma **4**:567, 1964.

77. Bayliss, W. M.: Is haemolysed blood toxic?, Brit. J. Exp. Path. **1**:1, 1920.

78. Beales, S. J.: Deaths from prolonged ingestion of phenacetin, Brit. J. Med. **65**:45, 1964.

79. Beall, A. C., Jr., Hall, C. W., Morris, G. C., Jr., and DeBakey, E. M.: Mannitol-induced osmotic diuresis during renal artery occlusion, Ann. Surg. **161**:46, 1965.

80. Becker, C. G., Becker, E. L., Maher, J. F., and Schreiner, G. E.: Nephrotic syndrome after contact with mercury: a report of five cases, three after the use of ammoniated mercury ointment, Arch. Intern. Med. **110**:178, 1962.

81. Beerman, H.: Fatalities due to bismuth in treatment of syphilis, Arch. Derm. Syph. **26**:797, 1932.

82. Beidleman, B.: Kidney damage from penicillin sensitivity, Med. Trial. Tech. Quart. **10**:39, 1964.

83. Beirne, G. J., Hansing, C. E., Octaviano, G. N., and Burns, R. O.: Acute renal failure caused by hypersensitivity to Polymyxin B Sulfate, J.A.M.A. **202**:62, 1967.

84. Beisel, W. R., Herndon, E. G., Myers, J. E., and Stones, L.: Acute renal failure as a complication of acute pancreatitis, Arch. Intern. Med. **104**:539, 1959.

85. Bell, E. T., and Knutson, R. C.: Extrarenal azotemia and tubular disease, J.A.M.A. **134**:441, 1947.

86. Bell, N. H., Andriole, V. T., Sabesin, S. M., and Utz, J. P.: On the nephrotoxicity of amphotericin B in man, Amer. J. Med. **33**:64, 1962.

87. Bell, N. H., and Bartter, F. C.: Transient reversal of hyperabsorption of calcium and of abnormal sensitivity to vitamin D in a patient with sarcoidosis during an episode of nephritis, Ann. Intern. Med. **61**:702, 1964.

88. Bell, W. N.: Proceedings of the 8th Congress International Society of Blood Transfusion, Basle, 1960.

89. Bernard, H., Gajdos, A., Gajdos-Torok, M., and Rambert, P.: Une intoxication aigue collective par le plomb, Sem. Hop. Paris **29**:785, 1953.

90. Benyajati, C., Keoplug, M., Beisel, W. R., Gangarosa, E. J., Sprinz, H., and Sitprija, V.: Acute renal failure in Asiatic cholera: clincopathologic correlations with acute tubular necrosis and hypokalemic nephropathy, Ann. Intern. Med. **52**:960, 1960.

91. Bereston, E. S., and Keil, H.: Membranous stomatitis associated with debilitation and with uremia, Arch. Derm. **44**:562, 1941.

92. Bergentz, S. E., Falkheden, T., and Olson, S.: Diuresis and urinary viscosity in dehydrated patients: influence of dextran-40,000 with and without mannitol, Ann. Surg. **161**:582, 1965.

93. Berglund, F., Ek, J., and Werko, L.: Acute anuria with special reference to renal function, Acta. Med. Scan. **144**:399, 1953.

94. Bergstrand, A.: Discussion du travail de A. Palmlov, Scan. J. Lab. Clin. Invest. **1**:308, 1949.

95. Bergstrand, H.: Comparison between kidney changes in case of "crush syndrome" and renal injury caused by sulfathiazole, Acta. Med. Scand. **124**:309, 1946.

96. Berlin, R.: Haff disease in Sweden, Acta. Med. Scand. **129**:560, 1948.

97. Berlyne, G. M., Janabi, K., and Shaw, A. B.: Dangers of resonium A in the treatment of hyperkalaemia in renal failure, Lancet **1**:167, 1966.

98. Berlyne, G. M., Janabi, K., Shaw, A. B., and Hocken, A. G.: Treatment of hyperkalaemia with a calcium-resin, Lancet **1**:169, 1966.

99. Berlyne, G. M., and Shaw, A. B.: Red eyes in renal failure, Lancet **1**:4, 1967.

100. Berylne, N., and Berlyne, G. M.: Acute renal failure following intravenous pyelography with hyopaque, Acta. Med. Scand. **171**:39, 1962.

101. Berman, L. B., and Schreiner, G. E.: Pressure flow relationship and urea dialysance: determinations in vivo in the twin-coil kidney. Trans. Amer. Soc. Artif. Intern. Organs **3**:12, 1957.

102. Berman, L. B., and Katz, S.: Kanamycin nephrotoxicity, Ann. N. Y. Acad. Sci. **76**:149, 1958.

103. Berman, L. B., and Tublin, I.: The nephropathies of sickle cell disease, Arch. Intern. Med. **103**:602, 1959.

104. Bernreiter, M., and Calovich, E. R.: Hyperpotassemia and hypopotassemia in case of anuria followed by severe diuresis: electrocardiographic changes, J.A.M.A. **147**:1036, 1951.

105. Bialestock, D., and Tange, J. D.: Acute necrotizing glomerulitis: the clinical features and pathology in nine cases, Aust. Ann. Med. **8**:281, 1959.

106. Bienenstock, J., and Harding, E. L.: Low-molecular-weight Dextran (Rheomacordex) in ischemic ulceration of the skin, Lancet **1**:524, 1964.

107. Biermer, V.: Ein ungewohnlicher fall von scharlach von Dr. Biermer, privatdocentin wurzbrg, Virchow's Arch. Path. Anat. **19**:537, 1860.

108. Bing, R. J.: The effect of hemoglobin and related pigments on renal functions of the normal and acidotic dog, Bull. Johns Hopkins Hosp. **74**:161, 1944.

109. Binger, C.: Toxicity of phosphates in relation to blood calcium and tetany, J. Pharm. Exp. Thera. **10**:105, 1917.

110. Bishop, W. B., Carlton, R. F., and Sanders, L. C.: Diffuse vasculitis and death after hyperimmunization with pertussis vaccine, N. Eng. J. Med. **274**:616, 1966.

111. Bjorklund, B., and Bjorklund, V.: Antigenicity of pooled human malignant and normal tissues by cyto-immunological technique: presence of an insoluble, heat-labile tumor antigen, International Arch. Allergy **10**:153, 1957.

112. Black, D. A. K.: Hyponatraemic syndromes: in essentials of fluid balance, Oxford, 1964, Blackwell Scientific Publications.

113. Black, D. A. K., and Howat, H. T.: Hepatitis and intermittent haemodialysis, Lancet **1:712** 1966.

114. Black, D. A. K., and Stanbury, S. W.: Renal insufficiency in terminal respiratory failure, Brit. Med. J. **1:872**, 1958.

115. Black, D. A. K., and Williams, R. T.: The use of hypertonic saline in patients with renal failure, Quart. J. Med., New Series **31:121**, 1962.

116. Blackburn, C. R. B., Hensley, W. J., Grant, D. K., and Wright, F. B.: Studies on intravascular hemolysis in man: pathogenesis of initial stages of acute renal failure, J. Clin. Invest. **33:825**, 1954.

117. Blagg, C. R., and Parsons, F. M.: Earlier dialysis and anabolic steroids in acute renal failure, Amer. Heart J. **61:287**, 1961.

118. Blalock, A.: Experimental shock: importance of local loss of fluid in production of low blood pressure after burns, Arch. Surg. **22:610**, 1931.

119. Blaufox, M. D., and Merrill, J. P.: Evaluation of renal transplant function by iodo-hippurate sodium 131, J.A.M.A. **202:123**, 1967.

120. Blegen, E. M., Enger, E., and Wendelbo, O.: Urinary microscopy, T. Norsk. Laege-foren **87:761**, 1967.

121. Block, M. A., Wakin, K. G., and Mann, F. C.: Effect of severe acute hemorrhage on kidney of rat, Arch. Path. **54:443**, 1952.

122. Bloodworth, J. M. B., Jr., and Sommers, S. C.: "Cirrhotic glomerulosclerosis," a renal lesion associated with hepatic cirrhosis, Lab. Invest. **8:962**, 1959.

123. Blount, R. E.: Management of chloroquine-resistant falciparum malaria, Arch. Int. Med. **119:557**, 1967.

124. Bluemle, L. W., Jr., Potter, H. P., and Elkinton, J. R.: Changes in body composition in acute renal failure, J. Clin. Invest. **35:1094**, 1956.

125. Bluemle, L. W., Jr.: Acute renal failure, GP **16:110**, 1957.

126. Bluemle, L. W., Jr., Webster, G. D., and Elkinton, J. R.: Acute tubular necrosis, Arch. Intern. Med. **104:180**, 1959.

127. Blythe, W. B., and Woods, J. W.: Acute renal insufficiency after ingestion of a gall-bladder dye: report of a case, N. Eng. J. Med. **264:1045**, 1961.

128. Boba, A., and Landmesser, C. M.: Renal complications after anesthesia and opera-tion, Anesthesiology **22:781**, 1961.

129. Boba, A., Gainor, J., and Powers, S. R., Jr.: The influence of mannitol on water and electrolyte excretion following trauma, Surgery **52:188**, 1962.

130. Boba, A., Landmesser, C. M., and Powers, S. R., Jr.: Prophylactic aspects of post-traumatic and postoperative renal failure, N. Y. S. J. Med. **63:812**, 1963.

131. Boen, S. T.: Kinetics of peritoneal dialysis, Medicine **40:243**, 1961.

132. Boen, S. T.: Peritoneal dialysis in clinical medicine, Springfield, Illinois, 1964, Charles C Thomas, Publisher.

133. Boen, S. T., Leijnse, B., and Gerbrandy, J.: Influence of serum calcium concentra-tion on Q.T. interval and circulation, Clin. Chim. Acta **7:432**, 1962.

134. Bomford, R. R., and Hunter, D.: Arseniuretted hydrogen due to the action of water on metallic arsenides, Lancet **2:1446**, 1932.

135. Bordley, J.: Reactions following transfusion of blood with urinary suppression and uremia, Arch. Intern. Med. **47:288**, 1931.

136. Borst, J. G. G.: De betekenis van het dieet en van de bestrijding van infecties bij de behandeling van uraemie, Nederl. Tijdschr. v. Geneesk. **91:2718**, 1947.

137. Borst, J. G. G.: Protein katabolism in uraemia: effects of protein-free diet, infections and blood transfusions, Lancet **1:824**, 1948.

138. Bouchard, C. J.: Lecons sur les auto-intoxications dans les maladies: recueillies et publiees par, Paris, 1887, Savy, ed.

139. Bourne, C. W., and Cerny, J. C.: The role of mannitol in acute trauma, University Michigan Medical Center J. **30:109**, 1964.

140. Boyce, F. F.: The role of the liver in surgery, Springfield, Illinois, 1941, Charles C Thomas, Publisher.

141. Boyette, D. D.: Bismuth nephrosis with anuria in an infant, J. Ped. **28:493**, 1946.

142. Bracey, D. W.: Acute renal failure: two cases treated by decapsulation and peritoneal dialysis, Brit. J. Surg. 38:482, 1951.

142a. Bradford, J. R., and Lawrence, T. W. P.: Endarteritis of the renal arteries, causing necrosis of the entire cortex of both kidneys, J. Path. and Bact. 5:195, 1898.

143. Bradford, H. A., and Shaffer, J. H.: Renal changes in a case of sulfadiazine anuria, J.A.M.A. 119:316, 1942.

144. Bradley, S. E., Bradley, G. P., Tyson, C. J., Curry, J. J., and Blake, W. D.: Renal function in renal diseases, Amer. J. Med. 9:766, 1950.

145. Brander, L., Kuhlback, B., Niemisto, M., and Riska, N.: The effect of massive doses of PAS on renal function and electrolyte balance, Scand. J. Lab. & Clin. Med. 15:38, 1963.

146. Brandt, J. L., Frank, N. R., and Lichtman, H. C.: Effects of hemoglobin solution on renal functions in man, Blood 6:1152, 1951.

147. Brain, M. C., Dacie, J. B., and Hourihane, D. O. B.: Microangiopathic haemolytic anemis: the possible role of vascular lesion on pathogenesis, Brit. J. Haemat. 8:358, 1962.

148. Brauninger, G. E., and Remington, J. S.: Nephropathy associated with methicillin therapy, J.A.M.A. 203:103, 1968.

149. Brest, A. N., and Moyer, J. H.: Renal failure: a symposium sponsored by Hahnemann Medical College, Philadelphia, 1967, J. B. Lippincott Co.

150. Bright, R.: Reports of medical cases selected with a view of illustrating the symptoms and cure of diseases by a reference to morbid anatomy, London, 1827, Longman, Rees, Brown and Green.

151. Broadbent, J. C., and Maher, F. T.: Extracorporeal hemodialysis in the management of acute renal failure, J.A.M.A. 166:608, 1958.

152. Brod, J., and Sirota, J. H.: Effects of emotional disturbance on water diuresis and renal blood flow in the rabbit, Amer. J. Physiol. 157:31, 1949.

153. Brooks, R. H., and Calleja, H. B.: Dermatitis, hepatitis, and nephritis due to phenindione (Phenylindandione), Ann. Intern. Med. 52:706, 1960.

154. Brown, K. A., Staubitz, W. J., Oberkircher, O. J., and Niesen, W. C.: A review of retroperitoneal fibrosis, J. Urol. 92:323, 1964.

155. Brown, J.: The philosophical transaction of the Royal Society, 3:248, 1685.

156. Brown, J. L., Samiy, A. H., and Pitts, R. F.: Localization of amino-nitrogen reabsorption in the nephron of the dog, Amer. J. Physiol. 200:370, 1961.

157. Brown, H. W., and Schreiner, G. E.: Prolonged hemodialysis with bath referigeration: the influence of dialyzer membrane thickness, temperature, and other variable of performance, Trans. Am. Soc. Artif. Int. Org. 8:187, 1962.

158. Brown, W. H., Thornton, W. B., and Wilson, J. S.: An evaluation of the clinical toxicity of sulfanilamide and sulfapyridine, J.A.M.A. 114:1605, 1940.

159. Bruck, E., Fearnley, M. D., Meanock, I., and Patley, H.: Phenylbutazone therapy: relation between toxic and therapeutic effects and blood level, Lancet 1:225, 1954.

160. Brun, C.: Acute anuria: a study based on renal function tests and aspiration biopsy of the kidney, Copenhagen, 1954, Ejnar Munksgaards.

161. Brun, C., Crone, C., Davidsen, H. G., Fabricius, J., Hansen, A. T., Lassen, N. A., and Munck, O.: Renal blood flow in anuric human subject determined by use of radioactive Krypton 85, Proc. Soc. Exp. Biol. Med. 89:687, 1955.

162. Brun, C., Crone, C., Davidsen, H. G., Fabricius, J., Hansen, A. T., Lassen, N. A., and Munck, O.: Renal interstitial pressure in normal and in anuric man: based on wedged renal vein pressure, Proc. Soc. Exp. Biol. Med. 91:199, 1956.

163. Brun, C., Gormsen, H., Hilden, T., Iversen, P., and Raaschou, F.: Kidney biopsy in acute glomerulonephritis, Acta Med. Scand. 160:155, 1958.

164. Brun, C., and Munck, K. O.: Lesions of the kidney in acute renal failure following shock, Lancet 1:603, 1957.

165. Bruno, M. S.: Fatal toxic nephrosis following administration of mercurial diuretics, New Eng. J. Med. 239:769, 1948.

166. Bryan, C. W., and Healy, J. K.: Acute renal failure in multiple mycloma, Amer. J. Med. **44**:128, 1968.

167. Bryer, M. S., Schoenbach, E. B., and Bliss, E. A.: Pharmacology of polymyxin, Ann. N. Y. Acad. Sc. **51**:935, 1949.

168. Buchanan, J. G.: Phenacetin-induced chronic interstitial nephritis, New Zealand Med. J. **60**:207, 1961.

169. Buck, R. W.: Mushroom toxins: brief review of literature, New Eng. J. Med. **265**:681, 1961.

170. Buckell, M.: Blood changes on intravenous administration of mannitol or urea for reduction of intracranial pressure in neurosurgical patients, Clin. Sci. **27**:223, 1964.

171. Bulger, R. J., Lindholm, D. D., Murray, J. S., and Kirby, W. M. M.: Effect of uremia on methicillin and Oxacillin blood levels, J.A.M.A. **187**:5, 1964.

172. Bull, G. M., Joekes, A. M., and Lowe, K. G.: Conservative treatment of anuric uremia, Lancet **2**:229, 1949.

173. Bull, G. M., Joekes, A. M., and Lowe, K. G.: Renal function studies in acute tubular necrosis, Clin. Sci. **9**:379, 1950.

174. Bull, G. M., Joekes, A. M., and Lowe, K. G.: Acute tubular necrosis of the kidney following abortion, Lancet **1**:186, 1956.

175. Bull, G. M., Joekes, A. M., and Lowe, K. G.: Acute renal failure following intravascular haemolysis, Lancet **2**:114, 1957.

176. Bull, G. M., Joekes, A. M., and Lowe, K. G.: Acute renal failure due to poisons and drugs, Lancet **1**:134, 1958.

177. Bulmer, F. M. R., Rothwell, H. E., Polack, S. S., and Stewart, D. W.: Chronic arsine poisoning among workers employed in the cyanide extraction of gold: report of 14 cases, J. Indust. Hyg. and Toxicol. **22**:111, 1940.

178. Burch, G. E., and Ray, C. T.: Lower nephron syndrome, Ann. Intern. Med. **31**:750, 1949.

179. Burmeister, W. H., and McNally, W. D.: Acute mercury poisoning: a parallel histological and chemical study of the renal and hepatic tissue changes as compared with the rapidity of absorption and the amount of mercury present in the circulating blood at the time such changes occur, J. Med. Res. **36**:87, 1917.

180. Burnett, C. H., Shapiro, S. L., Simeone, F. A., Beecher, H. K., Mallory, T. B., and Sullivan, E. R.: Renal function studies in the wounded, Surgery **22**:856, 1947.

181. Burnett, C. H., Shapiro, S. L., Simeone, F. A., Beecher, H. K., Mallory, T. B., and Sullivan, E. R.: Post-traumatic renal insufficiency, Surgery **22**:994, 1947.

182. Burns, R. O., Henderson, L. W., Hager, E. B., and Merrill, J. P.: Peritoneal dialysis: clinical experience, New Eng. J. Med. **267**:1060, 1962.

183. Burros, H. M., Borromeo, U. H. J., and Seligson, D.: Anuria following retrograde pyelography, Ann. Intern. Med. **48**:674, 1958.

184. Burston, J., Darmady, E. M., and Stranack, F.: Nephrosis due to mercurial diuretics, Brit. Med. J. **1**:1277, 1958.

185. Burwell, E. L., Kinney, T. D., and Finch, C. A.: Renal damage following intravascular hemolysis, New Eng. J. Med. **237**:657, 1947.

186. Butler, W. T., Bennett, J. E., Alling, D. W., Wertlake, P. T., Utz, J. P., and Hill, G. J.: Nephrotoxicity of amphotericin B: early and late effects in 81 patients, Ann. Intern. Med. **61**:175, 1964.

187. Butt, H. R., Allen, E. V., and Bollman, J. L.: A preparation from spoiled sweet clover 3,3'-Methylene-bis-(4-hydrocycoumarin) which prolongs coagulation and prothrombin time of blood, Proc. Staff Meeting, Mayo Clinic **16**:388, 1941.

188. Bywaters, E. G. L.: Ischemic muscle necrosis, crushing injury, traumatic edema, the crush syndrome, traumatic anuria, compresssion syndrome: a type of injury seen in air raid casualties following burial beneath debris, J.A.M.A. **124**:1103, 1944.

189. Bywaters, E. G. L., and Beall, D.: Crush injuries with impairment of renal function, Brit. Med. J. **1**:427, 1941.

190. Bywaters, E. G. L., Delory, G. E., Rimington, C., and Smiles, J.: Myohaemoglobin in urine of air raid casualties with crushing injury, Biochem. J. **35**:1164, 1941.

191. Bywaters, E. G. L., and Dible, J. H.: The renal lesion in traumatic anuria, J. Path. Bact. **54**:111, 1942.

192. Bywaters, E. G. L., and Dible, J. H.: Acute paralytic myohaemoglobinuria in man, J. Path. Bact. **55**:7, 1943.

193. Bywaters, E. G. L., and Joekes, A. M.: The artificial kidney: its clinical application in the treatment of traumatic anuria, Proc. Royal Soc. Med. **41**:420, 1948.

194. Bywaters, E. G. L., and McMichael, J.: Crush syndrome: In History of the Second World War, London, 1953, M.M.S.O.

195. Bywaters, E. G. L., and Stead, J. K.: Production of renal failure following injection of solutions containing myohaemoglobin, Quart. J. Exper. Physiol. **33**:53, 1944.

196. Callaway, J. J., and Roemmich, W.: Lower nephron nephrosis: development of hypokaliemia during recovery, Ann. Intern. Med. **37**:784, 1952.

197. Caller, A., and Garcia-Caceres, U.: Studies of tubular alterations in diffuse renal disease. III. Quantitative evaluation of cellularity and length of proximal convoluted tubules in the kidney of acute tubular necrosis, John Hopkins Med. J. **121**:333, 1967.

198. Cameron, J. S., Ogg, C., and Trounce, J. R.: Peritoneal dialysis in hypercatabolic acute renal failure, Lancet **1**:1188, 1967.

199. Camishion, R. C., and Fishman, N. H.: Effect of mannitol on renal blood flow and cardiac output in hemorrhagic shock, Circulation (Suppl.) **29**:130, 1962.

200. Campbell, S., and Carre, I. J.: Fatal haemolytic uraemic syndrome and idiopathic hyperlipaemia in monozygotic twins, Arch. Dis. Child. **40**:214, 1965.

201. Cannon, P. J., Stason, W. B., Demartini, F. E., Sommers, S. C., and Laragh, J. H.: Hyperuricemia in primary and renal hypertension, New Eng. J. Med. **275**:457, 1966.

202. Carayon, A.: Les formes anuriques de la fievre bilieuse hemoglobinurique: bases cliniques, anatomopathologiques et physiopathologiques du traitement, Med. Trop. **8**:432, 1948.

203. Carlstrom, B.: Uber du atiologie and pathogenese dir kreuzlihime des pferdes (H amsglobinamia paralytica), Scan. Arch. Physiol. **61**:161, 1931.

204. Caroli, J.: Les angiocholites ictero-uremigenes, Presse Med. **53**:142, 1945.

205. Carpenter, A. A., and Kunin, A. S.: Pheochromocytoma with acute tubular necrosis, New Eng. J. Med. **265**:986, 1961.

206. Carre, I. J., and Squire, J. R.: Anuria ascribed to acute tubular necrosis in infancy and early childhood, Arch. Dis. Child. **31**:512, 1956.

207. Casciano, A. D.: Acute methemoglobinemia due to aniline, J. Med. Soc. New Jersey **49**:141, 1952.

208. Castaigne, P.: Le'evolution du catabolisme proteique au cours des anuries, J. Urol. Med. Chir. **56**:794, 1950.

209. Castell, D. O., and Sparks, H. A.: Nephrogenic diabetes insipidus due to demethylchlortetracycline hydrochloride, J.A.M.A. **193**:237, 1965.

210. Castle, W. B., Ham, T. H., and Shen, S. C.: Observations on mechanism of hemolytic transfusion reactions occurring without demonstrable hemolysin, Trans. Ass. Amer. Physicians **63**:161, 1950.

211. Chamberlain, J. L., and Franks, R. C.: Nephropathy resulting from Bismuth, Southern Med. J. **56**:509, 1963.

212. Chambers, W. R.: Use of the cerebrospinal fluid system as an accessory kidney: preliminary note and report of a case, Ohio Med. J. **49**:696, 1953.

213. Chapman, E. M.: Observations on the effect of paint on the kidneys with particular reference to the role of turpentine, J. Indust. Hyg. Toxic. **23**:277, 1941.

214. Chervony, A. M., Biaua, C. G., Schwartz, M. A., and West, M.: Bilateral renal cortical necrosis, malignant hypertension, probable pituitary deficiency with survival, Amer. J. Med. **39**:147, 1965.

215. Chesley, L. C., and McCaw, W. H.: A physiologic study of acute renal failure with follow-up observations, Amer. J. Obstet. Gynec. **62**:1187, 1951.

216. Chevalier, H.: L'electrocardiogramme des troubles metaboliques, Arch. Mal. Coeur. **51**:233, 1958.

217. Christiansen, W. F.: Nephrotic syndrome after application of mercurial diuretics, Ugeskr. Laeger **121**:200, 1959.
218. Ciccantelli, M. J., Gallagher, W. B., Skemp, F. C., and Dietz, P. C.: Fatal nephropathy and adrenal necrosis after translumbar aortography, New Eng. J. Med. **258**:433, 1958.
218a. Clark, A. J.: Absorption from the peritoneal cavity, J. Pharmac. **16**:415, 1921.
219. Clark, J. E.: Prognosis in acute renal failure. In Brest, A. N. and Moyer, J. H., editors: Renal failure, Philadelphia, 1967, J. B. Lippincott Co.
220. Clausen, E., and Harvald, B.: Nephrotoxicity of different analgesics, Acta. Med. Scand. **170**:469, 1961.
221. Clausen, E., and Peterson, J.: Necrosis of renal papillae in rheumatoid arthritis, Acta. Med. Scand. **170**:631, 1961.
222. Clinton, M., Jr.: Toxic effects of gases and vapors: mechanisms of poisoning by volatile solvents, New Eng. J. Med. **238**:51, 1948.
223. Clute, K. F., and Fitzgerald, G. W.: Anuria following electric shock therapy, Canad. Med. Assoc. J. **59**:426, 1948.
224. Coester, V.: Vergiftung durch arsenwasserstaffgas mit todtlichem ansgang (haemoglobinuric lcterus, anuric), Berlin, klin. Wchnschr. **21**:119, 1884.
225. Cohen, H.: A clinical evaluation of peritoneal dialysis, Canad. Med. Assoc. J. **88**:932, 1963.
226. Cohen, T.: Nephropathy associated with the oral administration of zoxazolamine (Flexin): report of a case, New Eng. J. Med. **256**:1193, 1957.
227. Cole, J. J., Pollard, T. L., and Murray, J. S.: Studies on the modified polypropylene kiil dialyzer, Trans. Amer. Soc. Artif. Int. Org. **9**:67, 1963.
228. Collins, H. A., and Jacobs, J. K.: Acute arterial injuries due to blunt trauma, J. Bone Joint Surg. **43A**:193, 1961.
229. Colmers, D. R.: Ueber die durch das Erdbeden in Messina on 28 December, 1908, verursachten Verletzungen, Arch. Klin. Chir. **90**:701, 1909.
230. Conn, J.: Salt loading as a possible factor in the production of potassium depletion, rhabdomyolysis, and heat injury, J.A.M.A. **183**:775, 1963.
231. Conn, H. L., Jr., Wilds, L., and Helwig, J.: Study of renal circulation tubular function and morphology and urinary volume and composition in dogs following mercury poisoning and transfusion of human blood, J. Clin. Invest. **33**:732, 1954.
232. Conn, H. L., Jr., Wood, J. C., and Rose, J. C.: Circulatory and renal effects following transfusion of human blood and its components to dogs, Circulation Research **4**:18, 1956.
233. Cope, O., and Moore, F. D.: The redistribution of body water and fluid therapy of the burned patients, Ann. Surg. **126**:1010, 1947.
234. Corcoran, A. C., and Page, I. H.: Effects of hypotension due to hemorrhage and of blood transfusion on renal function in dogs, J. Exp. Med. **78**:205, 1943.
235. Corcoran, A. C., Taylor, R. D., and Page, I. H.: Immediate effects on renal function of the onset of shock due to partially occluding limb tourniquets, Ann. Surg. **118**:871, 1943.
236. Corcoran, A. C., Taylor, R. D., and Page, I. H.: Acute toxic nephrosis: clinical and laboratory study based on a case of carbon tetrachloride poisoning, J.A.M.A. **123**:81, 1943.
237. Corcoran, A. C., and Page, I. H.: Renal damage from ferroheme pigments: myoglobin, hemoglobin, hematin, Texas Rep. Biol. Med. **3**:528, 1945.
238. Corcoran, A. C., and Page, I. H.: Crush-syndrome: post-traumatic anuria: observations on genesis and treatment, J.A.M.A. **134**:436, 1947.
239. Corcoran, A. C., and Page, I. H.: Post-traumatic renal injury: summary of experimental observations, Arch. Surg. **51**:93, 1945.
240. Cottet, J., and Varay, A.: Dissociation de l'elimination de l'uree et de la P.S.P. dans un cas de lithiase par sulfathiazol, J. Urol. Med. Chir. **56**:818, 1950.
241. Councilman, W. T.: An anatomical and bacteriological study of 49 cases of acute and and subacute nephritis with special reference to the glomerular lesions, Med. Surg. Rep. (Boston City Hospital series) **8**:31, 1857.
242. Councilman, W. T.: Acute interstitial nephritis, J. Exp. Med. **3**:393, 1898.

243. Coventry, W. D., and Wells, A. H.: A review of 100 cases of renal failure, Minnesota Med. 31:1003, 1964.

244. Crawford, E. S., Beall, A. C., Moyer, J. H., and DeBakey, M. E.: Complications of aortography, Surg. Gynec. Obstet. 104:129, 1957.

245. Creevy, C. D.: Hemolytic reactions during transurethral prostatic resection, J. Urol. 58:125, 1947.

246. Creevy, C. D., and Webb, E. A.: A fatal hemolytic reaction following transurethral resection of prostate gland: a discussion of its prevention and treatment, Surgery 21:56, 1947.

247. Crook, A.: Communication on necrosis of the cortex of the kidney after labour, Proc. Rep. Soc. Med. (Section of Obst. and Gynec). 20:1249, 1926.

248. Crosby, W. H., and Stefanini, M.: Pathogenesis of plasma transfusion reaction with special reference to the blood coagulation system, J. Lab. Clin. Med. 40:374, 1952.

249. Crosnier, J.: Troubles des electrolytes et du metabolisme de l'eau au cours de l'insuffisance renale. Rapport au III. Symposium sur les Maladies du rein. Fribourg en Brisgau, 1954. Pathologische, Physiologie and Klinik der Nierensekretion, Berlin, 1955, Springer, Ed.

250. Crosnier, J. Dormont, J., Montera, H. de., and Rueff, B.: Les lesions du parenchyme renal au cours des septicemies. In Actualites Nephrologiques de l'Hopital Necker, Paris, 1962, Flammarion, ed.

251. Crosnier, J., Menegaux, J. C., Slama, R., Delzant, J. F., and Thervet, F.: A propos de six cas d'insuffisance renale post-trauma-tique observes a l'hopital Necker apres le tremblement de terre d'Agadir, J. Urol Med. Chir. 66:636, 1960.

252. Cumin, W.: Cases of severe burns with dissection and remarks, Edinburgh M.E.S. J. 19:337, 1823.

253. Cuppage, F. E., and Scarpelli, D. G.: Repair of the nephron following injury with mercuric chloride (abstract), Proc. Am. Assoc. Path. Bact. and Am. J. Path. 50:42a, 1967.

254. Currie, G. A., Little, P. J., and McDonald, S. J.: The localization of cephaloridine and nitrofurantoin in the kidney, Nephron 3:282, 1966.

255. Czerwinski, A. W., and Ginn, H. E.: Bismuth nephrotoxicity, Amer. J. Med. 37:969, 1964.

256. Dalgaard, O. Z., and Pedersen, J. J.: Renal tubular degeneration: electron microscopy in ischaemic anuria, Lancet 2:484, 1959.

257. Dalgaard, O. Z., and Pedersen, J. J.: Ultrastructure of the kidney in shock. In Ier Congres Int. Nephrologie, Geneve-Evian, 1961. Karger, Ed.

258. Daniell, H. W.: Vasopastic reaction to methysergide maleate simulating Leriche syndrome, Ann. Intern. Med. 60:881, 1964.

259. Daniels, W. B., Leonard, B. W., and Holtzman, S.: Renal insufficiency following transfusion; report of 13 cases, J.A.M.A. 116:1208, 1941.

260. Danzig, L. E.: Dynamics of thiocyanate dialysis: the artificial kidney in the therapy of thiocyanate intoxication, New Eng. J. Med. 252:49, 1955.

261. Darmady, E. M.: Renal anoxia and traumatic uraemia syndrome, Brit. J. Surg. 34:262, 1947.

262. Darmady, E. M.: Traumatic uraemia, a collective review, J. Bone and Joint Surg. 30B:309, 1948.

263. Darmady, E. M.: Renal lesions in relation to amino-aciduria and water diuresis. In Ciba Foundation Symposium on the kidney, London, 1954, Churchill, Ed.

264. Darrow, D. C., and Yannet, H.: The changes in the distribution of body water accompanying increase and decrease in extracellular electrolyte, J. Clin. Invest. 14:266, 1935.

265. Dausset, J.: Lower nephron nephrosis: report of treatment of 44 patients by repeated replacement transfusions, Arch. Int. Med. 85:416, 1950.

266. Davidov, M., Kalaviatos, N., and Finnerty, F. A., Jr.: Antihypertensive properties of furosemide, Circulation 36:125, 1967.

267. Davidson, C. S.: Plants and fungi as etiologic agents of cirrhosis, New Eng. J. Med. 268:1072, 1963.

268. Davies, D. D.: Toxicity of acetazolamide, Brit. Med. J. **63**:1204, 1964.
269. Davis, J. P., and Lennox, W. G.: A comparison of paradione and tridione in the treatment of epilepsy, J. Pediat. **34**:273, 1949.
270. Dawson, J. L.: Post-operative renal function in obstructive jaundice: effect of mannitol diuresis, Brit. Med. J. **5427**:82, 1965.
271. Dawson, J., and Findley, G. M.: Experiments on the relation of haemoglobinuria and anuria with reference to blackwater fever, Ann. Trop. Med. Parasit. **41**:306, 1947.
272. De, S. N., Sengupta, K. P., and Chanda, N. N.: Renal changes including total cortical necrosis in cholera, Arch. Path. **57**:505, 1954.
273. Defalco, A. J., Mundth, E. D., Brettschneider, L., Jacobson, Y. G., and McClenathan, J. A.: A possible explanation for transplantation anuria, Surg. Gynec. Obstet. **120**:748, 1965.
274. De Lapava, S., Nigogosyan, G., and Pickren, J. W.: Fatal glomerulonephritis after receiving horse anti-human-cancer serum, Arch. Intern. Med. **109**:67, 1962.
275. DeMaria, W. J. A., and Harris, J. S.: Effect of magnesium sulfate on alterations in renal dynamics induced by intravenous hemoglobin, Amer. J. Physiol. **182**:251, 1955.
276. DeNavasquez, S.: The histology and pathogenesis of bilateral cortical necrosis of the kidney in pregnancy, J. Path. Bact. **41**:385, 1935.
277. DeNavasquez, S.: The excretion of haemoglobin with special reference to the "transfusion" kidney, J. Path. Bact. **51**:413, 1940.
278. Denis, W., and Hobson, S.: A study of the inorganic constituents of the blood serum in nephritis, J. Biol. Chem. **55**:183, 1923.
279. Derbes, V. J., Dent, J. H., Forrest, W. W., and Johnson, M. F.: Fatal chlordane poisoning, J.A.M.A. **158**:15, 1955.
280. Derobert, L., Caby, Hadengue, A., Martin, R., and Pradut, J.: Deux cas d'hepatonephrite mortelle par inhalation de trichlorethylene, Ann. Med. Leg. **32**:282, 1952.
281. Derot, M.: La creatininemie, These. Med. 1932.
282. Derot, M., Bernier, J. J., Pignard, P., Miocque, M., and Legrain, M.: Le taux du potassium plasmatique au cours des nephrites anuriques: elude clinique, biologique et therapeutique, Sem. Hop. Paris **30**:4179, 1954.
283. Derot, M., Charlier, P., Mauge, F., and Legrain, M.: Traitement des oligo-anuries post-abortum par une charge osmotique au mannitol, J. Urol. Nephrol. **69**:632, 1963.
284. Derot, M., Kahn, J., Mazalton, A., and Peyrafort, J.: Nephrite anurique aigue mortelle apres traitement aurique, chysocyanose associee, Bull. Soc. Med. Hop. Paris **70**:234, 1954.
285. Derot, M., and Legrain, M.: La nephropathie hemolytique post-transfusionnelle: etude critique de 36 observations, Bull. Soc. Med. Hop. Paris **70**:1007, 1954.
286. Derot, M., Legrain, M., Bernier, J. J., and Pignard, P.: Nephrites aigues anuriques: etude de la diurese, Sem. Hop. Paris **28**:242, 1952.
287. Derot, M., Legrain, M., Jacobs, C., Prunier, P., and Hazebroucq, G.: Intoxication par l'hydrogene arsenie: etude des formes renales a propos d'une intoxication collective (5 cases), J. Urol. Nephrol. **69**:407, 1963.
288. Derot, M., Legrain, M., Pignard, P., Micoque, M., and Bernier, J. J.: Perturbations cliniques et hydro-electrolytiques survenant lors de la reprise de la diurese des nephropathies tubularies oligoanuriques, J. Urol. Med. Chir. **60**:351, 1954.
289. Derot, M., Nebout, R., Bernier, J. J., and Legrain, M.: Le traitement des nephritis aigues anuriques, La Presse Med. **57**:952, 1949.
290. Derot, M., and Pignard, P.: Variations du taux du magnesium sanguin au cours de certaines nephrites, Bull. Acad. Nat. Med. **135**:95, 1951.
291. Derot, M., Pignard, P., and Legrain, M.: Variations des protides seriques dans les tubulonephrites anuriques, La Presse Med. **64**:1307, 1956.
292. Derot, M., Pignard, P., and Mioque, M.: Nephropathie tubulaire anurique: crises de tetanie et pelade decalvante totale pendant la convalescence, Bull. Soc. Med. Hop. Paris **70**:319, 1954.
293. Derot, M., Pignard, P., Touraine, R., and Bernard, J.: Le potassium dans les nephropathies tubularies anuriques, La Presse Med. **61**:207, 1953.

294. Derot, M., Rathery, M., Dubrisay, J., and Roudier, R.: Anurie mortelle par choc apres intraveneuse de solution de para-aminosalicylate de sodium, Bull. Soc. Med. Hop. Paris **72**:904, 1956.

295. Derot, M., Tanret, P., Solignac, H., and Delaveau, P.: Hepato-nephrite hemolytique apres ingestion accidentelle de chlorate de sodium: guerison par la dialyse peritoneale et l'exsanguino-transfusion, Bull. Soc. Med. Hop. Paris **64**:1062, 1948.

296. Desmit, E. M., Hart, H. C., Helleman, P. W., and Tiddens, H. A. W. M.: Heparin treatment in a patient with haemolytic uraemic syndrome, Excerpta Medica Foundation, Amsterdam, 1966, Proceedings of the European Dialysis and Transplant Association.

297. Detmer, D. E., Zimmerman, J. M., and King, T. C.: Mannitol diuresis: the relationship of plasma volume to renal blood flow, J. Surg. Res. **5**:552, 1965.

298. Deutsch, E., and Kock, M.: Action of furosemide on the coagulability of blood, Wien. Med. Wschr. **117**:498, 1967.

299. Dinon, L. R., Kim, Y. S., and Vander Veer, J. B.: Clinical experience with chlorothiazide with particular emphasis on untoward responses: report of 121 cases studied over 15 month period, Amer. J. Med. Sci. **236**:533, 1958.

300. DiScala, V. A., Salomon, M., Grishman, E., and Churg, J.: Renal structure in myxedema, Arch. Path. **84**:474, 1967.

301. Doberneck, R. C., Reiser, M. P., and Lillehei, C. W.: Acute renal failure after open heart surgery utilizing extracorporeal circulation and total body perfusion, J. Thorac. Cardiovasc. Surg. **43**:441, 1962.

302. Dodd, K., Minot, A. S., and Arena, J. M.: Salicylate poisoning: explanation of more serious manifestations, Amer. J. Dis. Child. **53**:1435, 1937.

303. Doig, A. T.: Arseniuretted hydrogen poisoning in tank cleaners, Lancet **2**:88, 1958.

304. Domart, A.: Nephrites par inhalation de tetrachlorure de carbone, These. Med., Paris, 1938, Le Francois, Ed.

305. Domart, A.: Nephritis par inhalation de tetrachlorure da carbone, These. Med., Paris, 1938, Le Francois, Ed.

306. Doniach, I.: Uremic edema of the lungs, Amer. J. Roentgenol. **58**:620, 1947.

307. Doolan, P., Hess, W. C., and Kyle, L. H.: Acute renal insufficiency due to bichloride of mercury, New Eng. J. Med. **249**:273, 1953.

308. Doolan, P. D., Murphy, W. P., Wiggins, R. A., Carter, N. W., Cooper, W. C., Watten, R. H., and Alpen, E. L.: An evaluation of intermittent peritoneal lavage, Amer. J. Med. **26**:831, 1959.

309. Doolan, P. D., Shaw, C. C., Shreeve, W. W., and Harper, H. A.: Post-traumatic acute renal insufficiency complicated by hypernatremia, Ann. Intern. Med. **42**:1101, 1955.

310. Doolan, P. D., Theil, G. B., Wiggins, R. A., Lee, K. J., and Martinez, E.: Acute renal insufficiency following aortic surgery. Amer. Soc. Artif. Intern. Org. **5**:69, 1959.

311. Doolan, P. D., Wiggins, R. A., Thiel, G. B., Lee, K. J., and Martinex, E.: Acute renal insufficiency following aortic surgery, Amer. J. Med. **28**:895, 1960.

312. Dos Santos, R., Lamas, A., and Caldas, J. P.: Aortiographia da aorta e dos basos abdominais, Med. Contemp. **47**:93, 1929.

313. Dowds, J. H.: Poisoning by sodium bismuth tartrate injections, Lancet **2**:1039, 1936.

314. Dowling, H. F., Dumorr-Stanley, E., Lepper, M. H., and Sweet, L. K.: Relative toxicity of sulfamerazine and sulfadiazine, J.A.M.A. **125**:103, 1944.

315. Doyle, J. E.: Extracorporeal hemodialysis therapy in blood chemistry disorders, Springfield, Illinois, 1962, Charles C Thomas, Publisher.

316. Dubash, J., and Teare, D.: Poisoning by *Amanita phalloides,* Brit. Med. J. **1**:45, 1946.

317. Dubos, R. J., and Schaedler, R. W.: Nutrition and infection, J. Pediat. **55**:1, 1959.

318. Ducrot, H., and Slama, R.: Les insuffiisances renales associees a une pancreatite aigue, Rev. Med. Chir. Mal. Foie. **35**:199, 1960.

319. Dudley, S. F.: Toxemic anemia from arseniuretted hydrogen gas in submarine, J. Indust. Hyg. Toxicol. **1**:215, 1919.

320. Dufault, F. X., and Tobias, G. J.: Potentially reversible renal failure following excessive calcium and alkali intake in peptic ulcer therapy, Amer. J. Med. **16**:231, 1954.

321. Duff, G. L., and Murray, E. G. D.: Bilateral cortical necrosis of kidneys, Amer. J. Med. Sci. **201**:428, 1941.

322. Duff, G. L., and Murray, E. G. D.: Pathologic lesions following the administration of sulfonamide drugs, Amer. J. Med. Sci. **205**:439, 1943.

323. Duffy, J. L.: Fatal retroperitoneal fibrosis associated with hydramnios, J.A.M.A. **198**:993, 1966.

324. Duncan, G. G., Tocantis, L., and Cuttle, T. D.: Application in man of method for continuous reciprocal transfusion of blood, Proc. Soc. Exper. Biol. Med. **44**:196, 1940.

324a. Dunea, G., Muehrcke, R. C., Nakamoto, S., and Schwartz, F. D.: Thrombotic thrombocytopenic purpura with acute anuric renal failure, Amer. J. Med. **41**:1000, 1966.

325. Dunn, J. S., Gillespie, M., and Niven, J. S. F.: Renal lesions in two cases of crush syndrome, Lancet **2**:549, 1941.

326. Dunsky, I.: Potassium bromate poisoning, Amer. J. Dis. Child. **74**:730, 1947.

327. Duvoir, M., Guibert, and Desoille, H.: Les intoxications par le tetrachlorure de carbone, Ann. Med. Leg. **13**:1357, 1933.

328. Earley, L. E.: Extreme polyuria in obstructive uropathy: report of a case of "water-losing nephritis" in an infant, with a discussion of polyuria, New Eng. J. Med. **255**:600, 1956.

329. Easterling, R. E., and Forland, M.: A five year experience with prophylactic dialysis for acute renal failure, Trans. Amer. Soc. Artif. Int. Org. **10**:200, 1964.

330. Edelman, I. S., Leibman, J., O'Meara, M. P., and Birkenfeld, L. W.: Interrelations between serum sodium concentration, serum osmolarity and total exchangeable sodium, total exchangeable potassium and total body water, J. Clin. Invest. **37**:1236, 1958.

331. Edling, N. P. G., and Helander, C. G.: On renal damage due to aortography and its prevention by renal tests, Acta. Radiol. **47**:473, 1957.

332. Edling, N. P. G., Helander, C. G., Persson, F., and Asheim, A.: Renal function after aortography with large contrast media doses, Acta. Radiol. **50**:352, 1958.

333. Edwards, K. D. G.: Creatinine space as a measure of total body water in anuric subjects, estimated after single injection and hemodialysis, Clin. Sci. **18**:455, 1959.

334. Edwards, J. G.: The renal tubule (nephron) as affected by mercury, Amer. J. Path. **18**:1011, 1942.

335. Edwards, K. D. G., and Whyte, H. M.: Streptomycin poisoning in renal failure: an indication for treatment with an artificial kidney, Brit. M. J. **1**:752, 1959.

336. Einspruch, B. C., and Gonzales, V. V.: Clinical and experimental nephropathy resulting from use of neomycin sulfate, J.A.M.A. **173**:809, 1960.

337. Eisalo, A., and Talanti, S.: Observations on the effect of phenacetin and N-acetyl-p-aminophenol on rat kidneys, Acta. Med. Scand. **169**:655, 1961.

338. Eknoyan, G., and Matson, J. L.: Acute renal failure caused by aminopyrine, J.A.M.A. **190**:934, 1964.

339. Eliahou, H. E., and Bata, A.: The diagnosis of acute renal failure, Nephron **2**:287, 1965.

340. Eliasson, R.: Low-molecular-weight dextran: symposium held at Royal Society of Medicine, London, 1963, The Society.

341. Elkinton, J. R., Tarail, R., and Peters, J. P.: Transfers of potassium in renal insufficiency, J. Clin. Invest. **28**:378, 1949.

342. Elkinton, J. R., and Danowski, T. S.: The body fluids, basic physiology and practical therapeutics, Baltimore, 1955, The Williams & Wilkins Co.

343. Elliott, W.: Mushroom poisoning, Lancet **2**:630, 1961.

344. Elliott, W., Hill, M., Kerr, D. N. S., and Ashcroft, R.: The management of acute renal failure, Postgrad. Med. J. **36**:230, 1960.

345. Elwood, C. M., Lucas, G., and Muehrcke, R. C.: Acute renal failure associated with sodium colistimethate treatment, Arch. Intern. Med. **118**:326, 1966.

345a. Emmerson, B. T., and Pryse-Davies, J.: Studies of the nephrotoxic effect of neomycin, Australasian Ann. Med. **13**:149, 1964.

346. Emslie-Smith, D., Johnstone, J. H., Thomson, M. B., and Lowe, K. G.: Amino-aciduria in acute tubular necrosis, Clin. Sci. **15**:171, 1956.

347. Epstein, E., Shelp, W. D., and Weinstein, A. B.: Acute renal failure following retrograde pyelography, Invest. Urol. **2**:355, 1965.
348. Erlanson, P., and Lundgren, A.: Ototoxic side effects following treatment with antibiotics: connection with dosage and renal function, Acta. Med. **176**:147, 1964.
349. Erlenborn, J. W., and Pilz, C. C.: Paroxysmal myoglobinuria: associated with cardiomegaly and electrocardiographic abnormalities, J.A.M.A. **181**:1111, 1962.
350. Eskelund, V.: Necrosis of renal papillae following retrograde pyelography, Acta. Radiol. **26**:548, 1945.
351. Etheredge, E. E., Levitin, H., Nakamura, K., and Glenn, W. W. L.: Effect of mannitol on renal function during open-heart surgery, Ann. Surg. **161**:53, 1965.
352. Evans, B. M., Milne, M. D., Jones, N. C., and Yellowlees, H.: Ion exchange resins in treatment of anuria, Lancet **2**:1067, 1954.
353. Fabre, R., Truhaut, R., and Laham, S.: Toxicologie du tetrachlorure de carbone: etablissement d'une methode de dosage applicable aux atmospheres et aux milieux biologigues, Ann. Pharm. Franc. **9**:251, 1951.
354. Fahlgren, H., Hed, R., and Lundmark, C.: Myonecrosis and myoglobinuria in alcohol and barbiturate intoxication, Acta. Med. Scand. **158**:405, 1957.
355. Faloon, W. W., Downs, J. J., Duggan, K., and Prior, J. T.: Nitrogen and electrolyte metabolism and hepatic function and histology in patients receiving tetracycline, Amer. J. Med. Sci. **233**:653, 1957.
356. Fantl, P., and Simon, S. E.: Fibrinolysis following electrically induced convulsions, Aust. J. Exp. Biol. Med. Sci. **26**:521, 1948.
357. Farber, S., and Wilson, J. L.: The hyaline membrane in the lungs: A descriptive study, Arch. Path. **14**:437, 1932.
358. Favara, B. E., Vawter, G. F., Wagner, R., Kevy, S., and Porter, E. G.: Familial paroxysmal rhabdomyolysis in children, a myoglobinuric syndrome, Amer. J. Med. **42**:196, 1967.
359. Feigin, R. D., and Fiascone, A.: Hematuria and proteinuria associated with methicillin administration, New Eng. J. Med. **272**:903, 1965.
359a. Feingold, D. S.: Antimicrobial chemotherapeutic agents: The nature of their action and selective toxicity, New Eng. J. Med. **269**:900, 1963.
360. Fellers, F., and Craig, J.: Analgesic nephritis, J.A.M.A. **186**:610, 1963.
361. Fenn, G. K., Nalefski, L. A., and Lasner, J.: Transperitoneal lavage for twenty-six days in the treatment of azotemia, Amer. J. Med. **7**:35, 1949.
362. Ferguson, C., and Miller, C. D.: The heat factor as a cause of hemoglobinemia in transurethral resections, J. Urol. **69**:128, 1953.
363. Fey, B., and LeGrain, M.: Hyperchloremie plasmatique et lithiase renale, Rev. Franc. Etud. Clin. Biol. **1**:406, 1956.
364. Fidon, L., Gautier, Cl., and Martin, E.: Recherches physiologiques sur le sang des noyes, C. R. Soc. Biol. **65**:474, 1908.
365. Fifield, M. M.: Renal disease associated with prolonged use of acetophenetidin containing compounds, New Eng. J. Med. **269**:722, 1963.
366. Finckh, E. S.: The failure of experimental renal tubulonecrosis to produce oliguria in the rat, Australasian Ann. Med. **9**:283, 1960.
367. Finckh, E. S., Jeremy, D., and Whyte, H. M.: Structural renal damage and its relationship to clinical features in acute oliguric renal failure, Quart. J. Med. **31**:429, 1962.
368. Fine, J.: Peritoneal dialysis, Lancet **1**:120, 1947.
369. Fine, J., Frank, H. A., and Seligman, A. M.: The treatment of acute renal failure by peritoneal irrigation, Ann. Surg. **124**:857, 1946.
370. Fink, H. E., Jr., Roenigk, W. R., and Wilson, G. P.: An experimental investigation of the nephrotoxic effects of oral cholecystographic agents, Amer. J. Med. Sci. **247**:201, 1964.
371. Finkenstaedt, J. T., and Merrill, J. P.: Renal function after recovery from acute renal failure, New Eng. J. Med. **254**:1023, 1956.
371a. Finzer, K. H.: Lower nephron nephrosis due to concentrated lysol vaginal douches: a report of two cases, Canad. Med. Ass. J. **84**:549, 1961.

372. Fischer, H., and Rossier, P. H.: Starkstromunfalle mit schweren Muskelschadigungen und Myoglobinuria, Helvet. Med. Acta. **14**:212, 1947.

373. Fischermann, K., and Ostenfeld, J.: Death following intravenous urography, Nord. Med. **45**:240, 1951.

374. Fishberg, A. M.: Prerenal azotemia and the pathology of renal blood flow, Bull. N. Y. Acad. Med. **13**:710, 1937.

375. Fishberg, A. M.: Hypertension and nephritis, Philadelphia, 1954, Lea & Febiger.

376. Fisher, J. H., and Gilmour, J. R.: Encephalomyelitis following administration of sulfanilamide, with note on histological findings, Lancet **2**:301, 1939.

377. Fitzgerald, E. W., Jr.: Fatal glomerulonephritis complicating allergic purpura due to chlorothiazide, Arch. Intern. Med. **105**:305, 1960.

378. Flanagan, J. F.: Toxic nephrosis and massive hepatic necrosis produced by urethan, Arch. Intern. Med. **96**:277, 1955.

379. Flanigan, W. J., and Ackerman, G. L.: Site of action of ethacrynic acid, Arch. Int. Med. **118**:117, 1966.

380. Flanigan, W. J., and Oken, D. E.: Renal micropuncture study of the development of anuria in the rat with mercury-induced acute renal failure, J. Clin. Invest. **44**:449, 1965.

381. Flandin, C., Brodin, P., and Pasteur Vallery-Radot, L.: Un cas d'empoisonnement aigu par le sel d'oseille, Bull. Soc. Med. Hosp. Paris **30**:975, 1914.

382. Flink, E. B.: Blood transfusion studies: the relationship of hemoglobinemia and of the pH of the urine to renal damage produced by injection of hemoglobin solution into dogs, J. Lab. Clin. Med. **32**:223, 1947.

383. Flint, A.: Clinical report on hydro-peritoneum, based on an analysis of forty-six cases, Amer. J. Med. Sci. **45**:306, 1863.

384. Flipse, M. E., and Flipse, M. J.: Acute renal insufficiency, J. Florida Med. Assoc. **37**:149, 1950.

385. Floch, M. H., and Groisser, V. W.: Serum proteolytic activity in pancreatic disease, New Eng. J. Med. **263**:1129, 1960.

386. Fordham, C. C., and Huffines, W. D.: Headache powders and renal disease, Arch. Intern. Med. **113**:395, 1964.

387. Foreign Letter: Intermediate nephron nephrosis in crotalis poisoning, J.A.M.A. **153**:1376, 1953.

388. Foster, J. H., Adkins, R. B., Chamberlain, N. O., Symbas, P. N., and Harris, A. P.: The renal effects of lower abdominal aortic cross-clamping, J.A.M.A. **183**:155, 1963.

389. Foulon, P., and Busser, F. A.: A propos des lesions renales secondaires a la pyelographic retrograde, Ann. d'anat Pathol. **11**:416, 1934.

390. Foy, H., Altmann, A., Barnes, H. D., and Kondi, A.: Anuria, with special reference to renal failure in blackwater fever, incompatible transfusions, and crush injuries, Trans. Roy. Soc. Trop. Med. Hyg. **36**:197, 1943.

391. Frank, H. A., Seligman, A. M., and Fine, J.: Treatment of uremia after acute renal failure by peritoneal irrigation, J.A.M.A. **130**:703, 1946.

392. Frankenthal, L.: Uber Verschuttungen, Virchows Arch. **222**:332, 1916.

393. Frankenthal, L.: Die Folgen der verletzungen durch verschuttung, Bruns Beitrage zur Klin. Chir. **109**:572, 1918.

394. Franklin, S. S., and Merrill, J. P.: Medical progress: acute renal failure, New Eng. J. Med. **262**:711, 1960.

395. Franklin, S. S., and Merrill, J. P.: Medical progress: acute renal failure, New Eng. J. Med. **262**:761, 1960.

396. Frazier, D. B., and Carter, F. H.: Use of the artificial kidney in snakebite, Calif. Med. **97**:177, 1962.

397. Freeman, R. B., Maher, J. F., and Schreiner, G. E.: Hemodialysis for chronic renal failure. 1. Technical considerations, Ann. Intern. Med. **62**:519, 1965.

398. Freeman, R. B., Maher, J. F., Schreiner, G. E., and Mostofi, F. K.: Renal tubular necrosis due to nephrotoxicity of organic mercurial diuretics, Ann. Intern. Med. **57**:34, 1962.

399. Freeman, R. B., Sheff, M. F., Maher, J. F., and Schreiner, G. E.: The blood-cerebro-spinal fluid barrier in uremia, Ann. Intern. Med. **56**:233, 1962.

400. French, A. J.: Hypersensitivity in pathogenesis of histopathologic changes associated with sulfonamide chemotherapy, Amer. J. Path. **22**:697, 1946.

401. Fretheim, B., and Selvaag, O.: Peritoneal irrigation in uremia, Acta. Chir. Scand. **96**:461, 1948.

402. Friedman, E. A., Greenberg, J. B., Merrill, J. P., and Dammin, G. J.: Consequence of ethylene glycol poisoning, Amer. J. Med. **32**:891, 1962.

403. Friesen, S. R., Harsha, W. N., and McCroskey, C. H.: Massive generalized wound bleeding during operation with clinical and experimental evidence of blood transfusion reactions, Surgery **32**:620, 1952.

404. Friesen, S. R., and Nelson, R. M.: The occurence of massive generalized wound bleeding during operation with reference to the possibility of blood transfusion in its etiology, Ann. Surg. **17**:609, 1951.

405. Frimpter, G. W., Timpanelli, A. E., Eisenmenger, W. J., Stein, H. S., and Ehrlich, L. I.: Reversible "Fanconi syndrome" caused by degraded tetracycline, J.A.M.A. **184**:111, 1963.

406. Fudenberg, H., and Allen, F. H., Jr.: Transfusion reactions in absence of demonstrable incompatibility, New Eng. J. Med. **256**:1180, 1957.

407. Fulop, M., and Drapkin, A.: Potassium-depletion syndrome secondary to nepropathy apparently caused by "outdated tetracycline", New Eng. J. Med. **272**:986, 1965.

408. Funck-Brentano, J. L.: Contribution a l'etude du mechanisme physiopathologique de l'anurie au cours des nephropathies aigues, These. Med. Paris Impr. Cario. 1953.

409. Funck-Brentano, J. L., Amiel, Cl., and Mery, J. Ph.: Insuffisance renale aigue secondaire a l'ingestion d'opacifiants biliares, J. Urol. Nephrol. **68**:561, 1962.

410. Funck-Brentano, J. L., and Jungers, P.: Les accidents renaux de la transfusion sanguine: etude de 73 observations, La Presse. Med. **68**:860, 1960.

411. Funck-Brentano, J. L., Mery, J. Ph., Vantelon, J., and Watchi, J.: Les insuffisances renales aigues de l "angiocholite uremigene" (18 observations personnelles), La Presse. Med. **71**:1039, 1963.

412. Gabuzda, G. J., Gocke, T. M., Jackson, G. G., Grisby, M. E., Love, B. D., and Finland, M.: Some effects of antibiotics on nutrition in man, including studies of the bacterial flora of the feces, Arch. Intern. Med. **101**:476, 1958.

413. Galea, E. G., Young, L. N., and Bell, J. R.: Fatal nephropathy due to phenindione sensitivity, Lancet **1**:920, 1963.

414. Gamble, J. L.: Extracellular fluid and its vicissitudes, Bull. Johns Hopkins Hosp. **61**:151, 1937.

415. Gans, H., and Krivit, W.: Effect of endotoxic shock on the clothing mechanism of dogs, Ann. Surg. **152**:69, 1960.

416. Ganter, G.: Uber die beseitigung giftiger stoffe aus dem blute durch dialyse, Munch. Med. **70**:1478, 1923.

417. Garrett, J. J.: Acute renal failure in pregnancy, Illinois Med. J. **133**:699, 1968.

418. Garrod, L. P.: The toxicity of antibiotics, Med. J. Aust. **2**:947, 1964.

419. Garvin, C. F., and Van Wezel, N.: Bilateral cortical necrosis of the kidneys, a report of 3 cases, Arch. Int. Med. **62**:423, 1938.

420. Gasses, C., Gautier, E., Steck, A. Siebenmann, R. E., and Oechslin, R.: Hamolytisch-uramische Syndrome: Bilaterale Nieenrindennekrosen bei akuten erworbenen hamolytischen Anamien, Schweiz. Med. Wschr. **85**:905, 1955.

421. Gaultier, M., Fournier, E., Gervais, P., Gorciex, A., and Frejaville, J. P.: Intoxication aigue volontaire a la phenylbutazone: anurie: guerison, Bull. Soc. Med. Hop. Paris **113**:317, 1962.

422. Gebert, F.: Uber die Reaktion zurischen Arsenwasserstoff and Hamoglobin, Biochem. Z. **293**:157, 1937.

422a. Geigy, E.: Beitrag zur Kenntniss der arsenwassertoff-Vergiftung der Menschen, Inaug. Diss. Basil, 1890.

423. Geiling, E. M. K., and Cannon, P. R.: Pathologic effects of elixir of sulfanilamide (di-

ethylene glycol) poisoning: a clinical and experimental correlation: final report, J.A.M.A. 111:919, 1938.

424. Gelfand, M. L.: Renal colic associated with chlorothiazide and hydrochlorothiazide therapy, New Eng. J. Med. 265:129, 1961.

425. Gelin, L. E.: Effect of low viscous dextran in the early postoperative period, Acta. Chir. Scand. 122:333, 1961.

426. Gelin, L. E., and Ingelman, B.: Rheomacrodex: a new dextran solution for rheological treatment of impaired capillary flow, Acta. Chir. Scand. 122:294, 1961.

427. Gelin, L. E., Solvell, L., and Zederfeldt, B.: The plasma volume expanding effect of low viscous dextran and macrodex, Acta. Chir. Scand. 122:309, 1961.

428. Genkins, G., Uhr, J. W., and Bryer, M. S.: Bacitracin nephropathy: report of a case of acute renal failure and death, J.A.M.A. 155:894, 1954.

429. Germain, A., and Marty, J.: Hepato-nephrite aigue mortelle par inhalation de trichlorethylene, Bull. Soc. Med. Hop. Paris 63:1044, 1947.

430. Giles, R. B., and others: The sequelae of epidemic hemorrhagic fever, Amer. J. Med. 26:629, 1954.

431. Gilbert, A., and Lereboullet, P.: Des urines retardies (apsiurie) dons les cirrhoses, Compt. Rend. Soc. Biol. 53:276, 1901.

432. Gilman, A.: Analgesic nephrotoxicity: a pharmacological analysis, Amer. J. Med. 36: 167, 1964.

433. Cirksen, W. J., Bastian, R. C., Mallory, J. P., and others: Use of mannitol in exogenous and endogenous intoxications, New Eng. J. Med. 270:161, 1964.

434. Gjorup, S., and Thaysen, J. H.: Anabolic steroids in treatment of uremia, Lancet 2:886, 1958.

435. Gjorup, S., and Thaysen, J. H.: The effect of anabolic steroid (Durabolin) in the conservative management of acute renal failure, Acta. Med. Scand. 167:227, 1960.

436. Glaister, J.: Jurisprudence and toxicology, Edinburgh, 1950, E. & S. Livingstone, Ltd.

437. Glushein, A. S., and Fisher, E. R.: Renal lesions of sulfonamide type after treatment with acetazolamide (Diamox), J.A.M.A. 160:204, 1956.

438. Godman, G. C., and Churg, J.: Wegener's granulomatosis, Arch. Path. 58:533, 1954.

439. Goldblatt, S.: Acute mercurial intoxication: report of 38 cases, Amer. J. Med. Sci. 176: 645, 1928.

440. Goldring, W., and Graef, K.: Nephrosis with uremia following transfusion with incompatible blood, Arch. Intern. Med. 58:825, 1936.

441. Goldring, W., and Chasis, H.: Hypertension and hypertensive diseases, London, 1944, Commonwealth Fund.

442. Goodman, L. S., and Gilman, A.: The pharmacological basis of therapeutics, New York, 1955, The Macmillan Company.

443. Goodale, W. T., and Kinney, T. D.: Sulfadiazine nephrosis with hyperchloremia and encephalopathy, Ann. Int. Med. 31:1118, 1949.

444. Goodpastor, W. E., Levenson, S. M., Tagnon, H. J., Lund, C. C., and Taylor, F. H. L.: A clinical and pathologic study of the kidney in patients with thermal burns, Surg. Gynec. Obstet. 82:652, 1946.

445. Goodwin, W. E., Cason, J. F., and Scott, W. W.: Hemoglobinemia and lower nephron nephrosis following transurethral prostatic surgery, J. Urol. 65:1075, 1951.

446. Gonzales, T. A., Vance, M., Helpern, M., and Umberger, C. J.: Legal medicine: pathology and toxicology, New York, 1954, Appleton-Century-Crofts.

447. Goodwin, W. E., Sloan, R. D., and Scott, W. W.: The "trueta" renal vascular "shunt," J. Urol. 61:1010, 1949.

448. Goodyer, A. V. N., and Jaeger, C. A.: Renal response to non-shocking hemorrhage: role of autonomic nervous system and of renal circulation, Amer. J. Physiol. 180:69, 1955.

449. Gordillo, G.: Acute renal failure in newborns and infants, Proceedings of the Third International Congress of Nephrology, Washington, 1966.

450. Gormsen, H., Iversen, P., and Raachou, F.: Kidney biopsy in acute anuria with a case of acute bilateral cortical necrosis, Amer. J. Med. 19:209, 1955.

451. Gornel, D. L., and Goldman, R.: Acute renal failure following hexol-induced abortion, J.A.M.A. **203**:146, 1968.

452. Gosset, J.: Le maintien de l'equilibre hydrique et ionique chez les operes, Sem. Hop Paris **27**:2737, 1951.

453. Gottlieb, A., Spiera, H., and Gordis, E.: Fatal renal insufficiency after oral cholecystography, New Eng. J. Med. **267**:389, 1962.

454. Govaerts, P.: The ratio of creatinine clearance to urea clearance in toxic nephropathies, Stanford Med. Bull. **6**:71, 1948.

455. Govan, A. D. T., and MacGillivray, I.: Puerperal uremia due to acute upper-nephron nephrotis: report of 3 cases, Lancet **2**:128, 1950.

456. DeGowin, E. L., Hardin, R. C., and Alsever, J. B.: Blood transfusion, Philadelphia, 1949, W. B. Saunders Co.

457. DeGowin, E. L., Osterhagen, H. F., and Andersch, M.: Renal insufficiency from blood transfusion, Arch. Intern. Med. **59**:432, 1937.

457a. Graber, C. J., Tombusch, W. T., Rudnicki, A. P., and Vogel, E. H., Jr.: Generalized Shwartzman-like reaction following Serratia or arcescens septicemia in a fatal burn, Surg. Kynec. Obstet. **110**:443, 1960.

458. Graber, I. G., and Sevitt, S.: Renal function in burned patients and its relationship to morphological changes, J. Clin. Path. **12**:25, 1959.

459. Graham, E. A., and Cole, W. H.: Roentgenologic examination of gallbladder: preliminary report of new method utilizing intravenous injection of tetrabromphenolphthalein, J.A.M.A. **82**:613, 1924.

460. Graham, J. R., Suby, H. I., LeCompte, P. R., and Sadowsky, N. L.: Fibrotic disorders associated with methysergide therapy for headache, New Eng. J. Med. **274**:359, 1966.

461. Graham, W. H.: Simulation of "acute abdomen" in carbon tetrachloride poisoning, Lancet **1**:1159, 1938.

462. Grattan, W. A.: Hematuria and azotemia associated with administration of methicillin, J. Pediat. **64**:285, 1964.

463. Graubarth, J., Bloom, C. J., Coleman, F. C., and Solomon, H. N.: Dye poisoning in nursery: review of 17 cases, J.A.M.A. **128**:1155, 1945.

464. Green, H. N.: Shock-producing factor(s) from striated muscle: isolation and biological properties, Lancet **2**:147, 1943.

465. Greenberg, L. A.: An evaluation of reported poisonings by acetyl salicylic acid, New Eng. J. Med. **243**:124, 1950.

466. Greenberg, P. A., and Sanford, J. P.: Removal and absorption of antibiotics in patients with renal failure undergoing peritoneal dialysis, Ann. Intern. Med. **66**:465, 1967.

467. Greenhill, J. P.: The yearbook of obstetrics and gynecology, Chicago, 1956-1957, Year Book Medical Publishers, Inc.

468. Greenwald, I.: The estimation of lipoid and acidesoluble phosphorus in small amounts of serum, J. Biol. Chem. **21**:29, 1915.

469. Gregorie, F., Malmendier, C., and Lambert, P.: Syndrome nephrotique apres traitement aux sels d'or, J. Urol. **62**:140, 1956.

470. Grieve, J., and Lowe, K. G.: Anuria following retrograde pyelography, Brit. J. Urol. **27**:63, 1955.

471. Grimlund, K.: Phenacetic and renal damage at a Swedish factory, Acta. Med. Scand. **174**:1, 1963.

472. Griffith, L. S., Fresh, J. W., and Watten, R. H., and others: Electrolyte replacement in pediatric cholera, Lancet **1**:1197, 1967.

473. Grollman, A.: Acute renal failure, Springfield, Illinois, 1954, Charles C Thomas, Publisher.

474. Grollman, A., Turner, L. B., and McLean, J. A.: Intermittent peritoneal lavage in nephrectomized dogs and its application to the human being, Arch. Intern. Med. **87**:379, 1951.

475. Grollman, A., Turner, L. B., Levitch, M., and Hill, D.: Hemodynamic of bilaterally nephrectomized dog and subjected to intermittent peritoneal lavage, Amer. J. Physiol. **165**:167, 1951.

476. Grosby, D. S.: Malarial relapse induced by intravenous chologiography, Arch. Intern. Med. **118**:79, 1966.

477. Gross, J. E.: Fanconi syndrome (adult type) developing secondary to the ingestion of outdated tetracycline, Ann. Intern. Med. **58**:523, 1963.

478. Gross, M., and Greenberg, L. A.: The salicylates: a critical bibliographic review, New Haven, 1948, New Haven Hillhouse Press.

479. Gross, P., Cooper, F. B., and Scott, R. E.: Urolithiasis medicamentosa, Urol. Cutan. Rev. **44**:205, 1940.

480. Grossman, J., Weston, R. E., Lehman, R. A., Halperin, J. P., Ullmann, T. D., and Leiter, L.: Urinary and fecal excretion of mercury in man following administration of mercurial diuretics, J. Clin. Invest. **30**:1208, 1951.

481. Grossman, L. A., Ory, E. M., and Willoughby, D. H.: Anuria treated by peritoneal irrigation, J.A.M.A. **135**:273, 1947.

482. Gsell, O., Rechenberg, H. K., and Miescher, P.: Die primar chronische interstitielle nephritis; klinische, experimentelle und aetiologische untersuchungen, Deutsche Med. Wchnschr. **82**:1673, 1957.

483. Guild, W. R., Bray, G., and Merrill, J. P.: Hemopericardium with cardiac tamponade in chronic uremia, New Eng. J. Med. **257**:230, 1957.

484. Guild, W. R., Young, J. V., and Merrill, J. P.: Anuria due to carbon tetrachloride intoxication, Ann. Intern. Med. **48**:1221, 1958.

485. Haas, G. G.: Dialysieren des Stromenden blutes am lebenden, Klin. Wchnschr. **2**:1888, 1923.

486. Hackradt, A.: Uber acute todliche vasomotor-ische nephrosin noch verschuttung (Munchen), Worishofen, 1917, Wagner.

487. Hagelstom, L., Kuhlback, B., and Riska, N.: Renal failure after intravenous para-aminosalicylic acid administration in a case of intestinal and renal amyloidosis, Scand. J. Lab. Clin. Med. **15**:62, 1963.

488. Hager, E. B., and Merrill, J. P.: Peritoneal dialysis and acute renal failure, Surg. Clin. N. Amer. 1963.

489. Hagstrom, R. S.: Studies on fluid absorption during transurethral prostatic resection, J. Urol. **73**:852, 1955.

490. Hall, C. E., and Hall, O.: Polyvinyl alcohol nephrosis: relationship of degree of polymerization to pathophysiologic effects, Proc. Soc. Exper. Biol. Med. **112**:86, 1963.

491. Haller, J. A., Jr., Ransdell, H. T., Jr., Stowens, D., and Rubel, W. F.: Renal toxicity of polybrene in open heart surgery, J. Thorac. Cardiovasc. Surg. **44**:486, 1962.

492. Hamburger, H. J.: Uber die regelung der osmotischen spannkraft von flussigkeiten in Bauchund Pericardialhohle, Arch. f. Phys. 281, 1895.

493. Hamburger, J.: Physiologie de l'innervation renale, Paris, 1936, Masson & Cie, Ed.

494. Hamburger, J.: Le retentissement humoral de l'insuffisance renale aigue, Rapport au XXVIIIe Congres Francais de Medecine, tome 1, Bruxelles, 1951.

495. Hamburger, J.: Les anuries par inhalation de tetrachlorure de carbone, Paris, 1958, Acquisitions Medicales Recentes.

496. Hamburger, J.: Les accidents renaux post-operatories (analyse de 200 observations), Med. Acad. Chir. **85**:41, 1959.

497. Hamburger, J., Crosnier, J., Funck-Brentano, J. L., Rapin, M., and Masson, M.: Conditions d'apparition de l'hyperkaliemie et de l'hypokaliemie au cours de l'insuffisance renale, Sem. Hop. Paris **30**:3424, 1954.

498. Hamburger, J., Halpern, B., and Cruchaud, S.: Action preventive d'un antihistaminique derive de la thiodiphenylamine sur l'aedeme aigu du poumon experimental, Acta. Allerg. **1**:97, 1948.

499. Hamburger, J., Halpern, B., and Funck-Grentano, J. L.: Une variete d'anurie provoquee par l'hydratation excessive des cellules renales, La Presse Med. **62**:972, 1954.

500. Hamburger, J., Hepp, J., Crosnier, J., and Caroli, J.: Angiocholite lithiasique icterouremigene gravissime Rein artificiel: guerison, Rev. Med. Chir. Mal Foie **33**:181, 1958.

501. Hamburger, J., and Mathe, G.: Physiologie normale et pathologique du metabolisme de l'eau, Paris, 1952, Med. Flammarion, Ed.

502. Hamburger, J., and Mathe, G.: Lesyndrome d'hyperhydratation cellulaire, Schweiz. Med. Wschr. **83**:277, 1953.

503. Hamburger, J., and Mathe, G.: Fluid balance in anuria. In Ciba foundation symposium on the kidney, London, 1954, Churchill.

504. Hamburger, J., Mathe, G., Crosnier, J., and Cournot, L.: Syndromes de dystonie osmotique du plasma sanguin, Sem. Hop. Paris **26**:3929, 1950.

505. Hamburger, J., and Richet, G.: Sur un phenomene inedit de liberation d'eau endogene observe au cours de certaines anuries, Bull. Soc. Med. Hop. Paris **68**:368, 1952.

506. Hamburger, J., and Richet, G.: Enseignements tires de la pratique du rein artificiel pour l'interpretation des desordres electrolytiques de l'uremie aigue, Rev. Franc. Etud. Clin. Biol. **1**:39, 1956.

507. Hamburger, J., Richet, G., Cournot, L., Laham, S., and Roques, S.: Intoxications graves par inhalation de produits capillaires a base de tetrachlorure de carbone, Bull. Soc. Med. Hop. Paris **67**:385, 1951.

508. Hamburger, J., Richet, G., and Crosnier, J.: Techniques de reanimation medicale et controle de L'equilibre humoral, ed. 2, Paris, 1957, Flammarion.

509. Hamburger, J., Richet, G., and Crosnier, J.: Techniques de reanimation medicale et de controle de l'equilibre humoral en medecine d'urgence, ed. 4, Paris, 1964, Flammarion.

510. Hamburger, J., Richet, G., Crosnier, J., and Funck-Brentano, J. L.: L'insuffisance renale, Berlin, 1962, Springer.

511. Hamilton, A.: Hygienic control of the anilin dye industry in Europe, U. S. Month Labor Rev. **9**:1675, 1919.

512. Hamilton, P. B., Phillips, R. A., and Hiller, A.: Duration of renal ischemia required to produce uremia, Amer. J. Physiol. **152**:517, 1948.

513. Hampers, C. L., Streiff, R., Nathan, D. G., Snyder, D., and Merrill, J. P.: Megaloblastic hematopoiesis in uremia and in patients on long-term hemodialysis, New Eng. J. Med. **276**:551, 1967.

514. Handa, S. P., and Lazor, M. Z.: Acute tubular necrosis: a review of 44 necropsied cases, Amer. J. Med. Sci., **251**:67, 1966.

515. Hardaway, R. M., III, McKay, D. G., Wahle, G. H., Jr., Tartock, D. E., and Edelstein, A.: Pathologic study of intravascular coagulation following incompatible blood transfusion in dogs. I. Intravenous injections of incompatible blood, Amer. J. Surg. **91**:24, 1956.

516. Harkins, H. N.: The treatment of burns, Springfield, Illinois, 1952, Charles C Thomas, Publisher.

517. Harmon, E. L.: Human mercuric chloride poisoning by intravenous injection, Amer. J. Path. **4**:321, 1928.

518. Harris, H., McDonald, I. R., and Williams, W.: The electrolyte patterns in experimental anuria, Aust. J. Exp. Biol. Med. Sci. **30**:33, 1952.

519. Harrison, C. V., Loughridge, L. W., and Milne, M. D.: Acute oliguric renal failure in acute glomerulonephritis and polyarteritis nodosa, Quart. J. Med. New Series **33**:39, 1964.

520. Harrow, B. R., and Sloane, J. A.: Anuria and hydronephrosis following ureteral catheterization, J.A.M.A. **180**:415, 1962.

521. Harrow, B. R., Sloane, J. A., and Liedman, N. C.: Renal papillary necrosis in analgesics, J.A.M.A. **184**:445, 1963.

522. Harthorne, J. W., Marcus, A. M., and Kaye, M.: Management of massive imipramine overdosage with mannitol and artificial dialysis, New Eng. J. Med. **268**:33, 1963.

523. Harvald, B., and Clausen, E.: Nephrotoxicity of acetylsalicylic acid, Lancet **2**:767, 1960.

524. Harvald, B., Valdorf-Hansen, F., and Nielsen, A.: Effect on the kidney of drugs containing phenacetin, Lancet **1**:303, 1960.

525. Haury, V. G., and Cantarow, A.: Effect of magnesium sulfate on serum and peritoneal fluid calcium, magnesium, inorganic phosphorus, Proc. Soc. Exp. Biol. New York **43**:335, 1940.

526. Haymann, J. M., Jr., and Johnston, S. M.: The excretion of inorganic sulphates, J. Clin. Invest. **11**:607, 1932.

527. Haynes, B. W., Jr., and Bright, R.: Burn coma: a syndrome associated with severe burn wound infection, J. Trauma, **7**:464, 1967.

528. Healy, J. K.: Acute oliguric renal failure associated with multiple myeloma, Brit. Med. J. **1**:1126, 1963.

529. Heard, K. M., Posey, E. L., Jr., and Long, J. W.: Fulminating uremic penumonitis associated with acute ischemic nephropathy (lower nephron nephrosis), Amer. J. Med. **24**:157, 1958.

530. Hecker, R., and Sherlock, S.: Electrolyte and circulatory changes in terminal liver failure, Lancet **2**:1121, 1956.

531. Hegstrom, R. M., Murray, J. S., Pendras, J. P., Burnell, J. M., and Scribner, B. H.: Two years experience with periodic hemodialysis in the treatment of chronic uremia, Trans. Amer. Soc. Artf. Int. Org. **6**:266, 1962.

532. Heilman, D. H., Heilman, F. R., Hinshaw, H. C., Nichols, D. R., and Herrell, E. W.: Streptomycin absorption, diffusion, excretion and toxicity, Amer. J. Med. Sci. **210**:576, 1945.

533. Hellwig, C. A., and Reed, H. L.: Fatal anuria following sulfadiazine therapy, J.A.M.A. **119**:561, 1942.

534. Helmly, R. B., Bergin, J. J., and Shulman, N. R.: Quinine induced purpura, Arch. Intern. Med. **120**:59, 1967.

535. Helwig, F. C., and Schultz, C. B.: A liver kidney syndrome: clinical, pathological and experimental studies, Surg. Gynec. Obstet. **55**:570, 1932.

536. Hempstead, B. E., and Hench, P. S.: Uremic stomatitis, Trans. Amer. Laryng. Rhinol. Otol. Soc. **36**:510, 1930.

537. Henkin, R. I., Maxwell, M. H., and Murray, J. F.: Uremic pneumonitis: a clinical physiological study, Ann. Intern. Med. **57**:1001, 1962.

538. Hepler, O. E., and Simonds, J. P.: Experimental nephropathies. III. Calcification and phosphatase in the kidneys of dogs poisoned with mercury bichloride, potassium dichromate and uranyl nitrate, Arch. Path. **30**:37, 1945.

539. Heptinstall, R. H.: Pathology of the kidney, Boston, 1966, Little, Brown and Company.

540. Herman, L.: Clinical nephrosis, Surg. Clin. N. Amer. **16**:515, 1936.

541. Herndon, R. F., Meroney, W. H., and Pearson, C. M.: The electrocardiographic effects of alterations in concentration of plasma chemicals, Amer. Heart J. **50**:188, 1955.

541a. Herrick, J. B.: Peculiar elongated and sickle-shaped red blood corpuscles in a case of severe anemia, Arch. Intern. Med. **6**:517, 1910.

542. Herrick, W. W., and Tillman, A. J. B.: Toxemia of pregnancy: its relationship to cardiovascular and renal disease; clinical and necropsy observations with a long followup, Arch. Intern. Med. **55**:643, 1935.

543. Herring, P. T.: The development of the malpighian bodies of the kidney and its relationship to pathologic changes which occur in them, J. Path. Bact. **6**:459, 1900.

544. Herrmann, W. P., Hopfeld, G., and Berning, H.: Uber Nierenentzundungen Nach Irgaprin-Be Handlung (Nephritis After Irgapyrin Therapy) Z. Klin. Med. **154**:302, 1956.

545. Heusser, H., and Werder, H.: Untersuchungen uber peritoneal dialysis, Brune Beirtz Z. Klin. Chirurgie **141**:38, 1927.

546. Hewitt, W. L., Finegold, S. M., and Monzon, O. T.: Untoward side effects associated with methicillin therapy, Antimicrobial Agents and Chemotherapy, 1961.

547. Heymann, W.: Trimethadione (Tridione) nephrosis, Pediatrics **22**:614, 1958.

548. Hillenbrand, H. J., Hoeltzenbein, J., and Schmandt, W.: Neuer Hamodialysator (sog. kinstliche Niere), Urol. Internists **5**:60, 1957.

549. Hinshaw, L. B., Day, S. B., and Carlson, C. H.: Tissue pressure as a causal factor in the autoregulation of blood flow in the isolated perfused kidney, Amer. J. Physiol. **197**:309, 1959.

550. Hint, H.: Proceedings of Conference on evaluation of low-molecular-weight dextran in

shock. National Academy of Science, Division of Medical Sciences, National Research Council, U. S. A., pg. 48, 1963.

551. Hirsh, H. L., Vivino, H. A., and Dowling, H. F.: Streptomycin: a review of the basic principles and their clinical application, Med. Ann. District of Columbia 17:311, 1948.

551a. Hjort, P. F., and Rapaport, S. I.: The Shwartzman reaction: pathogenetic mechanisms and clinical manifestations, Annual Review of Medicine 2:135, 1965.

552. Hoffman, W. S., and Marshall, D.: Management of lower nephron nephrosis, Arch. Intern. Med. 83:249, 1949.

553. Hofle, K. H., and Schoop, W.: Akutes nephrotisches syndrom bei Mesantoin-Behandlung, Deutsche Med. Wchnschr. 84:837, 1959.

554. Hollander, D., and Manning, R. T.: The use of alkylating agents in the treatment of Wegener's granulomatosis, Ann. Intern. Med. 67:393, 1967.

555. Hollenberg, N. K., Epstein, M., Rosen, S. M., Basch, R. I., Oken, D. E., and Merrill, J. P.: Acute oliguric renal failure in man: evidence preferential renal cortical ischemia, Medicine 47:455, 1968.

556. Holman, R. L.: Complete anuria due to blockage of renal tubules by protein casts in a case of multiple myeloma, Arch. Path. 27:748, 1939.

557. Holmes, J. H.: Acute tubular necrosis and its management, Surg. Clin. N. Amer. 43: 555, 1963.

558. Holmes, K. K.: Toxicity of colistin and polymyxin B, New Eng. J. Med. 271:633, 1964.

559. Hope, J. W., and Michie, A. J.: Hydronephrosis following retrograde pyelography, Radiology 72:844, 1959.

560. Hopper, J., Jr., O'Connell, B. P., and Fluss, H. R.: Serum potassium patterns in anuria and oliguria, Ann. Intern. Med. 38:935, 1953.

561. Hopps, H. C., and Wissler, R. W.: Uremic pneumonitis, Amer. J. Path. 31:261, 1955.

562. Horn, H.: Experimental nephropathies, Arch. Path. 23:71, 1937.

563. Hostnik, W. J., Powers, S. R., Jr., and Bobam, A.: Observations on the effect of mannitol on renal hemodynamics and O_2 tension in the urine and renal vein, Surg. Forum 10:872, 1960.

564. Houck, C. R.: Possible renal vascular shunt in dogs during intravenous epinephrine, Fed. Proc. 9:63, 1950.

565. Howenstine, J. A.: Exertion-induced myoglobinuria and hemoglobinuria, J.A.M.A. 173: 493, 1960.

566. Hughes, W., and Levvy, G. A.: The toxicity of arsine solutions for tissue slices, Biochem. J. 41:8, 1947.

567. Hull, E., and Monte, L. A.: Acute mercury poisoning, New Orleans Med. Surg. J. 88: 455, 1936.

568. Hunter, D.: The disorders of occupations, London, 1957, English Universities Press.

569. Hunter, R. B., and Muirhead, E. E.: Prolonged renal salt wastage in "lower nephron nephrosis," Ann. Intern. Med. 36:1297, 1952.

570. Hunter, W. C.: Experimental study of acquired resistance of the rabbit's renal epithelium to mercuric chloride, Ann. Intern. Med. 2:796, 1929.

571. Hunter, W. C., and Roberts, J. M.: Glomerular changes in the kidneys of the rabbits and monkeys induced by uranium nitrate, mercuric chloride and potassium bichromate, Amer. J. Path. 8:665, 1932.

572. Hutt, M. P., and Holmes, J. H.: Pericardial effusion complicating acute tubular necrosis, Arch. Int. Med. 108:116, 1961.

573. Hutton-Leonetti, F. M.: Les insuffisances renales aigues post-partum, These. Med. Paris 1963.

574. Idbohrn, H.: Tolerance to contrast media in renal angiography, Acta. Radiol. 45:141, 1956.

575. Idbohrn, H., and Berg, N.: On the tolerance of rabbit's kidney to contrast media in renal angiography; a roentgenologic and histologic investigation, Acta. Radiol. 42: 121, 1954.

576. Inouye, W. Y., and Engelberg, J.: A simplified artificial dialyser and ultrafilter, Surg. Forum 4:438, 1953.

577. Iovine, G., Berman, L. B., Halikis, D. N., Mowrey, F. H., Chappelle, E. H., and Gierson, H. W.: Nephrotoxicity of amphotericin B, Arch. Int. Med. **112**:853, 1963.

578. Iversen, P., and Brun, C.: Aspiration biopsy of the kidney, Amer. J. Med. **11**:324, 1951.

579. Jackson, G. G., and McCabe, W. R.: Gram-negative bacteremia, Arch. Int. Med. **110**:83, 1962.

580. Jacobziner, H., and Raybin, H. W.: Activities of the poison control center, Arch. Pediat. **78**:357, 1961.

581. Jacobziner, H., and Raybin, H. W.: Turpentine poisoning, Arch. Pediat. **78**:357, 1961.

582. Jaffe, R. H., and Laing, D. R.: Changes of the digestive tract in uremia: a pathological anatomic study, Arch. Intern. Med. **53**:851, 1934.

583. Jawetz, E.: Laboratory and clinical observations on polymyxin B and E, Amer. J. Med. **10**:111, 1951.

584. Jeddeloh, B.: Haffkrankheit, Ergebn. Inn. Med. Kinderheilk **57**:138, 1939.

585. Jeghers, H., and Bakst, H. J.: The syndrome of extrarenal azotemia, Ann. Intern. Med. **11**:1861, 1938.

586. Jennings, R. B., and Earle, D. P.: Post-streptococcal glomerulonephritis: histopathologic and clinical studies of the acute, subsiding acute, and early chronic latent phases, J. Clin. Med. **40**:1525, 1961.

587. Joekes, A. M., and Rellan, D. R.: Radioactive renography in diagnosis and treatment of acute obstructive renal failure, Lancet **2**:96, 1965.

588. Johnson, W. J.: Principles of management of acute renal failure. In Brest, A. N., and Moyer, J. H.: Renal failure, Philadelphia, 1967, J. B. Lippincott Co.

589. Johnstone, B. I., Keith, H. M.: Toxicity of novasurol (merbaphen): its action on the kidney of the rabbit, Arch. Intern. Med. **42**:189, 1928.

590. Jones, N. W.: Arseniuretted hydrogen poisoning, J.A.M.A. **48**:1099, 1907.

591. Jones, R. A., McDonald, G. O., and Last, J. H.: Reversal of diurnal variation in renal function in cases of cirrhosis with ascites, J. Clin. Invest. **31**:326, 1952.

592. Jorgensen, H. E., Balslov, J. R., and Brun, C.: Efficiency of a modified Skeggs-Leonard's hemodialyzer, J. Lab. Clin. Med. **59**:932, 1962.

593. Juhel-Renoy, E.: De l'anurie precoce scarlatineuse, Arch. Gen. Med. **17**:385, 1886.

594. Kabat, E. A., Turino, G. M., Tarron, A. B., and Maurer, P. H.: Studies on the immunochemical basis of allergic reactions to dextran in man, J. Clin. Invest. **36**:1160, 1957.

595. Kober, G. M., and Hayhurst, E. R.: Industrial health, Philadelphia, 1924, P. Blackiston's Son & Co.

596. Kaden, W. S., and Friedman, E. A.: Obstructive uropathy complicating anticoagulant therapy, New Eng. J. Med. **265**:283, 1961.

597. Kanee, B., and Stoffman, I.: BAL in the successful treatment of mercury poisoning from gray powder, Canad. M. A. J. **60**:292, 1949 (Abstract); J.A.M.A. **140**:1359, 1949.

598. Kahn, H. S., and Brotchner, R. J.: A recovery from ethylene glycol (antifreeze) intoxication: a case of survival and two fatalities from ethylene glycol including autopsy findings, Ann. Intern. Med. **32**:284, 1950.

599. Kahn, M. H., and Berhulst, H. L.: Accidental poisoning in young children—hazards of iron medication, Amer. J. Dis. Child. **99**:688, 1960.

600. Kolten, R. J., Zaltzman, S., Coe, F. I., and Metcoff, J.: Hemodialysis in children: technique, kinetic aspects related to varying body size and application to salicylate intoxication, acute renal failure and some other disorders, Medicine **45**:1, 1966.

601. Kaplan, J. M., Wachtel, H. L., Czarnecki, S. W., and Sampson, J. J.: Lupus-like illness precipitated by procainamide hydrochloride, J.A.M.A. **192**:444, 1965.

602. Kaplan, K., Reisberg, B., and Weinstein, L.: Cephaloridine, Arch. Intern. Med. **121**:17, 1968.

603. Kaplan, K., and Weinstein, L.: Anaphylaxis to cephaloridine in a nurse who prepared solutions of the drug, J.A.M.A. **200**:75, 1967.

604. Kaplan, S. A., Foman, S. J., and Rapoport, S.: Effects of epinephrine and l-nor-epinephrine on renal excretion of solutes during mannitol diuresis in the hydropenic dog, Amer. J. Physiol. **169**:588, 1952.

308 *References*

605. Karafin, L., and Stearns, T. M.: Renal vein thrombosis in children, J. Urol. **92**:91, 1964.
606. Karelitz, S., and Freeman, A. D.: Hepatitis and nephrosis due to soluble bismuth, Pediatrics **8**:772, 1951.
607. Karlson, A. G., Gainer, U. H., and Feldman, W. H.: The effect of neomycin on tuberculosis in guinea pigs infected with streptomycin-resistant tubercule bacilli, Amer. Rev. Tuberc. **62**:345, 1950.
608. Kark, R. M.: Some aspects of nutrition and the kidney. In Wohl, M. G., and Goodhart, R. S., editors: Modern nutrition in health and disease, ed. 4, London, 1968, Henry Kimpton.
609. Kark, R. M., Lawrence, J. R., Pollak, V. E., Pirani, C. L., Muehrcke, R. C., and Silva, H.: A primer of urinalysis, ed. 2, New York, 1963, Harper & Row, Publishers.
610. Kass, E. H.: Pyelonephritis and bacteruria: a major problem in preventive medicine, Ann. Intern. Med. **56**:46, 1962.
611. Kass, E. H., and Schneiderman, L. J.: Entry of bacteria into the urinary tracts of patients with inlying catheters, New Eng. J. Med. **256**:556, 1957.
612. Katz, R.: Renal and possibly hepatic toxicity from coly-mycin, M. Ann. District of Columbia **32**:408, 1963.
613. Kaufman, J. J., Moloney, P. J., and Maxwell, M. H.: Urinary blockade after bilateral catheterization, New Eng. J. Med. **275**:412, 1966.
614. Kayser, F. F. O.: von Schjerning's Handbuch der arztlichen Erfahrungen im Weltkriege, Leipzig, 1922, Chirurgie.
615. Kegel, A. H., McNally, W. D., and Pope, A. S.: Methyl chloride poisoning from domestic refrigerators, J.A.M.A. **93**:353, 1929.
616. Keitzer, W. A., and Campbell, J. A.: Renal complications of sulfadiazine, J.A.M.A. **119**:701, 1942.
617. Keitzer, W. A., Ford, M. L., and Miller, E. W.: Clinical experience with the Skeggs-Leonards artificial kidney, J. Urol. **72**:629, 1954.
618. Kennedy, A. C., Luice, R. G., and Linton, A. L.: Dialysis disequilibrium syndrome. In Shaldon, S., and Cook, G. C., editors: Acute renal failure: a symposium, Philadelphia, 1964, F. A. Davis Co.
619. Kensler, C. J., Abels, J. C., and Rhoads, C. P.: Arsine poisoning: modes of action and treatment, J. Pharmacol. **88**:99, 1946.
620. Kent, G., Minick, O. T., Volini, F. I., and Orfei, E.: Autophagic vacuoles in human red cells, Amer. J. Path. **48**:831, 1966.
621. Kiil, F.: Development of a parallel flow artificial kidney in plastics, Acta. Chir. Scand. (suppl.) **253**:142, 1960.
622. Kiil, F., and Glover, J. F.: Parallel flow plastic hemodialyzer as a membrane oxygenator, Trans. Amer. Soc. Artif. Int. Org. **8**:45, 1962.
623. Kiley, J., and Hines, O.: Electroencephalographic evaluation of uremia, Arch. Intern. Med. **116**:67, 1965.
624. Kiley, J. E., Powers, S. R., Jr., and Beebe, R. T.: Acute renal failure: eighty cases of renal tubular necrosis, New Eng. J. Med. **262**:481, 1960.
625. Killen, D. A., and Lance, E. M.: Experimental appraisal of the agents employed as angiocardiographic and aortographic contrast media. II. Nephrotoxicity, Surgery **47**:260, 1960.
626. Killman, S. A., Gjorup, S., and Thaysen, J. H.: Fatal acute renal failure following intravenous pyelography in patient with multiple myeloma, Acta. Med. Scand. **158**:43, 1957.
627. Kimmelstiel, P.: Acute hematogenous interstitial nephritis, Amer. J. Path. **14**:737, 1938.
628. Kincaid, O. W., and Davis, G. D.: Abdominal aortography, New Eng. J. Med. **259**:1067, 1958.
629. Kincaid-Smith, P.: Cadaveric renal transplantation, Lancet **1**:51, 1968.
630. Kinney, V. R., Olsen, A. M., Hepper, N. G. G., and Harrison, E. G., Jr.: Wegener's granulomatosis, Arch. Intern. Med. **108**:159, 1961.

631. Kirby, W. M. M.: Vancomycin therapy of staphylococcal infection. In Second International Symposium on chemotherapy, Vol. 1, 1963.

632. Kirkland, K., Edwards, K. D. G., and Whyte, H. M.: Oliguric renal failure: a report of 400 cases including classification, survival and response to dialysis, Australasian Ann. Med. 14:275, 1965.

633. Kjellbo, H., Stakeberg, H., and Mellgren, J.: Possibly thiazide-induced renal necrotizing vasculitis, Lancet 1:1034, 1965.

634. Kleeman, C. R., and Maxwell, M. H.: The nephrotoxicity of antibiotics: a review. In Quinn, E. L., and Kass, E. H., editors: Biology of pyelonephritis, Boston, 1960, Little, Brown and Company.

635. Klutsch, K., Heidland, A., and Kammerer, H.: Nierenfunktion nach infusion von niedermolekularem Dextran, Med. Klin. 60:464, 1965.

636. Knochel, I. P., Clayton, C. E., Smith, W. L., and Barry, K. G.: Intraperitonal tham: an effective method to enhance phenobarbital removal during peritonal dialysis, J. Lab. Clin. Med. 64:257, 1964.

637. Knowles, H. C., and Kaplan, S. A.: Treatment of hyperkalemia in acute renal failure using exchange resins, Arch. Int. Med. 92:189, 1953.

638. Kobernick, S. D., More, J. R., and Wiglesworth, F. W.: Thrombosis of the renal veins with massive hemorrhagic infarction of the kidneys in childhood, Amer. J. Path. 27:435, 1951.

639. Kolff, W. J., and Berk, H. T. J.: The artificial kidney: a dialyser with great area, Acta. Med. Scand. 117:121, 1944.

640. Kolff, W. J.: New ways of treating uremia: the artificial kidney, peritoneal lavage, intestinal lavage, London, 1947, J. & A. Churchill Ltd.

641. Kolff, W. J.: Forced high caloric, low protein diet and the treatment of uremia, Amer. J. Med. 12:667, 1952.

642. Kolff, W. J.: Acute renal failure, causes and treatment, Med. Clin. N. Amer. 39:1041, 1955.

643. Kolff, W. J.: Experiences in the treatment of surgical patients having anuria and uremia, Surg. Gynec. Obstet. 101:563, 1955.

644. Kolff, W. J., and Berk, H. R. J.: The artificial kidney, a dialyzer with great areas, Acta. Med. Scand. 117:131, 1944.

645. Kolff, W. J., and Watschinger, B.: Further development of a coil kidney: disposable artificial kidney, J. Lab. Clin. Med. 47:969, 1956.

646. Koota, G. M., Schweinburg, F. B., and Rutenberg, A. M.: Role of kanamycin in the management of infections, New Eng. J. Med. 263:629, 1960.

647. Kravitz, S. C., Diamond, H. E., and Craver, L. F.: Uremia complicating leukemia chemotherapy: report of a case treated with triethylene malamine, J.A.M.A. 146:1595, 1951.

648. Krikler, D. M.: Paracetamol and the kidney, Brit. Med. J. 2:615, 1967.

649. Kuhn, W., Majer, H., Heusser, H., Rufinen, B. Z.: Kunstliche niere kapillarsystem fur den stoffaustausch, Experientia (Basel) 13:469, 1957.

650. Kunin, C. M.: A guide to use of antibiotics in patients with renal disease, Ann. Intern. Med. 67:151, 1967.

651. Kunin, C. M., Chalmers, T. C., Levy, C. M., Sebastyen, S. C., Lieber, C. S., and Finland, M.: Absorption of orally administered neomycin and kanamycin with special reference to patients with severe hepatic and renal disease, New Eng. J. Med. 262:380, 1960.

652. Kunin, C. M., and Finland, M.: Restrictions enforced on antibiotic therapy by renal failure, Arch. Int. Med. 104:1030, 1959.

653. Kunin, C. M., and Finland, M.: Persistence of antibiotics in blood of patients with acute renal failure. III. Penicillin, streptomycin, erythromycin and kanamycin, J. Clin. Invest. 38:1509, 1959.

654. Kunin, C. M., Glasko, A. J., and Finland, M.: Persistence of antibiotics in blood of patients with acute renal failure. II. Chloramphenicol and its metabolic products in

blood of patients with severe renal damage or hepatic cirrhosis, J. Clin. Invest. **38**:1498, 1959.

655. Kunin, C. M., Rees, S. B., Merrill, J. P., and Finland, M.: Persistence of antibiotics in blood of patients with acute renal failure: tetracycline and chloramphenicol, J. Clin. Invest. **38**:1487, 1959.

656. Kuntz, E.: Klinische untersuchungen zur nephrotoxicitat von kanamycin, Klin. Wchnschr. **40**:830, 1962.

657. Kuttner, H.: Beitrage zur kriegschirurgie der grossin blutize fassstomme. II. Die Verschultungsnekrose ganzer extremitaten, Bruns Beitrage Zur Klin. Chir. **112**:581, 1918.

658. Kupfer, S., and Rosenak, S.: A new parallel tube continous hemodialyzer, Trans. Amer. Soc. Artif. Int. Org. **5**:2, 1959.

659. Kurland, G. S., and Ravin, H. A.: Another case of nephrotoxicity associated with zoxazolamine, New Eng. J. Med. **261**:411, 1959.

660. Lakey, W. H.: Interstitial nephritis due to chronic phenacetin poisoning, Canad. Med. Ass. J. **85**:477, 1961.

661. Lamson, P. D., Minot, A. S., and Robbins, B. H.: The prevention and treatment of carbon tetrachloride intoxication, J.A.M.A. **90**:345, 1928.

662. Landsberg, M., and Gnoinski, H.: Recherches sur la diffusion de l'uree dans le peritonine sur le vivant, Compt. Rend. Soc. de Biol. **93**:787, 1925.

663. Landsteiner, E. K., and Finch, C. A.: Hemoglobinemia accompanying transurethral resection of the prostate, New Eng. J. Med. **237**:310, 1947.

664. Lang, P. A., and Jones, C. C.: Acute renal failure precipitated by quinine sulfate in early pregnancy, J.A.M.A. **188**:464, 1964.

665. Lange, K., Wasserman, E., and Slobody, L. B.: The significance of serum complement levels for the diagnosis and prognosis of acute and subacute glomerulonephritis and lupus erythematosus disseminatus, Ann. Intern. Med. **53**:635, 1960.

666. Lansing, A. M.: Arteriovenous shunts for chronic hemodialysis, Surg. Gynec. Obstet. **125**:775, 1967.

667. Lany, P.: Nephropathies par intolerance a la methicilline, Ann. Med. Nancy **2**:1489, 1963.

668. Laragh, J. H.: Ethacrynic acid and furosemide, Amer. Heart J. **75**:564, 1968.

669. Larsen, K., and Moller, C. E.: A renal lesion caused by abuse of phenacetin, Acta Med. Scand. **164**:53, 1959.

670. Larsson, H., and Palmlov, A.: Abdominal aortography with special reference to its complications, Acta. Radiology **38**:111, 1952.

671. Lassen, N. A., and Thomsen, A. C.: The pathogenesis of the hepatorenal syndrome, Acta. Med. Scand. **160**:165, 1958.

672. Latorraca, F.: Reperti anatomo-isto-patologici istochimici nell'intossicazione acuta sperimentale da sali di argento, Folia Med. **45**:1065, 1962.

673. Lattimer, J. K.: Plan for management of anuria, J. Urol. **54**:312, 1945.

674. Lauler, D. P., and Schreiner, G. E.: Bilateral renal cortical necrosis, Amer. J. Med. **24**:519, 1958.

675. Lauler, D. P., Schreiner, G. E., and David, A.: Renal medullary necrosis, Amer. J. Med. **29**:132, 1960.

676. Lawrence, H. S.: Uremia—nature's immunosuppressive device, Ann. Intern. Med. **62**:166, 1965.

677. Lawson, L. J., Blainey, J. D., Dawson-Edwards, P., and Tonge, S. M.: Dietary management of acute oliguric renal failure, Brit. Med. J. **2**:293, 1962.

678. Lawson, L. J., Blainey, J. D., Dawson-Edwards, P., and Dukes, D. C.: The minicoil artificial kidney, Lancet **2**:23, 1962.

679. Lear, H., and Oppenheimer, G. D.: Anuria following radiation therapy in leukemia, J.A.M.A. **143**:806, 1950.

680. Leathes, J. B., and Starling, E. H.: On the absorption of salt solutions from the pleural cavities, J. Physiol. **18**:106, 1895.

681. Leduc, E. H., and Holt, S. J.: "Hydroxpropyl methacrylate," a new water miscible embedding: medicines for electron microscopy, J. Cell Biology **26**:137, 1965.

781. Minami, S.: Uber nierenuerander ungen nach verschuttung, Virchons Arch. Path. Ann. **245**:247, 1923.

782. Mitchinson, M. J.: Systemic idiopathic fibrosis and systemic Weber-Christian disease, J. Clin. Path. **18**:645, 1966.

783. Moeschlin, S.: Phenacetinsucht und-schaden: innenkorperanamien und interstitielle nephritis, Schweiz Med. Wchnschr. **87**:123, 1957.

784. Moeschlin, S.: Zur Klinik und therapie der bleivergiftung mit bericht uber eine todliche toxische nephrose durch caedta (calciumversenat), Schweiz Med. Wchnschr. **87**:1091, 1957.

785. Montgomerie, J. G., Kalmanson, G. M., and Guze, L. B.: Renal failure and infection, Medicine **47**:1, 1968.

786. Moody, E. A.: The therapeutic use of peritoneal lavage for anuria caused by toxic nephritis, J. Pediat. **33**:710, 1948.

787. Moolten, S. E., and Smith, I. B.: Fatal nephritis in chronic phenacetin poisoning, Amer. J. Med. **23**:127, 1960.

788. Moore, C. A., and Dodson, C. C.: Reflex anuria: report of a case, U.S. Armed Forces Med. J. **5**:549, 1954.

789. Moore, D. V., and Lanier, J. E.: Observations on two plasmodium falciparum infections with an abnormal response to chloroquine, Amer. J. Trop. Med. **10**:5, 1961.

790. Moore, F. D.: Tris buffer, mannitol and low viscous dextran: 3 new solutions for old problems, Surg. Clin. N. Amer. **43**:577, 1963.

791. Moore, R. A., Goldstein, S., and Canowitz, A.: The mitochondria in acute experimental nephrosis due to mercuric chloride, Arch. Path. **8**:930, 1929.

792. Morgan, A. D., Loughridge, I. W., and Calne, R. Y.: Combined mediastinal and retroperitoneal fibrosis, Lancet **1**:67, 1966.

793. Morgan, I. O., Little, J. M., and Evans, W. A.: Renal failure associated with low molecular weight dextran infusion, Brit. Med. J. **2**:737, 1966.

794. Morin, Y., and Daniel, P.: Quebec beer-drinkers' cardiomyopathy: etiological considerations, Canad. Med. Ass. J. **97**:926, 1967.

795. Morrin, P. A. F., Handa, S. P., Valberg, L. S., Bencosme, S. A., Kipkir, G. F., and Wyllie, J. C.: Acute renal failure in association with fatty liver of pregnancy, Amer. J. Med. **42**:844, 1967.

796. Morse, K. M., and Setterlind, A. N.: Arsine poisoning in the smelting and refining industry, Arch. Indust. Hyg. **2**:148, 1950.

797. Morton, H. D.: Temporary suppression of urine following double pyelography, J. Urol. **10**:261, 1923.

798. Moschcovitz, E.: An acute febrile pleiochromic anemia with hyaline thrombosis of the terminal arterioles and capillaries: an undescribed disease, Arch. Intern. Med. **36**:89, 1925.

799. Moser, R. H.: Diseases of medical progress: progress report, Clin. Pharmacol. Therap. **2**:446, 1961.

800. Mostofi, F. K., Vorder Bruegge, C. F., and Diggs, L. W.: Lesions in kidneys removed for unilateral hematuria in sickle-cell disease, Arch. Path. **63**:336, 1957.

801. Moyer, C. A.: Acute temporary changes in renal function associated with major surgical procedures, Surgery **27**:198, 1950.

802. Movat, H. Z., Steiner, J. W., and Huhn, D.: The fine structure of the glomerulus in acute glomerulonephritis, Lab. Invest. **11**:117, 1962.

803. Moyer, J. H., Mills, L. C., and Yow, E. M.: Toxicity of polymyxin B. 1. Animal studies with particular reference to evaluation of renal function, Arch. Int. Med. **92**:238, 1953.

804. Muehlberger, C. W., Oevenhart, A. S., and O'Malley, T. S.: Arsine intoxication: a case of suspected poisoning in the steel industry, J. Indust. Hyg. **10**:137, 1928.

804a. Muehrcke, R. C.: Interstitial nephritis, Chicago Med. **71**:211, 1968.

805. Muehrcke, R. C., Kark, R. M., and Pirani, C. L.: Technique of percutaneous renal biopsy in the prone position, J. Urol. **74**:267, 1955.

805a Muehrcke, R. C., Kark, R. M., Pirani, C. L., and Pollak, V. E.: Renal biopsy, technique and clinical application, Proc. Royal Soc. Med. **49**:327, 1955.

806. Muehrcke, R. C., Pirani, C. L., and Kark, R. M.: Interstitial nephritis: a clinicopathological and renal biopsy study, Ann. Intern. Med. **66**:1052, 1967.

806a. Muehrcke, R. C., and Pirani, C. L.: Arsine-induced anuria: a correlative clinicpathological study with electron microscopic observations, Ann. Intern. Med. **68**:853, 1968.

807. Muehrcke, R. C., Rosen, S., Pirani, C. L., and Kark, R. M.: Renal lesions in patients recovering from acute renal failure (Abstract), J. Lab. Clin. Invest. **64**:888, 1964.

808. Mueller, C. B.: The pathogenesis of acute renal failure. In Brest, A. N., and Moyer, J. H., editors: Renal failure, Philadelphia, 1967, J. B. Lippincott Co.

809. Muirhead, E. E.: Incompatible blood transfusions with emphasis on acute renal failure, Surg., Gynec. Obstet. **92**:734, 1951.

810. Muirhead, E. E., Daniels, E. G., Pike, J. E., and Hinman, J. W.: Renomedullary antihypertensive lipids and the prostaglanins. Nobel Symposium, Interscience Publishers, New York, 1967.

811. Muirhead, E. E., Vanatta, J., and Grollman, A.: Acute renal insufficiency: a comparison of the use of an artificial kidney, peritoneal lavage and more conservative measures in its management, Arch. Intern. Med. **83**:528, 1949.

812. Mulinari, A., and Hegstrom, R. M.: Hemodialysis in acute renal failure. In Shaldon, S., and Cook, G. C., editors: Acute renal failure: a symposium, Philadelphia, 1964, F. A. Davis Co.

813. Munck, O.: Renal circulation in acute renal failure, Oxford, 1958, Blackwell Scientific Publications.

814. Munck, O., Lassen, N., Deetjen, P., and Kramer, K.: Evidence against renal hypoxia in acute haemorrhagia shock, Pflugers Arch. Ges. Physiol. **274**:356, 1962.

815. Munro, J. F., Geddes, A. M., and Lamb, W. L.: Goodpasture's syndrome: survival following acute renal failure, Brit. Med. J. **4**:95, 1967.

816. Murphy, F. D.: Acute toxic nephrosis, Postgrad. Med. **12**:3, 1952.

817. Murphy, F. D., Kuzma, J. F., Polley, T. Z., and Grill, J.: Clinicopathologic studies of renal damage due to sulfonamide compounds: a report of 14 cases, Arch. Intern. Med. **73**:433, 1944.

818. Murphy, G. P., Gagnon, J. A., Johnson, G. S., and Teschan, P. E.: Renal hemodynamics and function in experimental hemorrhagic hypotension: effects of osmotic diuresis, J. Urol. **93**:529, 1965.

819. Murray, J. S., Hegstrom, R. M., Pendras, J. P., Burnell, J. M., and Scribner, B. H.: Continuous flow hemodialysis and bypass cannulas in the management of acute renal failure, Trans. Amer. Soc. Artif. Int. Org. **7**:94, 1961.

820. Mustakallio, K. K., and Telkka, A.: Histochemical localization of the mercurial inhibition of succinic dehydrogenase in rat kidney, Science **118**:320, 1953.

821. Myers, J. K., Storrs, D., Miller, T. B., and Mueller, C. B.: The role of tubular flow in pathogenesis of traumatic renal failure, Surg. Gynec. Obstet. **123**:1243, 1966.

822. Myers, W. A.: Obstructive anuria, J.A.M.A. **85**:10, 1925.

823. Myhre, J. R., Brodwall, E. K., and Knutsen, S. B.: Acute renal failure following intravenous pyelography in cases of myelomatosis, Acta. Med. Scand. **156**:263, 1956.

824. Myler, R. K, Lee, J. C., Hopper, J.: Renal tubular necrosis caused by mushroom poisoning, Arch. Intern. Med. **114**:196, 1964.

825. Nahum, L. H.: Phenacetin nephritis, Medicine **27**:297, 1963.

826. Nakamoto, S., Dunea, G., Kolff, W. J., and McCormack, L. J.: Acute renal failure—oliguric: treatment of oliguric glomerulonephritis with dialysis and steroids, Ann. Int. Med. **63**:359, 1965.

827. Nathan, D. A., Meitus, M. L., Capland, L., and Lev, M.: Death following phenylbutazone (Butazolidin) therapy: report of case, Ann. Intern. Med. **39**:1096, 1953.

828. Nau, C. A.: Accidental generation of arsine gas in industry, South. Med. J. **41**:341, 1948.

829. Necheles, H.: Uber dialysieren des stromenden blutes am lebenden, Klin. Wchnschr. **2**:1257, 1923.

830. Nelson, A. A., Radomski, J. L., and Hogan, E. C.: Renal and other lesions in dogs and rats from intramuscular injection of neomycin, Fed. Proc. **10**:366, 1951.

831. Nelson, E.: Crystalluria potential of cholecystographic agents, New Eng. J. Med. **268**:1236, 1963.

832. Nelson, E., and Levy, G.: Precautions indicated with cholecystographic agents, Arch. Surg. **88**:921, 1964.

833. Neuwirtova, R., Chytil, M., Valek, A., Daum, A., and Valach, V.: Acute renal failure following an occupational intoxication with arsine (AsH$_3$) treated by the artificial kidney, Acta. Med. Scand. **170**:535, 1961.

834. Newburg, L. H., and Camara, A. A.: Lack of correlation between symptoms and degree of renal impairment, Ann. Intern. Med. **35**:39, 1951.

835. Niall, J. F., and Doyle, J. C.: Renal failure associated with dextran infusions. Proceedings of The Third International Congress of Nephrology, Washington, 1966.

836. Noltenius, H.: Observations historadiographiques avec 3H thymidine sur la regeneration renale apres intoxication au sublime chez le rat, Proceedings of the Second International Congress of Nephrology, Prague, 1963.

837. Nordenfelt, O., and Ringertz, N.: Phenacetin takers dead with renal failure: 27 men and 3 women, Acta. Med. Scand. **170**:385, 1961.

838. Nordyke, R. A., and Tonchen, A.: The radiohippuran renogram, J.A.M.A. **183**:144, 1963.

839. Oard, H. C., and Walker, G. I.: Clinical management of the anuric patient, Amer. J. Med. **18**:199, 1955.

840. Ober, W. B., Bruno, M. S., Weinberg, S. B., Jones, F. M., Jr., and Weiner, L.: Fatal intravascular sickling in a patient with sickle-cell trait, New Eng. J. Med. **263**:947, 1960.

841. Ober, W. E., Reid, D. E., Romney, S. L., and Merrill, J. P.: Renal lesions and acute renal failure in pregnancy, Amer. J. Med. **21**:781, 1956.

842. O'Connor, V. J.: Oliguria and auria, Ill. Med. J. **112**:105, 1957.

842a. O'Connor, V. J., Jr., Libretti, J. V., and Grayhack, J. T.: Early differential diagnosis of post-operative anuria using radioactive renogram: an experimental study, J. Urol. **86**:276, 1961.

843. Odel, H. M., and Ferris, D. O.: Treatment of acute renal insufficiency with peritoneal lavage, Proc. Staff Meet. Mayo Clinic **22**:305, 1947.

844. Odel, H. M., and Popp, W. C.: Lymphoblastoma with signs of renal involvement improved by roentgen therapy: report of three cases, Radiology **31**:687, 1938.

844a. O'Grady, J. A.: Bleeding tendency in uremia, J.A.M.A. **169**:1727, 1959.

845. Oliver, J.: Experimental nephritis in the frog. IV. Significance of the functional response to vascular and to parenchymal disturbances in the kidney, J. Exper. Med. **55**:295, 1932.

846. Oliver, J.: New directions in renal morphology: a method, its results, and its future, Harvey Lectures **40**:102, 1944-45.

847. Oliver, J.: Correlations of structure and function and mechanism of recovery in acute tubular necrosis, Amer. J. Med. **15**:535, 1953.

848. Oliver, J., and MacDowell, M.: The renal lesion in epidemic hemorrhagic fever, J. Clin. Invest. **36**:99, 1957.

849. Oliver, J., MacDowell, M., and Tracy, A.: The pathogenesis of acute renal failure associated with traumatic and toxic injury: renal ischemia, nephrotoxic damage, and the ischemuric episode, J. Clin. Invest. **30**:1307, 1951.

850. Ono, I.: Studies on myoglobin, Tohoku J. Exper. Med. **57**:273, 1953.

851. Orbison, J. L.: Morphology of a thrombotic thrombocytopenic purpura with demonstration of aneurysms, Amer. J. Path. **28**:129, 1952.

852. Ormond, J. K.: Bilateral ureteral obstruction due to envelopment and compression by inflammatory retroperitoneal processes, J. Urol. **59**:1072, 1948.

853. Osler, W.: The principles and practice of medicine, New York, 1892, Appleton-Century-Crofts, Inc.

854. Osler, W.: Principles and practice of medicine, ed. 2, New York, 1895, Appleton-Century-Crofts Company.

855. Osler, W.: The principles and practice of medicine, ed. 7, New York, 1909, Appleton-Century-Crofts.

318 *References*

856. Oulmont, P.: Deux cas d'esapoismnement suivis de mort par l'hydrogene servant a gonfler les ballons, Med. Mod. 1:933, 1890.

857. Owen, D.: Renal failure due to para-aminosalicylic acid, Brit. Med. J. 2:483, 1958.

858. Palmer, R. A., and Henry, E. W.: The clinical course of acute renal failure, Canad. Med. Ass. J. 77:1078, 1957.

859. Pappas, G., Davis, R. L., and Thomas, L.: Studies on the generalized Shwartzman reaction. VI. Appearance by electron microscopy of intravascular fibrinoid in the glomerular capillaries during the reaction, J. Exper. Med. 107:333, 1958.

860. Pappenheimer, J. R., and Kinter, W. B.: Hematocrit ratio of blood within Mammalian kidneys and its significance for renal hemodynamics, Amer. J. Physiol. 185:377, 1956.

861. Papper, S.: Role of kidney in Laennec's cirrhosis of liver, Medicine, 37:299, 1958.

862. Papper, S., Belsky, J. L., and Bleifer, K. H.: Renal failure in Laennec's cirrhosis of the liver. I. Description of clinical and laboratory features, Case reports 51:759, 1959.

863. Papper, S., and Saxon, L.: The diuretic response to administer water in liver disease. II. Laennec's cirrhosis. Arch. Int. Med. 103:750, 1959.

864. Parrish, A. E., Rubenstein, N. H., and Howe, J. S.: Acute renal insufficiency associated with respiratory infections, Amer. J. Med. 18:237, 1955.

865. Parrish, H. M., and Carr, C. A.: Bites by copperheads (*Ancistrodon contortrix*) in the United States, J.A.M.A. 201:927, 1967.

866. Parsons, F. M., and McCraken, B. H.: The use and function of the artificial kidney, Brit. J. Urol. 30:463, 1958.

867. Parsons, F. M., and McCracken, B. H.: The artificial kidney, Brit. Med. J. 1:740, 1959.

867a. Paterson, H. di C.: Acute encephalopathy associated with renal hemodialysis: The reverse urea effect, Neurology (Minneap.) 13:358, 1963.

868. Paterson, J. C. S., and Sprague, C. C.: Observations on genesis of crises in sickle cell anemia, Ann. Int. Med. 50:1502, 1959.

869. Pavy, F. W.: On the physiological effect of this substance on animals, Guy Hosp. Rep., Ser. 3, 6:505, 1860.

870. Pease, D. C.: Histological techniques for electron microscopy, ed. 2, New York, 1965, Academic Press.

871. Pendergrass, E. P., Chamberlain, G. W., Godfrey, W. E., and Burdick, E. D.: Survey of deaths in unfavorable sequelae following administration of contrast media, Amer. J. Roentgen. 48:741, 1942.

871a. Pendergrass, E. P., Hodes, P. J., Tondreau, R. E., Powell, C. C., and Burdick, E. D.: Further consideration of deaths and unfavorable sequelae following the administration of contrast media in urography in the United States, Amer. J. Roentgen. 74:262, 1955.

872. Peschel, E., McIntosh, H. D., Brown, I. W., Jr., and Murdaugh, H. V.: Acute tubular necrosis after transfusion reaction due to anti-Kell antibodies, J.A.M.A. 167:1736, 1958.

873. Pendras, J.: Ethylene glycol poisoning, an indication for hemodialysis, Clin. Res. 11:118, 1963.

874. Perilie, P. E., and Conn, H. O.: Acute renal failure after intravenous pyelography in plasma cell myeloma, J.A.M.A. 167:2186, 1958.

875. Perimutter, M.: Unusual cases of acute tubular necrosis, Ann. Intern. Med. 47:81, 1957.

876. Persky, L., and Chambers, D.: Calculus formation and ureteral colic following acetazolamide (Diamox) therapy, J.A.M.A. 161:1625, 1956.

877. Peters, G., and Hedwall, P. R.: Aristolochic acid intoxication: a new type of impairment of urinary concentrating ability, Arch. Int. Pharmacodyn. 145:334, 1963.

878. Peters, J. P., Eisenman, A. J., and Kydd, D. M.: Mercury poisoning, Amer. J. Med. Sci. 185:149, 1933.

879. Peters, J. T.: Oliguria and anuria due to increased intrarenal pressure, Ann. Intern. Med. 28:221, 1945.

880. Petersdorf, R. G., and Plorde, J. J.: Colistin, a reappraisal, J.A.M.A. 183:123, 1963.

881. Petersilge, C. L.: Prolonged anuria following single injection of bismuth preparation, J. Pediat. 31:580, 1947.

882. Phillips, R. A., and Hamilton, P. B.: The effect of 20, 60 and 120 minutes of renal ischemia on glomerular and tubular function, Amer. J. Physiol. 152:523, 1948.

883. Piazza, A., Chaname, W., Cauti, D., and Maya, L.: Acute renal failure due to spider bite (*Loxosceles laeta*), Washington, D.C., 1966, International Congress of Nephrology.

884. Pigeon, G., LeFebvre, R., Cartier, G. E., and Genest, J.: Unilateral renal damage after translumbar aortography, Canad. Med. Ass. J. **83**:69, 1960.

885. Pinto, S. S., Petronella, S. J., Johns, D. R., and Arnold, M. F.: Arsine poisoning, a study of thirteen cases, Arch. Hyg. Occup. Med. **1**:437, 1950.

886. Pitts, R. F.: Physiology of the kidney and body fluids, Chicago, 1963, Year Book Medical Publishers, Inc.

887. Pletscher, A., Studer, A., and Miescher, P.: Experimental investigations of erythrocytic and organ changes due to N-acetyl-p-aminophenol and phenacetin, Schwiez. Med. Wchnschr. **88**:1214, 1958.

888. Plummer, N., and Wheeler, C.: Toxicity of sulfadiazine; observations of 1357 cases, Amer. J. Med. Sci. **207**:175, 1944.

889. Pollak, V. E., and Nettles, J. B.: The kidney in toxemia of pregnancy, Medicine (Balt.) **39**:469, 1960.

890. Pollak, V. E., Pirani, C. L., Seskind, C., and Griffel, B.: Bilateral renal vein thrombosis: clinical and electromicroscopic studies of a case with complete recovery following anticoagulant therapy, Ann. Intern. Med. **65**:1056, 1966.

891. Pons, C. A., and Custer, R. P.: Acute ethylene glycol poisoning: A clinicopathologic report of 18 fatal cases, Amer. J. Med. Sci. **211**:544, 1946.

892. Porporis, A. A., Elliott, G. V., Fischer, C. L., and Mueller, C. P.: The mechanism of urokon excretion, Amer. J. Radiol. **72**:995, 1954.

893. Powell, L. W., and Hooker, J. W.: Neomycin nephropathy, J.A.M.A. **160**:557, 1956.

894. Powers, S. R., Jr., Boba, A., Hostnik, W., and Stein, A.: Prevention of postoperative acute renal failure with mannitol in 100 cases, Surgery **55**:15, 1964.

895. Pratt-Thomas, H. R., and Switzer, P. K.: Sicklemia: its pathological and clinical significance, Southern Med. J. **42**:376, 1949.

896. Price, J. D. E., and Palmer, R. A.: A function and morphological follow-up study of acute renal failure, Arch. Int. Med. (Chicago) **105**:114, 1960.

897. Pringle, H., Maunsell, C. B., and Pringle, S.: Clinical effects of ether anesthesia on renal activity, Brit. Med. J. **2**:542, 1905.

898. Putman, T. J.: The living peritoneum as a dialyzing membrane, Amer. J. Phys. **63**:548, 1922-23.

899. Pyrtek, L. J., and Bartus, S. A.: Hepatic pyemia, New Eng. J. Med. **272**:555, 1965.

900. Quinby, W. C., and Austin, G., Jr.: Suppression of urine complication pyelography, New Eng. J. Med. **221**:814, 1939.

901. Rackermann, F. M., Longcope, W. T., and Peters, J. P.: The excretion of chlorides and water and the renal function in serum disease, Arch. Intern. Med. **18**:496, 1916.

902. Rackley, C. E., Mengel, C. E., Pomerantz, M., and McIntosh, H. D.: Vascular complications with use of methysergide, Arch. Intern. Med. **117**:265, 1966.

903. Ramsay, A. G., and White, D. F.: Phenacetin nephropathy, Canad. Med. Ass. J. **92**:55, 1965.

904. Randall, R. E., Jr.: Renal failure following antibiotics, Ann. Intern. Med. **66**:1056, 1967.

905. Randall, R. E., Jr., Singh, R., Laster, J., Belle, C., and Setter, J. G.: Increased intracranial pressure from unsustained levels of plasma mannitol during hemodialysis, J. Lab. Clin. Med. **70**:129, 1967.

906. Raper, F. P.: Idiopathic retroperitoneal fibrosis involving the ureters, Brit. J. Urol. **28**:436, 1956.

907. Rapoport, A., White, L. W., and Ranking, G. N.: Renal damage associated with chronic phenacetin overdosage, Ann. Intern. Med. **57**:970, 1962.

908. Rath, C. E., Mailliard, J. A., and Schreiner, G. E.: Bleeding tendency in uremia, New Eng. J. Med. **257**:808, 1957.

909. Ravdin, I. S.: Vasodepressor substances in the liver: after obstruction of the common duct, Arch. Surg. **18**:2191, 1929.

910. Ravid, J. M., and Chesner, C.: A fatal case of hemolytic anemia and nephrotic uremia following sulfapyridine administration, Amer. J. Med. Sci. **199**:280, 1940.

911. Reid, R., Penfold, J. B., and Jones, R. N.: Anuria treated by renal decapsulation and peritoneal dialysis, Lancet **2**:749, 1946.

912. Reidbord, H. E., and Hawk, W. A.: Idiopathic retroperitoneal fibrosis and necrotizing vasculitis, Cleveland Clin. Quart. **32**:19, 1965.

913. Reidenberg, M. M., Powers, D. V., Sevy, R. W., and Bella, C. T.: Acute renal failure due to nephrotoxins, Amer. J. Med. Sci. **247**:25, 1964.

914. Reimann, H. A., and Sukaton, R. U.: Djenkol bean poisoning (Djenkolism), a case of hematuria and anuria, Amer. J. Med. Sci. **232**:172, 1956.

915. Rene, R. M., and Mellinkoff, S. M.: Renal insufficiency after oral administration of a double dose of a cholecystographic medium; report of two cases, New Eng. J. Med. **261**:589, 1959.

916. Rennie, I. D. B.: Acute renal changes after oral cholecystography, Lancet **2**:645, 1964.

917. Reuber, M. D., and Bradley, J. E.: Acute versenate nephrosis occurring as a result of treatment for lead intoxication, J.A.M.A. **174**:263, 1960.

918. Reubi, F. C., Gurtler, R., and Gossweiler, N.: A dye dilution method of measuring renal blood flow in man, with special reference to the anuric subject, Proc. Soc. Exp. Biol. Med. **111**:760, 1962.

919. Reynolds, E. S., Tomkiewicz, Z. M., and Dammin, G. J.: The renal lesion related to amphotericin B treatment for coccidioidomycosis, Med. Clin. N. Amer. **47**:1149, 1963.

920. Reynolds, T. B.: Phenacetin nephritis, Amer. Heart J. **67**:845, 1964.

921. Reynolds, T. B., and Edmondson, H. A.: Chronic renal disease and heavy use of analgesics, J.A.M.A. **184**:435, 1963.

922. Rhoads, J. E.: Peritoneal lavage in the treatment of renal insufficiency, Amer. J. Med. Sci. **196**:642, 1938.

923. Rich, A. R.: The role of hypersensitivity in periarteritis nodosa as indicated by 7 cases developing during serum sickness and sulfonamide therapy, Bull. Johns Hopkins Hosp. **71**:123, 1942.

924. Richards, A. N.: Direct observations of change in function of the renal tubule caused by certain poisons, Trans. Ass. Amer. Physicians **44**:64, 1929.

925. Richardson, J. H., and Alderfer, H. H.: Acute renal failure caused by phenylbutazone, New Eng. J. Med. **268**:809, 1963.

926. Richmond, G. H., and Beardsley, G. D.: Nitrogen mustard therapy complicated by acute renal failure due to uric acid crystallization, Ann. Intern. Med. **39**:1327, 1953.

927. Richmond, J., Sherman, R. S., Diamond, H. D., and Craver, L. F.: Renal lesions associated with malignant lymphomas, Amer. J. Med. **32**:184, 1962.

928. Ricketts, W. E.: Clinical manifestations of Carrion's disease. Arch. Intern. Med. **84**:751, 1949.

929. Riddle, M., Gardner, F., Beswick, I., and Filshie, I.: The nephrotic syndrome complicating mercurial diuretic therapy, Brit. Med. J. **1**:1274, 1958.

930. Riff, D. P., Wilson, D. M., Dunea, G., Schwartz, F. D., and Kark, R. M.: Renocortical necrosis: partial recovery after 49 days of oliguria, Arch. Intern. Med. **119**:518, 1967.

931. Ringertz, O., and Melen, B.: Hepatitis and the artificial kidney, Lancet **1**:151, 1966.

932. Robertson, H. R., and Rutherford, P. S.: Peritoneal irrigation in the treatment of renal failure due to transfusion reaction, J. Lab. Clin. Med. **32**:982, 1947.

933. Robin, E. D., Davis, R. P., and Rees, S. B.: Salicylate intoxication with special reference to the development of hypokalemia, Amer. J. Med. **26**:869, 1949.

934. Robinson, G. C., and Wong, I. C.: Acute tubular necrosis in infancy and childhood, J. Dis. Child. **95**:417, 1958.

935. Robson, J. S.: Drug-induced renal disease, Practitioner **181**:288, 1958.

936. Rocha, H., Guze, L. B., Freeman, L. R., and Beeson, P. B.: Experimental pyelonephritis. III. The influence of localized injury in different parts of the kidney on susceptibility to bacillary infection, Yale J. Biol. Med. **103**:109, 1956.

937. Rodin, A. E., and Crowson, C. N.: Mercury nephrotoxicity in the rat. I. Factors influencing the localization of the tubular lesions, Amer. J. Path. **41**:297, 1962.

938. Rodin, A. E., and Crowson, C. M.: Mercury nephrotoxicity in the rat. II. Investigation of the intracellular site of mercury nephrotoxicity by correlated serial time histologic and histoenzymatic studies, Amer. J. Path. **41**:485, 1962.

939. Rodriguez-Erdmann, F.: Pathogenes of bilateral renal cortical necrosis: production by means of exogenons fibrin, Arch. Path. (Chicago) **79**:615, 1965.

939a. Rogers, L.: Bowel diseases in the tropics. London, 1921, Hodder and Stoughton Ltd.

940. Rosen, A. P., and Scanlan, J. J.: Favism, New Eng. J. Med. **239**:367, 1948.

941. Rosen, S. M., O'Conner, K., and Shaldon, S.: Dialysis disequilibrium. In Shaldon, S., and Cook, G. C., editors: Acute renal failure: a symposium, Philadelphia, 1964, F. A. Davis Co.

942. Rosenbaum, J. L.: Differential diagnosis of acute renal failure. In Brest, A. N., and Moyer, J. H., editors: Renal failure, ed. 1, Philadelphia, 1967, J. B. Lippincott Co.

943. Rosenbaum, J. L., and Black, M. W.: Hemodialysis for acute carbon tetrachloride poisoning, J. Albert Einstein Med. Center **12**:200, 1964.

944. Rosenblum, J., Sonnenschein, H., and Minsky, A.: Trimethadione (Tridione) nephrois, Amer. J. Dis. Child. **97**:790, 1959.

945. Rosin, R. D.: Cantharides intoxication, Brit. Med. J. **2**:33, 1967.

946. Roy, A. D.: Acute renal failure after aortography, Lancet **2**:16, 1957.

947. Rubini, M. E.: Renal residuals of acute epidemic hemorritagic fever, Arch. Intern. Med. **106**:378, 1960.

948. Rush, B. F., Fishbein, R., and Wilder, R. J.: Effect of operative trauma upon renal function in older patients, Ann. Surg. **162**:863, 1965.

949. Russell, K. P., MaHarry, J. F., and Stehly, J. W.: Acute renal failure as an obstetric complication, J.A.M.A. **157**:15, 1955.

950. Rutenburg, A. M.: The clinical use of sulfisomidine in urinary tract infections, Ann. N. Y. Acad. Sci. **69**:389, 1957.

951. Salisbury, P. F.: Timely versus delayed use of the artificial kidney, Arch. Intern. Med. **101**:690, 1958.

951a. Salisbury, P. F.: Recovery from acute renal failure and acidosis in sickle-cell disease, J.A.M.A. **174**:356, 1960.

952. Sanford, W. G., Rasch, J. R., and Stonehill, R. B.: A therapeutic dilemma. The treatment of disseminated coccidioidomycosis with amphotericin B, Ann. Int. Med. **56**:553, 1962.

953. Sanghvi, L. M., Sharma, R., Mirsa, S. N., and Samuel, K. C.: Sulfhemoglobinemia and acute renal insufficiency after copper sulfate poisoning; report of two fatal cases, Arch. Path. **63**:172, 1957.

954. Sarre, H., and Knorr, R.: Fuhrt die sog. osmotische nephrose oder zuckerspeicherniere zur niereninsuffizienz?, Klin. Wchnschr. **41**:311, 1963.

955. Sartorius, H.: Our experience with the disposable Kolff-coil kidney, Trans. Amer. Soc. Artif. Intern. Organs **3**:74, 1957.

956. Savino, F. M.: Dialyzer chamber with capillary system for artificial kidney, J. Urol. **83**:867, 1960.

957. Schaar, F. E., and LaBru, J. W.: Gleason, D. F.: Paroxysmal myohemoglobinuria with fatal renal tubular injury, J. Lab. Clin. Med. **34**:1744, 1947.

958. Schachter, D., and Manis, J. G.: Salicylate and salicyl conjugates. Fluorometric estimation, biosynthesis and renal excretion in man, J. Clin. Invest. **37**:800, 1958.

959. Schaefer, A. E., Parry, W. L., and Mueller, C. B.: Experimental studies of acute renal failure. III. Histopathology of the renal lesion produced by methemoglobin, J. Surg. Res. **6**:247, 1966.

960. Schatz, A., Bugie, E., and Waksman, S. A.: Streptomycin, a substance exhibiting antibiotic activity against gram-positive and gram-negative bacteria, Proc. Soc. Exper. Biol. Med. **55**:66, 1944.

961. Schechter, A. J., Cary, M. K., Carpentier, A. L., and Darrow, D. C.: Changes in composition of fluids injected into the peritoneal cavity, Amer. J. Dis. Child. **46**:1015, 1933.

962. Scheitlin, W., and Jeanneret, P.: Uber akute nierenschadigungen unter phenylbutazontherapie, Schweiz. Med. Wchnschr. **87**:881, 1957.

963. Schindel, L.: Unexpected reactions to kanamycin, Israel Med. J. 23:131, 1964.

964. Schloerb, P. R.: Management of uremia by perfusion of isolated jejunum segment: with observation on dynamics of water and electrolyte exchange in human jejunum, J. Clin. Invest. 37:1818, 1958.

965. Schmidt, P. J., and Holland, P. V.: Pathogenesis of the acute renal failure associated with incompatible transfusion, Lancet 2:1169, 1967.

966. Schmidt, P. J., Peden, J. C., Brecher, G., and Baranovsky, A.: Thrombocytopenia and bleeding tendency after extracorporeal circulation, New Eng. J. Med. 265:1181, 1961.

967. Schnall, C., and Wiener, J. S.: Nephrosis occurring during tolbutamide administration, J.A.M.A. 167:214, 1958.

968. Schoeffel, M. E., Arean, V. M., and Gravenstein, J. S.: Liver and kidney after anesthesia, Southern Med. J. 58:198, 1965.

969. Schoenbach, E. B., Bryer, M. S., and Lang, P. H.: The clinical use of polymyxin, Ann. N. Y. Acad. Sci. 51:987, 1949.

969a. Schonlein, J. L.: Allgemeine erud speciello. Pathologie erud therapie, Herisan Lit. Compt. 2:45, 1837.

970. Schourup, K., Orskow, I., Orskov, F., and Bartels, E. D.: Phenacetin as the cause of kidney damage in rabbits, Danish Med. Bull. 10:85, 1963.

971. Schreiner, G. E.: Treatment of acute renal insufficiency, Med. Ann. D. C. 22:531-535, 1953.

972. Schreiner, G. E.: The role of hemodialysis (artificial kidney) in acute poisoning, Arch. Intern. Med. 102:896, 1958.

973. Schreiner, G. E.: The nephrotoxicity of analgesic abuse, Ann. Int. Med. 57:1047, 1962.

974. Schreiner, G. E.: Toxic nephropathy, Med. Ann. D.C. 33:287, 1964.

975. Schreiner, G. E., and Berman, L. B.: The clinical spectrum of postpartum acute renal insufficiency, Ann. Intern. Med. 43:1230, 1955.

976. Schreiner, G. E., and Maher, J. F.: Dialysis of poisons, Acad. Med. New J. Bull. 6:310, 1960.

977. Schreiner, G. E., and Maher, J. F.: The patient with chronic renal failure and surgery, Amer. J. Cardiol. 12:317, 1961.

978. Schreiner, G. E., and Maher, J. F.: Uremia: Biochemistry, pathogenesis and treatment, Springfield, Ill., 1961, Charles C Thomas, Publisher.

979. Schreiner, G. E., and Maher, J. F.: Toxic nephropathy, Amer. J. Med. 38:409, 1965.

980. Schreiner, G. E., Maher, J. F., and Golden, A.: Nephrotoxicity of analgesic abuse. In Excerpta Medica International Congress, Series No. 78, Proceedings of Second International Congress of Nephrology, Prague, 1963.

981. Scribner, B. H.: Syllabus for the course on fluid and electrolyte balance, Seattle, 1953, Fluid Research Fund.

982. Scribner, B. H., Caner, J. E. Z., Buri, R., and Quinton, W.: The technique of continuous hemodialysis, Trans. Amer. Soc. Artif. Intern. Organs. 6:88, 1960.

983. Scribner, B. H., Korenski, W. R., Marr, T. A., and Burnell, J. M.: Gastrodialysis in the treatmen of acute renal failure, Trans. Amer. Soc. Artif. Intern. Organs. 4:32, 1958

984. Schrier, R. W., Henderson, H. S., Tisher, C. C., and Tannen, R. L.: Nephropathy associated with heat stress and exercise, Ann. Intern. Med. 67:356, 1967.

985. Schroeder, H. A.: Renal failure associated with low extracellular sodium chloride, the low salt syndrome, J.A.M.A. 141:117, 1949.

986. Schulz, E. G., and Murphy, F. D.: Treatment of acute renal failure, Arch. Intern. Med. 103:453, 1959.

987. Schwartz, F. D., and Dunea, G.: Progression of retroperitoneal fibrosis despite cessation of treatment with methysergide, Lancet 1:955, 1966.

988. Schwartz, W. B., Bennett, W., Curelop, S., and Bartter, F. C.: A syndrome of renal sodium loss and hyponatremia probably resulting from inappropriate secretion of antidiuretic hormone, Amer. J. Med. 23:529, 1957.

989. Schweinburg, F. B., Frank, H. A., Frank, E. D., Heimberg, F., and Fine, J.: Trans-

mural migration of intestinal bacteria during peritoneal irrigation in uremic dogs, Proc. Soc. Exp. Biol. Med. **71**:150, 1949.

990. Scott, J. T., Denman, A. M., and Dorling, J.: Renal irritation caused by salicylates, Lancet **1**:344, 1963.

991. Scudi, J. V., and Antopol, W.: Some pharmacologic characteristics of bacitracin, Proc. Soc. Exp. Biol. Med. **64**:503, 1947.

992. Sebesin, S. M., and Bethesda, M. D.: Renal failure and disseminated candidiasis, Arch. Intern. Med. **110**:172, 1962.

993. Selkurt, E. E.: The changes in renal clearance following complete ischemia of the kidney, Amer. J. Physiol. **144**:395, 1945.

994. Setter, J. G., Maher, J. F., and Schreiner, G. E.: Acute renal failure following cholecystography, J.A.M.A. **184**:102, 1963.

995. Sevitt, S.: Distal tubular and proximal tubular necrosis in the kidneys of burned patients, J. Clin. Path. **9**:279, 1956.

996. Sevitt, S.: Pathogenesis of traumatic uraemia, Lancet **2**:135, 1959.

997. Shackman, R., Milne, M. D., and Struthers, N. W.: Oliguric renal failure of surgical origin, Brit. Med. J. **2**:1473, 1960.

998. Shaffer, B., Burgoon, C. F., and Gosman, J. H.: Acute glomerulonephritis following administration of rhus toxin. Report of a fatal and near fatal case, J.A.M.A. **146**:1570, 1951.

999. Shaldon, S., Rosen, S. M., Silva, H., Rae, A. I., Pomeroy, J., and Ryder, J.: Effects of chlorothiazide on renal ammonia production, plasma electrolytes and acid-base balance in acute renal failure, Proc. Soc. Exp. Biol. Med. **113**:983, 1963.

1000. Shaldon, S., Silva, H., Pomeroy, J., Rae, A. I., and Rosen, S. M.: Percutaneous femoral venous catheterization and reusable dialyzer in the treatment of acute renal failure, Trans. Amer. Soc. Artif. Intern. Organs **10**:133, 1964.

1001. Shannon, J. A., and Winton, F. R.: The renal excretion of inulin and creatinine by the anesthetized dog in the pump lung kidney preparation, J. Physiol. **98**:97, 1940.

1002. Shapiro, J. H., Ramsay, C. G., Jacobson, H. G., Botstein, C. C., and Allen, L. B.: Renal involvement in lymphomas and leukemias in adults. Amer. J. Roentgen. **88**:928, 1962.

1003. Sheedy, J. A., Froeb, H. F., Batson, H. A., Conley, C. C., Murphy, J. P., Hunter, R. B., Cugell, D. W., Giles, R. B., Bershadsky, S. C., Vester, J. W., and Yoe, R. H.: The clinical course of epidemic hemorrragic fever, Amer. J. Med. **26**:619, 1954.

1004. Sheehan, H. L., and Moore, H. C.: Renal cortical necrosis and the kidney of concealed accidental hemorrhage. Springfield, Ill., 1953, Charles C Thomas, Publisher.

1005. Sheehy, T. W.: Malaria in servicemen from Vietnam, Ann. Int. Med. **66**:447, 1967.

1006. Shelley, W. B., and Resnik, S. S.: Methysergide induced degranulation of basophil leucocyte in man, J. Invest. Dermat. **43**:491, 1964.

1007. Shibolet, S., Fisher, S., Gilat, T., Bank, H., and Heller, H.: Fibrinolysis and hemorrhages in fatal heatstroke, New Eng. J. Med. **266**:169, 1962.

1008. Shils, M. E.: Renal disease and the metabolic effects of tetracycline, Ann. Intern. Med. **58**:389, 1963.

1009. Shorr, E.: Hepatorenal vasotropic factors in experimental cirrhosis. In conference on Liver Injury, Transactions, 1947, Josiah Macy, Jr. Foundation, New York.

1010. Shwartz, S. O., and Motto, S. A.: The diagnostic significance of "Burr" red cells, Amer. J. Med. Sci. **218**:563, 1949.

1011. Shwartzman, G.: Phenomenon of local tissue reactivity, London, 1937, Humphrey Milford, Oxford University Press.

1012. Sigler, M. H.: Oliguric renal failure and acute tubular necrosis, Med. Clin. N. Amer. **47**:1023, 1963.

1013. Silva, H. B., Brito, T., Lima, P. R., Penaa, D. O., Almeida, S. S., and Mattar, E.: Acute anuric renal insufficiency (ARI) due to snake, waxbee and spider bites. Clinical and pathological observations in 8 cases, Washington, D. C., 1966, International Congress of Nephrology.

1014. Silva, H., Pomeroy, J., Rae, A. I., Rosen, S. M., and Shalton, S.: Haemodialysis in "hypercatabolic" acute renal failure, Brit. Med. J. **2**:407, 1964.

1014a. Simkin, E. P., Chir, M., and Wright, F. K.: Perforating injuries of the bowel complicating peritoneal catheter insertion, Lancet 1:64, 1968.

1015. Simonds, J. P., and Hepler, O. E.: Experimental nephropathies. I. A method of producing controlled selective injury of renal units by means of chemical agents, Arch. Path. **39**:103, 1945.

1016. Simpson, B., Cook, A. T., Dimond, A. H., Brown, M., and Thin, R. N. T.: Renal function after leptospirosis, Brit. Med. J. **2**:472, 1967.

1017. Sirota, J. H., Narins, L.: Acute urinary suppression after ureteral catheterization, New Eng. J. Med. **257**:1111, 1957.

1017a. Sirota, J. H.: Carbon tetrachloride poisoning in man. I. Mechanisms of renal failure and recovery, J. Clin. Invest. **28**:1412, 1949.

1018. Sitprija, V., and Holmes, J. H.: Preliminary observations on the change in intracranial pressure and intraocular pressure during hemodialysis. Trans. Amer. Soc. Artif. Intern. Organs. **8**:300, 1962.

1018a. Sitprija, V., Indraprasit, S., Pochanugool, G., Benyajati, C., and Piyaratn, P.: Renal failure in malaria, Lancet **1**:185, 1967.

1019. Skeggs, L. T., Jr., and Leonards, J. R.: Studies on an artificial kidney. I. Preliminary results with a new type of continuous dialyzer, Science **108**:212, 1948.

1020. Skimming, L. H., Knies, P. T., Anthony, M. A., and Melarango, E. S.: Hemolytic anemia caused by sulfamethoxypyridazine; report of a case successfully treated by hemodialysis, Ohio Med. J. **57**:280, 1961.

1021. Smith, E. W., and Conley, C. L.: Sicklemia and infarction of spleen during aerial flight: electrophoresis of hemoglobin in 15 cases, Bull. Johns Hopkins Hosp. **96**:35, 1955.

1022. Smith, W.: The kidney, structure and function in health and disease, New York, 1951, Oxford University Press.

1023. Smith, J. P.: Pathology of ferrous sulfate poisoning, J. Path. Bact. **64**:467, 1950.

1024. Smith, K., Browne, J. C. M., Shackman, R. and Wrong, O. M.: Acute renal failure of obstetric origin: an analysis of 70 patients, Lancet **2**:351, 1965.

1025. Smith, K., McClure, J. C., Shackman, R., Wrong, O. M., Lond, M. B., and Oxon, D. M.: Acute renal failure of obstetric origin, Lancet **2**:351, 1965.

1026. Smith, L. H., Jr., Post, R. S., Teschan, P. E., Abernathy, R. S., Davis, J. H., Gray, D. M., Howard, J. M., Johnson, K. E., Klopp, E., Mundy, R. L., O'Meara, M. P., and Rush, B. F., Jr.: Post-traumatic renal insufficiency in military casualties. II. Management, use of an artificial kidney, Prognosis; Surg. Res. Team, Army Med. Serv. Grad. School, Washington, D. C., Amer. J. Med. **18**:187, 1955.

1027. Smith, P. K., Gleason, H. L., Stoll, C. G., and Ogorzalek, S.: Studies on the pharmacology of salicylates. J. Pharmacol. Exper. Therap. **87**:237, 1946.

1028. Snapper, I.: Management of acute renal failure, Bull. N. Y. Acad. Med. **25**:199, 1949.

1029. Snapper, I., and Schaeffer, L. E.: Treatment of 2 patients with hepatorenal syndrome and acute renal failure by exsanguinotransfusion, Ann. Int. Med. **34**:692, 1951.

1030. Solomon, A., Waldmann, T. A., Fahey, J. L., and McFarlene, A. S., Metabolism of Bence Jones proteins, J. Clin. Invest. **43**:103, 1964.

1031. Solomon, M., Galloway, N. C., and Patterson, R.: The kidney and tetracycline toxicity, Missouri Med. **62**:283, 1965.

1032. Solsona Conillera, J.: Linfogranulomatosis maligna: forma monoganglionar Y nefrosica, Med. Clin. (Barc.) **20**:37, 1953.

1033. Sorenson, A. W.: Phenacetin consumption in relation to 24 endogenous creatinine clearances, Scand. J. Clin. Lab. Invest. **13**:337, 1961.

1034. Spink, W. W.: Effects of vaccines and bacterial and parasitic infections on eosinophilia in trichinous animals, Arch. Int. Med. **54**:805, 1934.

1035. Spink, W. W.: Endotoxin shock, Ann. Intern. Med. **57**:538, 1962.

1036. Spolyar, L. W., and Hager, R. N.: Arsine poisoning: epidermologic studies of an outbreak following exposure to gases from metallic dross, Arch. Indust. Hyg. **1**:419, 1950.

1037. Sporn, N., Lancestremere, R. G., and Papper, S.: Differential diagnosis of oliguria in aged patients, New Eng. J. Med. **267**:130, 1962.

1038. Sprunt, D. H.: Renal damage following administration of merbaphen (Novasurol), Arch. Int. Med. **46**:494, 1930.

1039. Spuhler, O., and Zollinger, H. U.: Die chronischinterstitielle nephritis, Ztschr. Klin. Med. **151**:1, 1953.

1040. Staemmler, M., and Karhoff, B.: Die akute nephrosen. Nierenschaden durch antibiotica, Arch. Path. Anat. **328**:481, 1956.

1041. Starling, E. H., and Tubby, A. H.: On absorption from and secretion into the serous cavities, J. Physiol. **16**:140, 1894.

1042. Steiness, I., and Thaysen, J. H.: Bilateral traumatic renal-artery thrombosis, Lancet **1**:527, 1965.

1043. Steinmetz, P. R., and Kiley, J. F.: Renal tubular necrosis following lesions of the brain, Amer. J. Med. **29**:268, 1960.

1044. Sternheimer, R., and Malbin, B.: Clinical recognition of pyelonephritis, with a new strain for urinary sediments, Amer. J. Med. **11**:312, 1951.

1045. Stewart, J. H.: Haemolytic anaemia in acute and chronic renal failure, Quart. J. Med. **36**:85, 1967.

1046. Stewart, J. H., Tuckwell, L. A., Sinnett, P. F., Edwards, K. D. G., and Whyte, H. M.: Peritoneal and haemodialysis: A comparison of their morbidity and of the mortality suffered by dialysed patients, Quart. J. Med. **35**:407, 1966.

1047. Stock, R. J.: Acute urine suppression, observations in 22 patients, Amer. J. Med. **7**:45, 1949.

1048. Strauss, M. B.: Acute renal insufficiency due to lower nephron nephrosis, New Eng. J. Med. **239**:693, 1948.

1049. Strauss, M. B., and Raisz, L.: Clinical management of renal failure, Springfield, Ill., 1956, Charles C Thomas, Publisher.

1050. Strauss, M. B., and Welt, L. G.: Diseases of the kidney, Boston, 1963, Little, Brown and Company.

1051. Strean, G. J., Korenberg, M., and Portnuff, J. C.: Acute uremia treated by peritoneal irrigation, J.A.M.A. **135**:278, 1947.

1052. Studer, A., and Zbinden, G.: Experimenteller beitrag zur frage von nierenschaden bei abusus von phenacetinhaltigen schmerzmitteln, Experientia **11**:450, 1955.

1052a. Sullivan, M. B., Morgan, J. M., and Johnson, I. M.: Tubular necrosis with sustained urinary output, J. Trauma **4**:373, 1964.

1053. Summerlin, W. T., Walder, A. I., and Moncrief, J. A.: White phosphorus burns and massive hemolysis, J. Trauma **7**:476, 1967.

1054. Sussman, R. M., and Kayden, II. J.: Renal insufficiency due to paroxysmal cold hemoglobinuria, Arch. Intern. Med. **82**:598, 1948.

1055. Swan, H., and Gordon, H. H.: Peritoneal lavage in the treatment of anuria in children, Pediatrics **4**:586, 1949.

1056. Swan, R. C., and Merrill, J. P.: The clinical course of acute renal failure, Medicine **32**:215, 1953.

1057. Swann, H. G., Hink, B. W., Koestler, H., Moore, V., and Princ, J. M.: The intra-renal venous pressure, Science **115**:64, 1952.

1057a. Swanson, M. A., and Schwartz, R. S.: Immunosuppressive therapy. The relation between clinical response and immunologic competence. New Eng. J. Med. **277**:163, 1967.

1058. Taddei, C., Gamma, G. B., Caluzzi, F., Laugeri, V., Besse, C., Vercellone, A., Angelino, P. F., Piccoli, G., and Varese, D.: Primi risultati sperimentali e clinici di un nuovo apparechii per emodialisi extracorporea (Rene artificiale Dogliotti A.M. Battezzati-Taddei), Min. Chir. **13**:1549, 1958.

1059. Tait, G. B.: Nephropathy during phenindione therapy, Lancet **2**:1198, 1960.

1060. Takacs, F. J., Tomkiewicz, Z. M., and Merrill, J. P.: Amphotericin B nephrotoxicity with reversible renal failure, Ann. Intern. Med. **59**:716, 1963.

1061. Talamo, R. C., and Crawford, J. D.: Trimethadione nephrosis treated with cortisone and nitrogen mustard, New Eng. J. Med. **269**:15, 1963.

1062. Tan, F. H., Rabbino, M. D., and Hopper, J., Jr.: Is phenacetin a nephrotoxin? A report on 23 users of the drug, Calif. Med. **101**:73, 1964.

1063. Taplin, G. V., Meredith, O. M., Jr., Kade, H., and Winter, C. C.: The radioisotope renogram; external test for individual kidney function and upper urinary tract patency, J. Lab. Clin. Med. **48**:886, 1956.

1064. Tapp, E., and Lowe, B.: Tetracycline toxicity in haemoglobinuria, Brit. Med. J. **1**:143, 1966.

1065. Tauxe, W. N., and Hunt, J. C.: Evaluation of renal function by isotope techniques. Med. Clin. N. Amer. **50**:937, 1966.

1066. Tauxe, W. N., Hunt, J. C., and Burbank, M. K.: The radioisotope renogram (ortho-iodohippurate-I-131): Standardization of technic and expression of data, Amer. J. Clin. Path. **37**:567, 1962.

1067. Tellem, M., Rubenstone, A. I., and Frumin, A. M.: Renal failure and other unusual manifestations in sickle-cell trait, Arch. Path. **63**:508, 1957.

1068. Terplan, K. L., and Javert, C. T.: Fatal hemoglobinuria with uremia from quinine used as abortifacient, New Eng. J. Med. **238**:120, 1948.

1069. Teschan, P. E.: Treatment of acute renal insufficiency, Mod. Treatm. **1**:19, 1964.

1070. Teschan, P. E., and Lawson, N. L.: Studies in acute renal failure—prevention by osmotic diuresis, and observations on the effect of plasma and extracellular volume expansion, Nephron **3**:1, 1966.

1071. Teschan, P. E., and Mason, A. D.: Mechanism of renal lesions induced by shock: hemodynamic data. In Richet, G., editor: Proceedings of the First International Congress of Nephrology, Basel, 1961, S. Karger, AG.

1072. Teschan, P. E., and Mason, A. D.: Studies in acute renal failure, J. Clin. Res. **3**:442, 1963.

1073. Teschan, P. E., and others: Post-traumatic renal insufficiency in military casualties. I. Clinical characteristics, Amer. J. Med. **18**:172, 1955.

1074. Thalhimer, W.: Experimental exchange transfusions for reducing azotemia: use of the artificial kidney for the purpose, Proc. Soc. Exper. Biol. Med. **37**:641, 1938.

1075. Thaysen, J. H., Gjorup, S., and Killman, S. A.: Acute renal failure: experiences with conservative and hemodialytic treatment of 32 consecutive cases, Danish Med. Bull. **4**:73, 1957.

1076. Thiele, K. G., Muehrcke, R. C., and Berning, H.: Nierenerkrankungen durch Medipamente, Deutsche Med. Wschr. **36**:1632, 1967.

1077. Tholen, H., Voegtli, J., Renschler, H., and Schaeffer, A.: Ein beitrag'zur genese der interstitiellen nephritis, Schweiz. Med. Wchnschr. **86**:946, 1956.

1078. Thomas, D. P., Wessler, S., and Reimer, S. M.: The relationship of activated factor XII (Hageman) and bacterial endotorin hypercoagulability, Federation Proc. **21**:61, 1962.

1079. Thomas, G. W.: Incidence and significance of sickle cell disease in deaths subject to medicolegal investigation, Amer. J. Med. Sci. **226**:412, 1953.

1080. Thomas, L., and Good, R. A.: Studies on generalized Shwartzman reaction, general observations concerning phenomenon, J. Exp. Med. **96**:605, 1952.

1081. Thompson, J.: Ferrous sulfate poisoning: its incidence, symptomatology, treatment and prevention, Brit. Med. J. **1**:645, 1950.

1082. Thomson, W. G., Buchanan, A. A., Doak, P. B., and Peart, W. S.: Hypercatabolic acute renal failure, Brit. Med. J. **1**:932, 1964.

1083. Thorburn, G. D., Kopald, H. H., Herd, J. A., Hollenberg, M., O'Morchoe, C. C. C., and Barger, A. C.: Intrarenal distribution of nutrient blood flow determined with Krypton$_{85}$ in the unanesthetized dog, Circulation Res. **13**:290, 1963.

1084. Thurlbeck, W. M., and Castleman, B.: Atheromatous emboli to the kidneys after aortic surgery, New Eng. J. Med. **257**:442, 1957.

1085. Tomb, J. W.: Cholera and uraemia, J. Trop. Med. **44**:80, 1941.

1086. Tomlin, E. M., and Quilter, T. N.: Reflex anuria, U. S. Armed Forces Med. J. **4**:1211, 1953.

1087. Trinkle, J., and Kiser, S.: Acute renal failure: diagnosis of etiology by radioisotope renography, J. Urol. **91**:199, 1961.

1088. Trueta, J., Barclay, A. E., Daniel, P. M., Franklin, K. J., and Pritchard, M. M.L.: Studies of the renal circulation, Oxford, 1947, Blackwell Scientific Publications.

1089. Tu, W. H.: Plasma renin activity in acute tubular necrosis and other renal diseases associated with hypertension, Circulation **31**:686, 1965.

1090. Twiss, E. E., and Kolff, W. J.: Treatment of uremia by perfusion of an isolated intestinal loop: survival for forty-six days after removal of the only functioning kidney, J.A.M.A. **146**:1019, 1951.

1091. Tyler, H. R.: Neurological complications of acute and chronic renal failure. In Merrill, J. P., editor: The treatment of renal failure, New York, 1965, Grune & Stratton, Inc.

1092. Ullrich, G.: Verlauf und Behandlung einer "akuten toxischen Niereninsuffizienz" nach Arsenwasserstoffvergiftung, Wiener Klin. Wachenschrift **70**:538, 1958.

1093. Unger, A. M., and Nemuth, H. I.: Penicillinase treatment of acute renal insufficiency due to penicillin hypersensitivity, J.A.M.A. **167**:1237, 1958.

1094. Utz, D. C., Rooke, E. D., Spittel, J. A., Jr., and Bartholomeu, L. G.: Retroperitoneal fibrosis in patients taking methysergide, J.A.M.A. **191**:983, 1965.

1095. Valek, A.: Acute renal insufficiency in intoxication with mercury compounds, Acta Med. Scand. **177**:63, 1965.

1096. Vallery-Radot, P.: Premiere observation de nephrite aigue azotemique indiscutablement querie par la methode de Bessis, Bull. Mem. Soc. Med. Hop. Paris **64**:908, 1948.

1097. Van Dyke, H. B.: The toxic effects of sulfonamides, Ann. New York Acad. Sci. **44**:477, 1943.

1098. Van Slyke, D. D., Phillips, R. A., Hamilton, P. B., Archibald, R. M., Dole, V. P., and Emerson, K., Jr.: Effect of shock on the kidney, Tr. Ass. Amer. Physicians **58**:119, 1944.

1099. Vartan, C. K., and Discombe, G.: Death from quinine poisoning, Brit. Med. J. **1**:525, 1940.

1100. Vertel, R. M., and Knochel, J. P.: Acute renal failure due to heat injury: an analysis of ten cases associated with a high incidence of myoglobulinuria, Amer. J. Med. **43**:435, 1967.

1101. Vilter, C. F., and Blankenhorn, M. A.: The toxic reactions of the new sulfonamides, J.A.M.A. **126**:691, 1944.

1102. Vogt, W., and Cottier, H.: Nekrotisierende nephrose nach behandlung einer subakut-chronischen bleivergiftung mit versenat in hohen dosen Schweiz, Med. Wchnschr. **87**:665, 1957.

1103. Von Recklinhausen, F.: Hamorrhagische niereninfarkte, Virchows Arch. **20**:205, 1861.

1104. Wachstein, M.: Histochemical staining reactions of the normally functioning and abnormal kidney, J. Histochem. **3**:246, 1955.

1105. Wachstein, M., and Meisel, E.: A comparative study of enzymatic staining reactions in the rat kidney with necrobiosis induced by ischemia and nephrotoxic agents (mercuhydrin and DL-Serin), J. Histochem. Cytochem. **5**:204, 1957.

1106. Wackerm, W. E. C., and Merill, J. P.: Uremic pericarditis in acute and chronic renal failure, J.A.M.A. **156**:764, 1954.

1107. Wagoner, R. D., Holley, K. E., and Johnson, W. J.: Accelerated nephrosclerosis and postpartum acute renal failure in normotensive patients, Ann. Intern. Med. **69**:237, 1968.

1108. Waife, S. O., and Pratt, P. T.: Fatal mercurial poisoning following prolonged administration of mercurophylline, Arch. Intern. Med. **78**:42, 1946.

1109. Waisbren, B. A., and Spink, W. W.: A clinical appraisal of neomycin, Ann. Intern. Med. **33**:1099, 1956.

1110. Wakim, K. G.: Symposium on fundamental aspects of disease of the kidney: physiological basis for anuria, Staff Meetings of the Mayo Clinic **29**:66, 1954.

1111. Wallach, J. B., Scharfman, S. B., and Angrist, A. A.: Uremia due to replacement of renal parenchyma by tumor, J. Urol. **67**:623, 1952.

1112. Walton, E. W.: Giant-cell granuloma of the respiratory tract (Wegener's granulomatosis), Brit. Med. J. **2**:265, 1958.

1112a. Ward, P. A., and Kibukamusoke, J. W.: Evidence for soluble immune complexes in the pathogenesis of the glomerulonephritis of quartan malaria, Lancet **1**:283, 1969.

1113. de Wardener, H. E.: Intrarenal pressure in experimental tubular necrosis, Lancet **1**:580, 1955.

1114. Warren, S. A., and Gross, W. V., Jr.: Clinical recovery following prolonged anuria in an infant 2 months of age, Pediatrics **5**:954, 1950.

1115. Waugh, D., and Beschel, H.: Infraglomerular epithelial reflux in the evolution of serotonin nephropathy in rats, Amer. J. Path. **39**:547, 1961.

1116. Waugh, D., Schlieter, W., and James, A. W.: Infraglomerular epithelial reflux: an early lesion of acute renal failure, Arch. Path. **77**:93, 1964.

1117. Wegener, F.: Uber eine eigenartige rhinogene granulomatose mit besonderer beteiligung des arteriensystems und der nieren, Beitr. Path. Anat. **102**:36, 1939.

1118. Wegienka, L. C., and Weller, J. M.: Renal tubular acidosis caused by degraded tetracycline, Arch. Intern. Med. **114**:232, 1964.

1119. Wegner, G.: Chirugische bemerkungen uber die periton calhrhle mit bisonderer beruchsich fegung der ovariotomic, Arch. F. Klin. Chir. **20**:51, 1877.

1120. Wehinger, D., and Konzer, P.: Haemolytic-uraemic syndrome, Lancet **2**:1394, 1968.

1121. Weinig, E., and Schwerd, W.: Gefahren bei der behandlung der bleiintoxikation mit calciumversenat ("mosatil komplexon"), Munchen. Med. Wchnschr. **100**:1788, 1958.

1122. Weinstein, I.: Fatalities associated with analbis suppositories, J.A.M.A. **133**:962, 1947.

1123. Weinstein, L., and Ehrenkranz, M. J.: Streptomycin and dihydrostreptomycin: antibiotics monographs, New York, 1958, Medical Encyclopedia.

1124. Weinstein, L., Madoff, M. A., and Samet, C. M.: The sulfonamides, New Eng. J. Med. **263**:793, 1960.

1124a. Weissmann, G., Pras, M., and Hirschorn, R.: A common mechanism for the fungicidal and nephrotoxic effect of amphotericin-B, J. Clin. Invest. **45**:1084, 1968.

1125. Welch, W. H.: An experimental study of glomerulonephritis, Trans. Ass. Amer. Physicians **1**:171, 1886.

1126. Wennberg, J. E., Okun, R., Hinman, E. J., Northcutt, R. C., Greip, R. J., and Walker, W. G.: Renal toxicity of oral cholecystographic media, J.A.M.A. **186**:461, 1963.

1127. Westervelt, F. B., and Schreiner, G. E.: Carbohydrate intolerance of uremic patients, Ann. Intern. Med. **57**:266, 1962.

1128. Whitehouse, F. W., and Root, H. F.: Necrotizing renal papillitis and diabetes mellitus, J.A.M.A. **162**:444, 1956.

1129. Wieland, T., and Wieland, O.: Chemistry and toxicology of toxins of amanita phalloides, Pharmacol. Rev. **11**:87, 1959.

1130. Willis, R. A.: Arsine gas poisoning—report of a case, Indust. Med. **17**:208, 1948.

1131. Wilson, R., Jr., and Magum, G. H.: Acute hemolytic anemia in fertilizer workers: new industrial hazard, South. Med. J. **36**:212, 1943.

1132. Wilson, S. A. K.: Neurology, Baltimore, 1941, The Williams & Wilkins Co.

1133. Winfield, M., Crisp, G. O., Maxwell, M. H., and Kleeman, C. R.: Nephrotoxic effects of kanamycin: a preliminary report, Ann. New York Acad. Sci. **76**:149, 1958.

1134. Winton, P. R.: The pressures and flows of blood and urine within the kidney. In modern views on the secretion of urine. London, 1956.

1135. Wolf, A. V., Remp, D. G., Kiley, J. E., and Currie, G. D.: Artificial kidney function: kinetics of hemodialysis, J. Clin. Invest. **30**:1062, 1951.

1136. Wolin, L. H.: Arteriovenous shunts for prolonged intermittent hemodialysis, J.A.M.A. **202**:99, 1967.

1137. Wolinsky, E., and Henis, J. D.: Neurotoxic and nephrotoxic effects of colistin in patients with renal disease, New Eng. J. Med. **266**:759, 1962.

1138. Wolthuis, F. H.: Balance studies on protein metabolism in normal and uraemic man, Amsterdam, 1961, Scheltema and Holkema N.V.

1138a. Wolthius, F. H.: Balance studies on protein metabolism in normal and uremic men, Acta. Med. Scand. **373**:1, 1962.

1139. Woods, W. W.: The changes in the kidneys in carbon tetrachloride poisoning and their resemblance to those in the "crush syndrome," J. Path. Bact. **58**:767, 1946.

1140. Wright, D. O., and Kinsey, R. E.: Renal complications due to sulfadiazine, J.A.M.A. **120**:1351, 1942.
1141. Wynn, V., and Rob, C. G.: Water intoxication: differential diagnosis of the hypotonic syndromes, Lancet **1**:587, 1954.
1142. Yates-Bell, J. G.: Renal colic and anuria from acetazolamide, Brit. Med. J. **2**:1392, 1958.
1143. Yorke, W., and Nauss, R. W.: The mechanism of the production of suppression of urine in blackwater fever, Ann. Trop. Med. and Parasitol. **5**:287, 1911.
1144. Young, A. G., Muehlberger, C. W., and Meek, W. J.: Toxicological studies of acute anilin poisoning. I. Experimental studies of acute anilin poisoning, J. Pharm. Exp. Ther. **27**:101, 1926.
1145. Young, J. V., Haydon, G. B., and Gray, C. P.: Nephropathy associated with the use of analgesic medications, Ann. Intern. Med. **62**:727, 1965.
1146. Yow, E. M.: Observations on the use of sulfisoxazole in 1,000 consecutive patients with particular reference to the frequency of undesirable side effects, Amer. Pract. and Digest. Treat. **4**:521, 1953.
1147. Yow, E. M., Moyer, J. H., and Smith, C. P.: Toxicity of polymyxin B. II. Human studies with particular reference to evaluation of renal function, Arch. Int. Med. **92**:248, 1953.
1148. Yow, E. M., and Abu-Nasser, H.: Kanamycin: a re-evaluation after three years experience, 2nd International Symposium Chemotherapy **1**:148, 1963.
1149. Yuile, C. L., Gold, M. A., and Hinds, E. G.: Hemoglobin precipitation in renal tubules: a study in its causes and effects, J. Exp. Med. **82**:361, 1945.
1150. Zabludovitch, S., and Milman, F.: Anuria por fenibutazone, Prensa Med. Argentina **45**:3035, 1958.
1151. Zeek, P. M.: Periarteritis nodosa and other forms of necrotizing angiitis, New Eng. J. Med. **248**:764, 1953.
1152. Zeman, F. D.: Toxic effects ascribed to prolonged abuse of acetophenetidin (Phenacetin), J. Chron. Dis. **16**:1085, 1963.
1153. Zilberg, B.: Anuria following penicillin administration, South African Med. J. **32**:350, 1958.
1154. Zollinger, H. U.: Relationship of renal toxicity of drugs to pyelonephritis: biology of pyelonephritis, Boston, 1960, Little, Brown and Company.
1155. Zuelzer, W W., Kurnetz, R., and Charles, S.: Circulatory diseases of kidneys in infancy and childhood: symmetrical cortical necrosis, Amer. J. Dis. Child. **81**:2, 1951.

Subject index